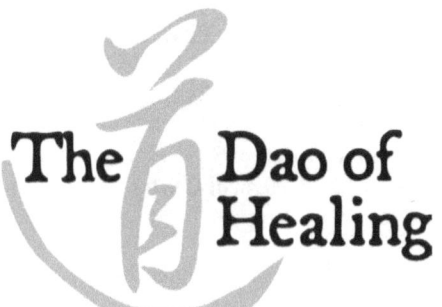

The 道 Dao of
Healing

"There has been much misconception and polarising controversy over Chinese medicine. This well-researched book with its robust theological framework challenges us to reconsider the immense depth, contribution and role of Chinese medicine in our complex world today. A brilliant book with confident clarity!"

Dr Goh Wei Leong
Chairman & Co-Founder, Healthserve
General Practitioner, Manhattan Medical Centre

"Lai Pak-Wah carefully distinguishes between the classical, with the folk or religious, presentations of Chinese medicine to understand its essence, or *Dao*. He does this to be fair to classical Chinese medicine, and shows that not only is this medicine as robust in its methodology as Western medicine, it is not incompatible with Christian anthropology. His detailed analysis is a fine example of contextualisation of this important area of medicine and healing. Hence, this book will be of interest not only to those who wonder whether or not they can seek healing from Chinese medicine, but also for anyone who seeks to relate the Christian faith with Chinese culture."

Dr Kwa Kiem Kiok
Lecturer, Missiology and Interdisciplinary Studies
Biblical Graduate School of Theology

"In *The Dao of Healing*, Pak-Wah Lai introduces us in a wonderfully lucid and respectful way to why it is okay for Christians to use Chinese medicine. In the process, he walks us along the paths taken over the millennia by both Western and Chinese medicine, then dips more deeply into the influence on those paths of the metaphors that shaped them. His is a deceptively simple account that speaks directly and persuasively to the concerns of lay Christians."

Professor Wendy Mayer
Australian Lutheran College, University of Divinity
Fellow of the Australian Academy of the Humanities

"This book is certainly one of a kind. Skilfully integrating interdisciplinary approaches such as medical historiography (of the West and China), philosophy, theology and cognitive linguistics, Lai provides the readers with an informative, thoughtful, trustworthy and accessible introduction for understanding and appreciating Chinese medicine from a Christian perspective. It not only informs but also guides the readers to fairly and critically engage both Western biomedicine and Traditional Chinese Medicine (TCM) in their respective historical and cultural contexts with a robust constructive theology. Regardless of the reader's religious orientation, however, one will come away with an enlightened perspective on understanding and evaluating TCM."

Prof. Helen Rhee
Professor of Church History, Westmont College

"History, the philosophy of healing, assumptions and myths in so-called 'Western' medicine—all these issues and more have been rolled into a scholarly but very readable book. Among the scholarly essays, there are accounts and vignettes of therapy and practice that are shared by Dr Diarra Boubacar. Knowing that Dr Diarra is an outstanding TCM physician whose heart is for the patient and community makes me applaud the publication of this book all the more."

Dr Tan Lai Yong
Director for Outreach & Community Engagement & Senior Lecturer
at the College of Alice & Peter Tan, NUS

"There is often this conflict between the practice and philosophies of TCM and Judeo-Christian worldviews. In Asia, these conflicts are often more acute because Western medicine predominates as the main healthcare provider. This is an especial problem for Asian Christians who often reject TCM as 'unbiblical'. Dr Pak-Wah Lai has written an excellent book in which he uses a scholarly approach to examine this complex issue and presents to the readers his well-reasoned conclusions."

Dr Alex Tang, MD, PhD, FRCPE
Consultant Paediatrician, Associate Professor of Paediatrics, Monash University
Malaysia, and Practical Theologian, Kairos Spiritual Formation Ministries

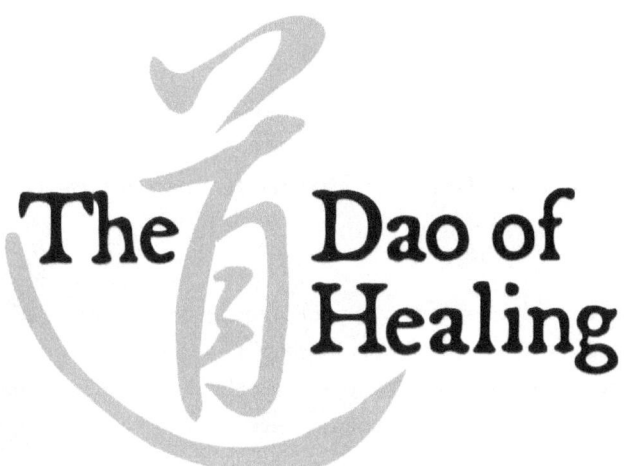

The 道 Dao of Healing

Written by
Pak-Wah Lai, PhD

Medical Consultant
Diarra Boubacar Thiemoke, PhD

GRACEW☐RKS

Published by: Graceworks Private Limited
                  22 Sin Ming Lane
                  #04-76 Midview City
                  Singapore 573969
                  Tel: 67523403
                  Email: enquiries@graceworks.com.sg
                  Website: www.graceworks.com.sg

Scripture quotations marked "NIV" are taken from *The Holy Bible, New International Version*®. NIV®. Copyright © 1973, 1978, 1984, 2011 by International Bible Society. Used by permission of Zondervan. All rights reserved.

Scripture quotations marked "ESV" are taken from *The Holy Bible, English Standard Version*. Copyright © 2000; 2001 by Crossway Bibles, a division of Good News Publishers. Used by permission. All rights reserved.

Cover design: Choo Graphic Design Workshop
Body text typeset in Arno Pro 12.5/16.5 pts

ISBN: 978-981-11-6663-1

2 3 4 5 6 7 8 9 10 • 25 24 23 22 21 20 19

CONTENTS

FOREWORD

This is a pioneer work, yet it is also exhaustive and comprehensive. If "truth is history", then this is "truthful" indeed! As a teaching textbook in medical schools, it will also re-introduce the Christian origins of modern medicine into our secular universities. For, like modern science, both have Christian ontological origins in the 17th century. The author is apologetic about the authorial regime of Singapore, where he teaches. But he needs to be reminded that the University of Singapore was strongly staffed in the pre-war era by Christian professors of medicine, mainly from London hospitals, under the aegis of the Christian Medical Fellowship.

It is commonly, and somewhat arrogantly assumed in Western medicine, that Chinese doctors have a lot to learn from modern medical practice; this is only partially true. For Western physicians will be surprised in reading this book, to find that psychosomatic symptoms and prescriptions were already being treated in the first century AD, in the Han dynasty. Acupuncture is now being used for the relief of intense pain for Western patients, while the new medical science of Osteoporosis—some 40 years old—has still to be studied comparatively with Chinese practices for blood circulation of the feet.

After an introductory survey of apologetic/theological concerns, and constructing a theological analytical framework, chapters 4 to 9 then survey the history, philosophy and linguistic differences of Western and Chinese medicine to elucidate why they are different.

Invasive surgery "has had its day" in the West, but non-invasive surgery, which ironically has always reigned supreme in Chinese medicine, is the future of Western medicine! Richly historic, this work is somewhat prophetic for the future of medicine, an unusual medical textbook indeed! As a historian of ideas, I know of no book like this, to read, reflect, and inwardly digest!

Prof. James M Houston
Founding Principal & Emeritus Professor of Spiritual Theology
Regent College, Vancouver, British Columbia

ACKNOWLEDGEMENTS

C. S. Lewis once remarked that if a person wants to be a writer, it is best for him to write about a subject he is interested in. In many ways, this is a book I have been looking for, but could not find—a book that takes seriously the rich teachings of the Christian tradition, and, at the same time, the complex histories and philosophies of both Western and Chinese medicine.

Although this book is by no means comprehensive, it has answered quite a number of questions I have asked about Chinese medicine, both as a Christian, and also as a Chinese. I pray that what I have discovered may be helpful not only for Christians asking similar questions, but also for those interested in finding out more about Chinese medicine, and how it relates to Western medical traditions. As it turned out, my journey required me to address several philosophical, historical and linguistic issues about comparative medicine which a medical physician should find helpful, even if we do not share a common faith.

There's an African proverb that says, "it takes a whole village to raise a child". The same, I think, can be said about this book. I am indebted to so many colleagues, friends, and loved ones for the fruition of this project. My gratitude goes, first of all, to Dr Diarra Boubacar Thiemoke, my Chinese medical consultant for this book. He not only reviewed the manuscript and gave helpful comments for improvements, but also allowed me to observe his clinical practice in Yunnan for two weeks in 2016. Indeed, without his assured support,

I would not have dared to embark on a project like this! I am thankful also for Prof. Jim Houston, who first impressed on me the importance of the Christian tradition, particularly, that of the church fathers. It was he who set me on the path of becoming a patristics scholar, and has now kindly written the Foreword. The same can be said of my supervisors, Prof. Andrew Louth and Prof. Carol Harrison, and former PhD colleagues at Durham University (2007–2010). It was our numerous discussions about the church fathers' appropriation of Graeco-Roman culture that sowed the seeds for this project. For it was through the fathers' experience of cultural contextualisation that I first saw the possibility of employing Chinese learning (including Chinese medicine) for Christian theological reflections. Particular appreciation also goes to Dr Wendy Mayer for her mentoring and encouragement. Her own studies of the fathers' reception of Hippocratic psycho-medicio therapy have provided many helpful insights for this project. Similar thanks go also to Prof. Pauline Allen and our colleagues at the Australian Catholic University (ACU), Brisbane, who kindly hosted my Sabbatical research in 2016. If not for this opportunity, I would not have been able to access the wide range of theological and medical resources within the ACU library.

On a more personal note, I would like to thank Vincent Ooi, for his fellowship at Durham, and his willingness to entertain my initial ventures into inter-disciplinary thinking. The same must be said of Leo Li, who first introduced me to the works of Geoffrey Lloyd. Prof. Lloyd's comparative studies of ancient Greek and Chinese sciences, as we shall see, provided me with a helpful framework for comparing Western and Chinese medicine. My deep appreciation also goes to my BGST colleagues, Philip Satterthwaite, Quek Tze-Ming and Tan Seng-Kong, who were ever so supportive of this project. BGST students, particularly those at the *Christian Perspectives of Chinese Medicine* seminar, also contributed invaluable feedback. I am grateful also for my editor, Bernice Tan, who had the courage to take on such an unorthodox Christian book proposal, and for the reviewers of the manuscript, Benjamin Grandey, Yam Tim Wing and Nigel Fong. As a medical doctor, Nigel was so helpful in fact-checking, updating, and, at times, correcting my knowledge about biomedicine.

I thank God for Rina, my ever-supportive wife, and children, Fide and Isaiah. They have accompanied me throughout my entire theological journey, and have, of course, borne the brunt of my reflections on Chinese medicine. Finally, I would like to express my appreciation to all colleagues and friends whom I am unable to mention, but who nevertheless contributed to this endeavour. All mistakes in this book, however, remain my own.

Pak-Wah Lai, PhD
Vice-Principal, Biblical Graduate School of Theology
Lecturer in Church History and Historical Theology

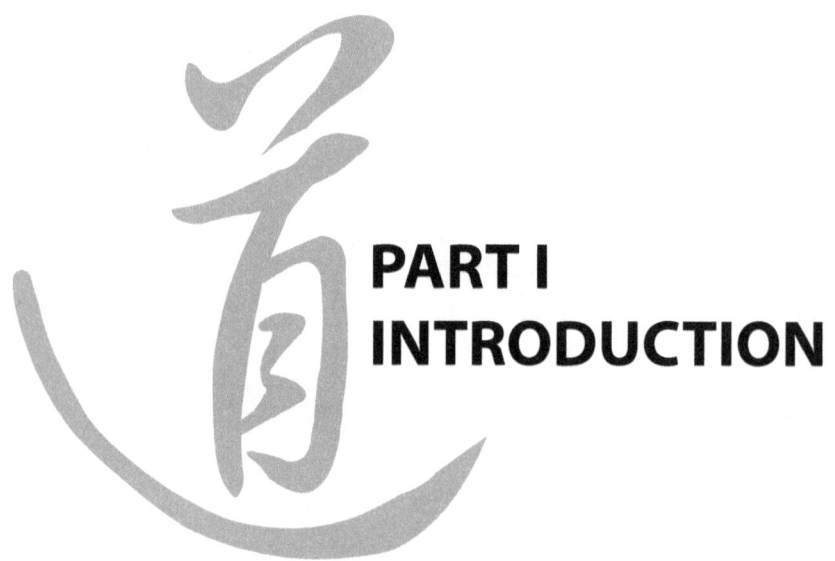

PART I
INTRODUCTION

1

INTRODUCTION

Chinese Medicine: To Use or Not to Use?

In his essay, *Call to Arms* (*Nahan* 呐喊), famous Chinese literary critic, Lu Xun (鲁迅, 1881–1936) reminisced about a childhood experience. As a child, he frequented a Chinese medicine shop where he had to procure herbs for his father. Besides the herbs' exotic names, what impressed him most was the fact that, after taking so much Chinese medication, his father did not recover but died from his illness. Years later, when Lu studied in Nanjing, he came into contact with Western science. This was when he concluded that Chinese medicine paled in comparison to its Western counterpart. "Chinese medicine," as he put it, "is but a lie, either intentionally or out of ignorance" (中医不过是一种有意或无意的骗子).

During the same period, however, a certain Secretary Qi in Shenyang had a different experience. In 1918, he read a Chinese medical journal called *Assimilation of Western to Chinese in Medicine* (*Yixue Zhongzhong Canxilu* 医学衷中参西录) and came across a diagnosis of syndromes that fit those experienced by his friend's wife: swollenness of the tummy, a lack of appetite, stomach cramps and so on. After recommending her the prescription, *Lizhong* Decoction (理中汤), they were delighted that she recovered only after ten doses of medication. Impressed by this success, Secretary Qi promptly invited the magazine's author, Zhang Xichun (张锡纯, 1860–1933) to Shenyang to establish what would become the first Chinese Medical

Hospital in China—*Li Da* hospital (立达医院). Zhang would go on to become one of the most significant figures in modern Chinese medicine, whose influence has yet to be surpassed.[1]

The last 50 years have seen the popularity of Chinese medicine grow by leaps and bounds. In China, Korea, Japan and Singapore, Chinese medicine has been incorporated into their healthcare systems to varying degrees.[2] In the West, it is no longer uncommon for patients to consult Chinese medical doctors, many of whom are non-Chinese.[3] More recently, the ancient practice appeared in the limelight after tennis world champion, Novak Djokovic, attributed his success to a diet informed by Chinese medical principles, and several members of the US Rio Olympics team, including Michael Phelps, received cupping treatments. The same year also saw Chinese physician, Tu Youyou (屠呦呦), being awarded a Nobel Prize for discovering, from the pages of Chinese medical classics, the potency of Artemisinim for combating malaria.[4] Despite these developments, criticisms of Chinese medicine have remained unabated. In 2011, Andy Ho, Senior Writer of *The Straits Times*, lambasted the Singapore Medical Council for permitting doctors to refer patients to

1   "中医名家张锡纯的影响_生活养生网", accessed December 30, 2015, http://www.shenghuoqq.com/zyys1/585.html.

2   Volker Scheid and Hugh MacPherson, *Integrating East Asian Medicine into Contemporary Healthcare* (Edinburgh; NY: Churchill Livingstone Elsevier, 2012), 61–62.

3   Many of these Western practitioners, such as Volker Scheid, Ted Kaptchuk and Giovanni Maciocia, have gone on to publish books on Chinese medicine. See, for example, Giovanni Maciocia, *The Foundations of Chinese Medicine: A Comprehensive Text for Acupuncturists and Herbalists* (Edinburgh: Elsevier Churchill Livingstone, 2005); Ted J. Kaptchuk, *Chinese Medicine: The Web That Has No Weaver* (London: Rider, 2000). Scheid and MacPherson, *Integrating East Asian Medicine into Contemporary Healthcare*.

4   "Tennis Wiz Novak Djokovic Uses Holistic Chinese Medicine to "Serve to Win" | Examiner.com", accessed January 1, 2016, http://www.examiner.com/article/tennis-wiz-novak-djokovic-uses-holistic-chinese-medicine-to-serve-to-win.; Kate Lyons, "Interest in Cupping Therapy Spikes after Michael Phelps Gold Win", *The Guardian*, August 8, 2016, sec. Sport, http://www.theguardian.com/sport/2016/aug/08/cupping-therapy-interest-spikes-michael-phelps-rio-olympics.; "Is the 2015 Nobel Prize a Turning Point for Traditional Chinese Medicine?", accessed January 1, 2016, http://theconversation.com/is-the-2015-nobel-prize-a-turning-point-for-traditional-chinese-medicine-48643.

Chinese Medicine practitioners. This, he charged, was a setback for "evidence-based medicine" since acupuncture is nothing more than a superstitious practice, used not by "the Chinese physician in days of yore" but by "the shamans and blood letters". More seriously, Chinese medical philosophy is based primarily on what he regards as a flawed Chinese cosmology, and an unverifiable notion of *qi*—a numinous force that supposedly animates all life.[5] Not surprisingly, Ho's article stirred up much response from both doctors and the general public, who wrote either in favour of or against the ancient medical practice.[6]

Among Christians, a similar disagreement is being played out, both in the East and the West. Generally speaking, Western Christians are doubtful about the legitimacy of Chinese medical practice.[7] It is, as they put it, a pseudo-science "based upon an ancient, limited and error-filled understanding of anatomy and physiology." Their concern, however, is more than just the scientific illegitimacy of the medicine. Rather, they fear contact with and use of Chinese medicine may expose Christians to unruly Daoist or religious teachings. Neil Anderson and Michael Jacobson, for example, suggest that Chinese medicine could well be one of the many "spiritually counterfeit health paradigms" conjured by Satan and his demons and so should not be

---

5   Notwithstanding Ho's skepticism, the Singapore Health Ministry has come out in support of TCM practice and allocated S$5 million for TCM research from 2017–2022. Andy Ho, "Pinning down Acupuncture: It's a Placebo," *The Straits Times*, 2011; "Traditional Chinese Medicine to Play Important Role as Singapore Population Ages: PM Lee", *Channel NewsAsia*, accessed October 30, 2017, http://www.channelnewsasia.com/news/singapore/traditional-chinese-medicine-to-play-important-role-as-singapore-9244600.

6   Such public skirmishes between TCM and biomedical physicians still persist. For a more recent episode, see 郑心锦, "中医是哪门子科学？," 联合早报网, May 31, 2017, http://www.zaobao.com.sg/forum/views/opinion/story20170531-766526. and 王修齐, "对医学的误解," 联合早报网, June 7, 2017, accessed July 4, 2018, http://www.zaobao.com.sg/forum/views/opinion/story20170607-769141.

7   Neil T. and Michael Jacobson Anderson, *The Biblical Guide to Alternative Medicine* (Ventura, CA: Regal, 2003), 178–93; Paul C Reisser, Dale Mabe, and Robert Velarde, *Examining Alternative Medicine: An inside Look at the Benefits & Risks* (Downers Grove, IL: InterVarsity Press, 2001), 78–99; Donald and Walt Larimore O'Mathuna, *Alternative Medicine: The Christian Handbook* (Grand Rapids, MI: Zondervan, 2001), 279–82; Robina Coker and Christian Medical Fellowship, *Alternative Medicine: Helpful or Harmful?* (Crowborough: Monarch, 1995).

judged "merely upon the appearance of success".[8] Such concerns are not uncommon among Christians in Asia. Daniel Tong, for example, argues likewise that Chinese medical theories (particularly the concepts of *yinyang* and *qi*) are not only unscientific and unattested to by biblical teachings, but are also tainted by Daoist philosophy. For these reasons, Christians should not consult, let alone practise Chinese medicine.[9]

This being said, not all Christians perceive Chinese medicine in such a negative light. In her biography of Pastor Xi Shengmo (席胜魔, 1830–1896), one of the earliest Chinese converts to the Protestant faith, Geraldine Taylor (1865–1945), noted that Xi was a Confucian scholar well-versed in Chinese herbs. He put this knowledge to good use when he opened a Chinese drugstore to provide work for unemployed Christians. Later, the same knowledge also came into play when Xi set up rehabilitation centres ("Refuges") for opium addicts. This time round, claimed Xi, God actually revealed a Chinese medical formula to him that would prove effective for helping the addicts wean themselves off their odious habit.[10] It appears then that both Xi and Taylor saw no conflict between his Chinese medical practice and their Christian faith.[11] Decades later, in 1984, a Malian Christian would arrive in China to advance his training in Western

---

8   Anderson, *Biblical Guide to Alternative Medicine*, 190–93. Things have not improved much since the early 2000s. See Liuan Huska, "Heal Me—Body, Mind, and Soul," *CT Women*, accessed March 7, 2018, http://www.christianitytoday.com/women/2014/march/heal-me-body-mind-and-soul.html. For a more balanced view see "Acupuncture—a Christian Assessment," *Christian Medical Fellowship* — cmf.org.uk, accessed March 5, 2018, http%3A%2F%2Fwww.cmf.org.uk%2Fresources%2Fpublications%2Fcontent%2F%3Fcontext%3Darticle%26id%3D759.

9   Daniel Tong, *A Biblical Approach to Chinese Traditions and Beliefs* (Singapore: Genesis, 2003), 108–24.

10   Taylor was a China Inland Missions (now known as OMF International) missionary and the daughter-in-law of Hudson Taylor. Geraldine Taylor, *Pastor Hsi (of North China): One of China's Christians* (London: Morgan & Scott, 1904), 43, 64.

11   Xi cannot be accused of theological naiveté or religious syncretism here. Elsewhere, the biography also notes how he increasingly realised that the upkeep of ancestral tablets was tantamount to idolatry and should, therefore, be abandoned by Chinese Christians. Taylor, 26–28.

biomedicine. When his plans did not materialise, he too received instructions from God in a vision. In his case, he was told to study Chinese medicine because "it was also a legitimate form of medicine" (中医也是医学). Thirty years on, Dr Diarra Boubacar Thiemoke is now a senior consultant in the Chengdu Chinese Medical Hospital and the first foreigner to obtain a PhD in Chinese Medicine. He has also contributed much to Chinese welfare by volunteering his medical skills in various social and medical philanthropic causes.[12]

In Singapore, a less dramatic but nevertheless similar project also takes place regularly in a Pentecostal Church. Every Wednesday and Friday, free Chinese medical services are offered by Bethel Assembly of God, as part of its outreach to its community. The clinic's doctor is no less than Ps. Moses Pi, pastor of Bethel's Mandarin service who has a doctorate in Chinese medicine.[13] For those familiar with Chinese churches in Singapore, Malaysia, Hong Kong and Taiwan, the experiences of Xi, Diarra and Pi are not exceptions to the norm. Rather, many Chinese-speaking Christians still use Chinese medicine regularly and see no contradiction between their faith and the ancient medical tradition.

Chinese Medicine or Traditional Chinese Medicine?

All these beg the question: is Chinese medicine a legitimate form of medicine for Christians? How shall we go about assessing it? By now, readers may have noticed how I often refer to our subject as "Chinese Medicine", rather than by its more popular name: "Traditional Chinese Medicine" or TCM. This is intentional and some clarification is called for here.

Prior to the arrival of the colonial powers in China, medicine was

---

12   "Malian Doctor All for TCM Healing—Global Times", accessed January 4, 2016, http://www.globaltimes.cn/content/828560.shtml.
13   "TCM Service | Bethel Community Services", accessed January 4, 2016, http://www.bethelcs.org.sg/services/tcm-service/.

simply known as *yi* (医). The term, however, was quite heterogeneous in Chinese minds since it was applied to both popular healers like religious ritualistic healers, travelling healers (*jianghu yi*, 江湖医), toothworm removers (*xiaoyachong*, 消牙蟲) and bone setters, and also to the practitioners of classical Chinese medicine.[14] The latter is generally regarded as the predecessor of TCM and is based largely on the Chinese philosophies of *qi* (气), *yinyang* (阴阳) and the five phases (*wuxing*, 五行), and medical classics such as the *Yellow Emperor's Inner Canon* (*Huangdi Neijing*, 黄帝内经) and the *Treatise on Cold Diseases* (*Shanghan Lun*, 伤寒论).

This being said, classical Chinese medicine was more pluralistic than what is conveyed by the term, TCM. Rather, there have been different traditions or, as Volker Scheid coins it, "currents of learning" (*xuepai*, 学派) in the history of Chinese medicine. Each is characterised by its peculiar doctrinal emphasis (*xueshuo*, 学说), medical scholars (*yijia*, 医家), medical works (*yizhu*, 医著) and case records (*yian*, 医案). Some of the more prominent "currents" include the cold pathogen disorder current of learning (*shanghan xuepai*, 伤寒学派), the warm pathogen disorder current (*wenbing xuepai*, 温病学派), and the *Menghe* current (孟河学派), all of which were sometimes at odds with one another.[15]

Nineteenth-century contact with the West, however, compelled Chinese intellectuals to compare Chinese medicine with its Western counterpart. This led to some, like Lu Xun, rejecting the former, while others, like Zhang Xichun, attempting to assimilate the two. The term, Chinese medicine (*zhongyi*, 中医), thus came into use as a means of differentiating it from Western medicine (*xiyi*, 西医).

---

14   Bridie Andrews, *The Making of Modern Chinese Medicine, 1850–1960* (Vancouver: UBC Press, 2014), 33–44.

15   This may be likened to the different Protestant denominations, such as the Anglicans, Baptists, Methodists and Presbyterians. While most of their doctrines are similar (such their beliefs in the Trinity, Christ's salvation and Christ's resurrection), they also differ in their doctrinal emphases, and some secondary doctrines, for example, whether one should baptise by sprinkling or immersion, and whether churches should be ruled by bishops or a council of elders.

After the communist takeover, the Maoist government established a dual health-care system in the 1950–60s and mandated the modernisation of Chinese medicine by integrating it with Western medicine (中西医结合).[16] With this policy change, traditional modes of learning that emphasised the reading and memorising of classical medical texts, and long clinical apprenticeships with one's teacher, gave way to a new medical pedagogy.[17] Thenceforth, Chinese medical theories and traditions were homogenised and condensed systematically into textbooks, and taught in a classroom format.[18] Western anatomy and biomedical concepts were also incorporated into this new curriculum.[19] Interestingly, this was also the period when the West became disenchanted with modernity and began to look eastwards "for sacred knowledge and enlightenment."[20] To appeal to this new interest in ancient traditions, Chinese foreign language publications began to adopt the term "TCM" in the 1960s to denote this modernised version of Chinese medicine. The term has held sway till this day.[21]

For the purpose of this book, we will focus primarily on classical or secular Chinese medicine, rather than folk or religious medicine.[22] In view of the fact that TCM does not quite represent the breadth and form of classical Chinese medicine in terms of its traditional

---

16   Volker Scheid, *Currents of Tradition in Chinese Medicine, 1626–2006* (Seattle: Eastland Press, 2007), 4, 11–12.

17   This emphasis on the mastery of the classics is standard Confucian pedagogy and dates back to the Han period. G. E. R. Lloyd, *Disciplines in the Making: Cross-Cultural Perspectives on Elites, Learning, and Innovation* (Oxford: Oxford University Press, 2009), 12.

18   Volker Scheid, *Chinese Medicine in Contemporary China: Plurality and Synthesis* (Durham, NC ; Oxford: Duke University Press, 2002), 72–74.

19   For example, the concept of bacteria (*xijun*, 细菌) did not exist in Chinese medical theory prior to its communist modernisation. The fact that it is commonly used among present day TCM doctors is a clear demonstration of the communists' success in re-making Chinese medicine.

20   Scheid, *Currents*, 5.

21   Scheid, *Chinese Medicine in Contemporary China*, 3.

22   The two words, "classical" and "secular" will be used interchangeably henceforth to denote the non-religious mainstream Chinese medicine.

doctrines, plurality and pedagogy, I have opted for the more general term "Chinese medicine" to refer to our subject instead. "TCM" will be used only when I refer to its modern counterpart.

How Then Should We Evaluate Chinese Medicine?

This short re-telling of modern Chinese medical history is instructive as it demonstrates the inter-disciplinary issues involved in a proper study and theological critique of Chinese medicine. To begin, apart from having a good grasp of Chinese medical history, some knowledge of Chinese culture, philosophy and science is called for in this project. This is not all. Most Christian critiques of Chinese medicine evaluate it by the norms of Western biomedicine and thus presume the legitimacy and superiority of the latter. Judging by the rhetoric and discourses of these writers, it is, perhaps, not unfair to conclude that some even take Western biomedicine to be *Christian* in some way. The rationale for this is not entirely clear, however. More importantly, such an assumption can only be justified, if it is grounded in some way in the Church's historical engagement with Western science and medicine.

This brings us to the problems prevalent in many of the Christian critiques of Chinese medicine. Judging by their arguments and the paucity of their bibliographies, it is evident that many have not engaged in critical scholarship pertaining to the histories and philosophies of both Chinese and Western medicine.[23] The net result is that the authors often betray an ignorance of how Western (or, in particular, Greek) epistemology has shaped their understanding of medicine, and how this philosophical framework may distort their interpretation of Chinese medicine which is based on a rather

---

23   Several of the Christian critiques of Alternative Medicine (and Chinese medicine) were written between the late 1990s and early 2000s. Since then, interest in the histories and comparative studies of Western and Chinese medicine have grown significantly in the English-speaking world. This new research would prove valuable for our present study.

different epistemic paradigm.[24] Furthermore, the existing studies rarely, if ever, examine the early Christians' engagement with Western medical traditions. The fact that Hippocratic medicine could dominate the West right until the 18th century is due in no small measure to Christianity. As we shall see in Chapter 3, it was the Church which adopted, safeguarded and transmitted this Greek medicine throughout Europe during the medieval period.[25] In the medieval mind, therefore, *Christian* medicine was none other than Hippocratic-Galenic medicine. Most present-day Christians would distance themselves from this stance, of course. Yet surely, the early Christians' adoption of Hippocratic medicine offers valuable lessons for our evaluation of Chinese medicine. At the very least, it suggests that just because a medical tradition is based on a non-Christian philosophy does not necessarily disqualify it from Christian usage.

Given these manifold challenges, how then should we evaluate Chinese medicine from a *Christian* perspective? We begin, in Chapter 2, with the question of methodology. Here, we shall argue that there are three aspects to such an inter-cultural engagement. The first is the ethics of love and respect for the community (Matt. 5:44, 22:35–40) we are dialoguing with, in this case, the users and practitioners of Chinese medicine. This leads us to our second point. Such an ethical concern compels us to adopt an inter-disciplinary approach towards understanding Chinese medicine, so that we may represent it accurately. The third is to tap on our rich Christian traditions—biblical, theological and historical—and what they may teach us about engaging indigenous cultures and medical traditions.

The first two methodological concerns will occupy most of this book. Chapters 3 and 4 will survey the history of Western medicine,

---

24   For the epistemic differences in Greek and Chinese medical approaches, see Shigehisa Kuriyama, *The Expressiveness of the Body and the Divergence of Greek and Chinese Medicine* (New York: Zone Books, 1999).

25   More will be said about Greek Hippocratic medicine in Chapter 2. W. F. Bynum, *History of Medicine: A Very Short Introduction* (Oxford; New York: Oxford University Press, 2008), 69–86.

from the inception of Hippocratic-Galenic medicine to the rise of modern medicine, or biomedicine.[26] In the course of our survey, we shall consider the theological principles which the early Christians used in their evaluation of Greek medicine, before they adopted it for their use and ministry. Chapter 5 will consider the epistemologies assumed by Western medical traditions, and how they shape our beliefs about the norms and legitimacy of medical science.[27] The aim of Chapters 3–5 is basically self-knowledge. We presume most readers to be users of biomedicine, but unfamiliar with its history, let alone its philosophical biases. Unfortunately, this lack can mislead many to assume Western medical epistemology to be the norm by which they judge all other forms of indigenous medicines. As we shall see, this premise is not justifiable since such assumptions were influenced by the historical, social and geopolitical circumstances of Greek and later Western societies.

Chapters 6–8 will see us doing the same for Chinese medicine. After surveying the historical and philosophical developments of Chinese medicine (Chapters 6–7), we shall look at how the epistemological differences between Chinese medicine and biomedicine inform their conception of health, disease and therapy (Chapter 8). The discipline of cognitive linguistics, particularly the contemporary theory of metaphors, will be employed here to elucidate the differences between Western and Chinese medical discourses in these areas. Chapter 8, however, is an optional stop in your journey through this book. While the chapter will add to your understanding of the epistemological differences between Chinese medicine and biomedicine, there will not be a gap in the meta narrative if you choose to skip it.

---

26   For the rest of this book, we shall use the terms "modern medicine" and "biomedicine" interchangeably.

27   Epistemology, or the theory of knowledge, is a branch of philosophy that examines the assumptions and methods by which we arrive at the knowledge of any discipline, and the limits of such knowledge.

Chapter 9 will introduce readers to the theories and practice of Chinese medicine, while Chapter 10 will explore how the two medical traditions can dialogue profitably. This involves an evaluation of the assumptions and limits of the benchmark of biomedical efficacy: clinical trials. The concluding chapter is an exercise in constructive theology. Here, we shall reflect on the theological norms that should be assumed when we engage any indigenous medical traditions, and consider what this may mean for Chinese medicine. It is here that we shall also take up the common objections for the Christian use of Chinese medicine.

Objectives of Our Study

When one visits the Yunnan Hospital of Traditional Chinese Medicine (云南省中医医院) in Kunming, it becomes quite apparent how pervasive Chinese medicine is in China. Surrounding the hospital are rows of Chinese drug stores, filled with herbs grown largely in the province. Scattered among these shops are Chinese medical clinics, often run by master physicians, or *Lao Zhongyi* (老中医), with their attendant long queues of patients. For such Chinese and the millions of others throughout China, the legitimacy of Chinese medicine is beyond doubt. To call this esteemed tradition into question, especially by the West, would be regarded as no less than a form of cultural imperialism. Sheer numbers alone, of course, do not justify one's case. Nonetheless, this observation is important: it is a sober reminder for Christians to take our engagement with Chinese medicine and culture carefully, lest we create an unnecessary stumbling block to the Gospel, and the Christian faith is deemed by the unreached as nothing but a Western religion. Apologetics is therefore the first concern for this book. The second is plain. If Chinese medicine, according to its practitioners and users, has garnered a wealth of wisdom that can prove helpful for the sick, establishing the legitimacy of this tradition then becomes a matter of life and death for many people.

The third and final aim of this book is an exercise in contextual theology. Throughout the history of the Church, Christians have found it beneficial to engage with non-Christian sources of wisdom, both as a means of articulating and contextualising their faith.[28] The same should be expected when we dialogue with Chinese culture, as expressed through its medical tradition. This reflection, as mentioned earlier, will be undertaken in the final chapter of our book.

Finally, while this book is written primarily for a Christian audience, most of its contents (Chapters 3–10) should be helpful for non-Christians interested in finding out more about and assessing the validity of Chinese Medicine. Such readers are more than welcome, of course, to also engage the Christian perspectives expounded in Chapter 2, the second half of Chapter 3, and Chapter 11.

---

28   The best biblical example is, perhaps, John the Evangelist's appropriation of the Greek notion of *logos* (John 1:1–18) to describe the mystery of the Incarnation.

2

ENGAGING CHINESE MEDICINE:

METHODS AND APPROACHES

Galileo's Trial: Pitfalls and Lessons

In popular imagination, Galileo Galilei (1564–1642) is often esteemed as a martyr for science, due to his persecution by the Catholic authorities for his support of Copernicus' (1473–1543) Heliocentric astronomy. For the critics of Christianity, Galileo's inquisition was the archetypal example of how religion has always been opposed to scientific progress. Yet when we delve into the details of Galileo's life and trial, the truth turns out to be more complex, and rather different. For a start, Copernicus' model was but one of the many astronomical theories proposed in the 16th century. Intriguingly, it was not a popular one due mostly to its convoluted presentation in Copernicus' *On the Revolutions of the Heavenly Sphere* (1530). This was despite the support of Cardinal Schoenberg, an influential confidant of three popes. Thus, when Galileo defended the Heliocentric model, he was not so much so defending scientific truth, but arguing for one of the many astronomical theories that were being contested in the 16th to 17th centuries.

The early 1600s saw Galileo inventing the telescope, which provided the first empirical evidence for Heliocentrism. While the new findings strengthened Galileo's faith in Copernicus' theory, they did not convince the Jesuit astronomers.[1] Nonetheless, their

---

1   For an overview of the Jesuits' scientific endeavours, particularly in astronomy, see

disagreement, at this stage, was largely scientific, and Galileo's relationship with the Jesuits and the Catholic leaders remained cordial. As to how Galileo eventually landed in trouble with the papal authorities, the reasons were three-fold.

First of all, his later writings often criticised the Jesuit astronomers, which inevitably estranged these former allies. Second, and more seriously, was his attack on Aristotelian astronomy. This offended the Aristotelian philosophers greatly and it was *they*, not the astronomers or the theologians, who petitioned for Galileo's inquisition. Finally, Aristotelian philosophy had, by this time, became such an edifice of Catholic teaching that "an attack on Aristotle was tantamount to an attack on the church itself". To be sure, if the trial had been conducted on a different occasion, it could have amounted to nothing, due to Galileo's popularity. Unfortunately, 1615 was a time when the Catholics were engaged in a bitter quarrel with the Protestants regarding a Christian's right to interpret the Bible for himself. The Catholics were thus in no mood for further dissent. It was the confluence of these factors, therefore, that caused the downfall of Galileo.[2] More importantly, in Galileo's mind, his inquisition was never a case of religion opposing science. Rather, it was the sad example of how obtuse readers read their "fancies" into Scriptures and, in so doing, distorted the "right meaning of Scripture".[3]

The above controversy is instructive in so many ways. To begin, it warns us against reacting too quickly to an issue or topic of contention solely on the basis of popular opinion.[4] Unfortunately, such sentiments are often caricatures of more complex

---

Augustin Udias, *Jesuit Contribution to Science* (Place of publication not identified: Springer, 2016), 23–53.

2   Denis Alexander, *Rebuilding the Matrix: Science and Faith in the 21st Century* (Grand Rapids, MI: Zondervan, 2003), 108–24; Stillman Drake, *Galileo: A Very Short Introduction* (Oxford; NY: Oxford University Press, 2001), 40–62.

3   Galileo, *Letter to the Grand Duchess Christina*, 189.

4   This is particularly the case when we live in an era where false news abounds in the social media.

realities, which can mislead rather than inform us. Sometimes, they are even strawmen constructed for the sole purpose of attacking an opposing viewpoint. Certainly, this is how Galileo's trial has been frequently presented by the critics of religion: as the archetypal conflict between religion and science. The truth, however, is quite a different story. Galileo's trial was much more a conflict between science and Aristotelian philosophy, and one that was due, in no small measure, to Galileo's lack of tact. Beyond these, the Catholics' bias for Aristotelianism should also caution us that contemporary culture and philosophy can influence our readings of Scripture in ways far greater than we realise. Consequently, we sometimes end up mistaking human ideas as biblical truths. To be able to discern such errors is no easy matter, however. This is because our tacit beliefs are usually so self-evident that they are difficult to spot.

The pitfalls that beset our understanding of Galileo's trials are similar for our present task: a Christian evaluation of Chinese medicine. For Western Christians brought up in the Western or Greek philosophical traditions, the philosophy of Chinese medicine and its patterns of thinking are likely to be unfamiliar, to say the least. If "the past is a foreign country", as Leslie P. Hartley reminds us, ancient Chinese medical philosophy can only be even more opaque and impenetrable. This is not helped by the fact that these philosophical paradigms are also assumed in Daoist beliefs, which renders them more suspicious to Christian ears. More seriously, most Christians, including the Chinese, have been brought up with modern scientific learning. Taking for granted the norms of modern scientific epistemology, we inevitably find it hard to grasp the logic of Chinese medicine, let alone evaluate it. Given such challenges, how then should we proceed?

Loving Thy Neighbour and the Need for Inter-Disciplinary Studies

Our starting point, I believe, should be ethics. Namely, to engage the Chinese medical community and their users by Christ's great commandment: to love these neighbours like ourselves (Mark 12:31). Practically speaking, this means avoiding misrepresentation of their teachings or, worse, creating caricatures of Chinese medicine. Rather, we should seek to present Chinese medical teachings accurately, in such a way that the Chinese medical community would agree with our portrayals.

The approach that is called for should be familiar to most Christians. When we study the Scriptures, our starting point is always ascertaining the meaning of biblical passages in their original contexts. While this is not exactly rocket science, the actual process can be quite demanding. This is because it requires a familiarity with the biblical readers' original contexts, such as their histories, cultures, socio-economic contexts, literary and linguistic approaches, and philosophies. The same can be said for Chinese medicine. If we are to present this discipline accurately, we must likewise acquire some familiarity with a broad range of non-theological disciplines, such as Sinology (or Chinese studies), Chinese philosophy, Chinese linguistics, Chinese medical historiography, and, of course, Chinese medical theory. In other words, we must adopt an inter-disciplinary approach to our study.

At this juncture, some Christians may ask, "are these academic disciplines not mere human ideas? Would they not be erroneous and misleading?" While this is a valid concern, it is not a tension that can be easily resolved. As those engaged in biblical and theological studies already know, our study of the Scriptures and Christian tradition already requires us to interact with, and consult extra-biblical or non-Christian sources and disciplines. For example, if one wants to find out the range of meanings for the word *logos*, in John 1:1, one will have to consult Greek lexicons or dictionaries, such as the Liddell-Scott-Jones (LSJ) or the Bauer-Danker Lexicon of the New Testament and Early Christian Literature (Bauer). The way by which these authors ascertain the semantic fields of the different Greek words is by a careful study of their usage in (non-biblical and biblical) Greek literature. In other words, the interpretation and translation of Scriptures is possible only with the help of *non-Christian* or secular disciplines, in this case, Greek philology. If this is assumed in the field of theological studies, surely the need to consult Sinology and other related disciplines in our study of Chinese medicine should be acceptable. The only caution we should take here is to proceed as all good scholars should: by ensuring that the scholarship we consult presents accurate and unbiased accounts of their subjects. In doing this, we are following a venerable tradition. The best teachers of our Christian faith, such as Augustine, the Cappadocian Fathers, Philip Melanchthon, John Calvin, Jonathan Edwards and others, had no qualms dialoguing with and learning from their non-Christian contemporaries. Neither should we.

Theological Perspectives on Human Knowing

This is not to say that there is no theological basis for the appropriation of secular disciplines in theological studies or, indeed, for our understanding of the world in general. There are theological grounds for doing so, and it is important to spend some time reflecting on this question.

We begin with the observation that intellectual history, be it in the East or the West, has, for the most part, assumed two sources of knowledge: namely, knowledge should be based on either some form of empirical study, or transcendental truths, or both.[5] Where we differ is how we go about justifying the legitimacy of our empirical approaches or transcendental ideas. Debates, fights, and

5   Transcendental ideas are also known as first principles of knowledge. They are principles to be assumed if we are to know something, but these principles cannot be proven in themselves. For example, the shortest distance between two dots is a straight line, or for every effect, we believe there is a cause(s) to it. With regards to empirical study, we certainly have in mind here the modern empirical sciences. Nevertheless, our understanding of empiricism is broader here as it refers to the cumulative experience that one gathers as one's human senses engage the warp and woof of Creation.

even wars have been waged as a result of such disagreements. From a theological perspective, the reason for such differences boils down to our human nature, or the nature of the knowers ourselves: we are all made in the image and likeness of God (Genesis 1:26). As God's image bearers, we cannot help but aspire after the Absolute or God Himself. Or to put it differently, we all need some kind of absolute claims in our knowledge and lives.[6] Is this not why philosophers are still seeking for an overarching metaphysical explanation of the world, a theory of everything, as they put it? For the same reason, physicists continue to search relentlessly for a grand unified theory that will explain all the different types of physical phenomena in the universe.[7]

Despite all these good intentions, we human beings face a severe constraint as images of God. Simply put, we are limited creatures, operating forever in a relative realm (we are not the absolute Creator!). Our conceptualisations of knowledge must always be partial, constrained by our individual abilities, experiences, communities, cultures and, ultimately, our environments.[8] Practically, the sum of all these factors plays a crucial role in how we frame our questions, and thus dictate the results we arrive at. Consequently, we see certain aspects of a subject clearly, but are completely blindsided with regards to its other characteristics. This is also why Geoffrey Lloyd, the historian of comparative sciences, speaks of the "multidimensionality", or a plurality of styles in the human inquiry or search for knowledge.[9] As we shall see, this is certainly the case for the

---

6   This applies even for relativists, who must make the absolute claim that "all things are relative".

7   "A Long Way from Everything: The Search for a Grand Unified Theory", accessed 7 November 2017, https://newatlas.com/einstein-quantum-field-theory-relativity-gravity/42389/.

8   We can also categorise these various elements broadly as "culture" of a particular society. Seen from this perspective, culture is everything that human beings do with, make of, and cultivate or nurture from nature. John Stackhouse, *Making the Best of It: Following Christ in the Real World* (Oxford ; NY: Oxford University Press, 2011), 14–15.

9   G. E. R. Lloyd, *Being, Humanity, and Understanding: Studies in Ancient and Modern Societies* (Oxford: Oxford University Press, 2012), 44.

Greeks and the Chinese. Their intellectual inquiry took place in very different geopolitical and cultural environments. This, in turn, gave rise to their rather different conceptions of the world, and their divergent approaches to both science and medicine. The West was guided by its ontological concerns, while the Chinese by their attentiveness towards relationships between entities. These differences will become clear when we explore the histories and philosophies of each medical tradition in the subsequent chapters.

Besides the doctrine of the image of God, Christians have also found it helpful to conceptualise one aspect of human knowledge— our knowledge of the divine, through another perspective. This is the doctrine of revelation, which outlines the ways and means by which we can know God. Ever since the Age of Enlightenment (18th century), Christian theologians have sub-divided this divine knowledge into two: Special versus General Revelation.

Broadly speaking, Special Revelation refers to God's self-disclosure in the salvation history of Israel and the person of Jesus Christ. Particularly, it refers to the modes by which God revealed Himself to Israel, such as visions, casting of lots, audible voices, dreams, prophetic messages and the Incarnation. More importantly, it refers to the teachings of the Bible, whose records and interpretations have now become for us the primary means by which we receive this Special Revelation.[10]

This biblical revelation, in turn, is also the basis by which we discern God's particular guidance and work in our lives. The latter, of course, takes different forms depending on the Christian traditions we come from. For the most part, such divine guidance is understood as illumination, that is, the insights we gain as we reflect on the teachings of Scripture. It is also made available to us whenever Christians share our wisdom with one another in church communities, seminaries, monasteries, and the like. On occasions, such guidance may also be

---

10   Gerald McDermott, *A Trinitarian Theology of Religions: An Evangelical Proposal* (Oxford: Oxford University Press, 2014), 88–90.

manifested as signs and wonders, such as visions, prophecies, healings or even mystical visions.[11]

General revelation, on the other hand, refers to God's revelation of Himself through His Creation, including human reason and culture.[12] As John Calvin put it in his *Institutes*, "there are innumerable evidences both in heaven and on earth that declare His wonderful wisdom". These can be observed not only through the natural sciences, such as astronomy and medicine, and the liberal arts, but also through the historical processes and our human conscience (Rom. 2:14–15). As Calvin saw it, such revelation was possible only because there was, in the first place, an inherent awareness of divinity, a *sensus divinitatis*, planted in our human nature.[13] It is noteworthy that the different disciplines Calvin mentioned above—natural sciences, humanities and ethics—all employ, in varying degrees, empirical studies and some kind of transcendental ideas in their theories. Experiments must be conducted, or manuscripts examined, before a scientific or historical theory can be proposed. Likewise, without the assumption of axiomatic ideas, geometry, economic models and a whole host of other disciplines will not be able to progress far. In other words, General Revelation is understood as presupposing and employing these two sources of knowledge, rather than standing in opposition or antithesis to them.

Furthermore, the contents of these disciplines on their own do not constitute General Revelation. For example, none of us would regard the laws of classical mechanics or anatomical knowledge as Gen-

---

11   While all Christians concur on the primacy of biblical illumination, and the importance of guidance from fellow Christians, they often disagree on the validity of signs and wonders. Generally speaking, the Pentecostals and Charismatics are more bullish about such signs and wonders, while the more Reformed-minded Christians are far more skeptical, or even reject such supernatural signs outright.

12   This distinction was first conceived during the Enlightenment period as an apologetic to the English Deists. McDermott, *A Trinitarian Theology of Religions*, 86–87.

13   John Calvin, *Institutes of Christian Religion*, 1.5.2; 1.18; 1.3.1.

14   This is not to say that God is not involved in the process of knowledge acquisition. As the

eral Revelation *per se*.[14] For such human knowledge to operate as elements within General Revelation, they must reveal to us something about God, including His purposes for humanity and Creation. Take, for example, the laws of classical mechanics. The equations governing time, velocity and acceleration tell us much about how projectiles work, or how aeroplanes can fly safely! On their own, however, they tell us dreadfully little about the nature of God, or His purposes for Creation. They only contribute to General Revelation when, collectively, they imply that there is an order in the Universe, and this order suggests the possible existence of a Creator-God. To this example, we may add other forms of human knowledge that may count as General Revelation: beliefs in monotheism, the idea that sacrifices are necessary for the propitiation of sins, and the transcultural esteem for virtues such as love, humility and compassion.

Having said this, there is much in human knowledge and practices that we do not count as General Revelation: cannibalism, greed, lust, pride and so on. The reason is simple: these ideas are contrary to biblical teachings. This distinction is instructive. It means that human knowledge of the divine only counts as General Revelation when it parallels with, is similar to, or analogous with what God has revealed through His Special Revelation. Seen diagrammatically, General Revelation is a sub-set of human knowledge and overlaps with Special Revelation. Nonetheless, there is much knowledge, such

Humanly Derived Knowledge	
General Revelation	Special Revelation

Creator and Sustainer of the cosmos, God is the source of all knowledge. If one is to discern the truth of the cosmos, even by approximation, it has to occur with the aid of the Holy Spirit. It is more appropriate, however, to count this aid or illumination as a grace that God gives commonly to humanity, rather than to regard it as a revelatory knowledge that points us to God. The fact of the matter is, due to our human limitations and sin, human knowledge is often terminal and does not reveal God to us. Roland Chia, "Vestiges of the Divine", *Ethos Institute for Public Christianity*, November 2016, http://ethosinstitute.sg/vestigesofthedivine/.

as the Incarnation, the Trinity and so on, that is unique to Special Revelation. For this reason, they exist outside the "realm" of humanly derived knowledge.

Thus far, we have seen how the limitations of our human nature constrain our ability to know God accurately. There is yet a more serious limitation to our epistemic ability. This is none other than the human propensity to sin, which darkens or perverts our ability to perceive clearly. We encounter this problem every day. Men and women regularly make bad decisions in their work, businesses and even relationships because we, in our pride and biases, refuse to explore other possibilities or heed advice from others. Likewise, some scientists, even when they acknowledge the remote possibility for intelligent life, and observe the intricate design in biological life, still refuse to acknowledge the possibility, let alone, affirm the existence of a Creator. Human sin, therefore, introduces an additional veil to human knowledge and, oftentimes, separates us further from the truth.

Having outlined the theological principles underlying the nature of human knowing, we can now ask what they might mean for our study of Greek, modern or Chinese medicine. To begin, we must recognise that all forms of human knowledge, including medicine, are perspectival. That is, they are construed on the basis of linguistic, cultural and philosophical assumptions peculiar to the cultures that gave rise to such knowledge.[15] This constraint is, of course, bound up with the limits of our human nature, not to mention the influence of sin. The net effect of all these is that our medical knowledge will never be complete or absolute, but always partial.

Furthermore, a large part of medical tradition, be it its theories, practices or philosophies, is religiously neutral and has no bearing on our knowledge of God. For example, while the disciplines of

---

15   This will become clear when we examine the histories and philosophies underlying the Western and Chinese medical traditions.

orthopaedics, epidemiology, and oncology are extremely useful for their patients, they teach them nothing about God's nature or character. This being said, some aspects of a medical tradition may have a bearing on divine knowledge. As we shall see, this is largely on the philosophical level, that is, how a medical tradition conceptualises the world (cosmology), the nature of things (ontology), human beings (anthropology) and disease. It is these aspects that require our theological attention. This brings us to our next section: the theological models that can guide our dialogue with Western and Chinese medicine.

Theological Models for Cross-Cultural Engagement

Over the last 2,000 years, Christian theologians have developed different approaches for theological reflection and engagement. These principles have been summarised helpfully in what Methodist scholar, Albert C. Outler, calls the Wesleyan Quadrilateral, or the theological method credited to the great evangelist, John Wesley (1701–1793). According to the founder of Methodism, any theological reflections must consult and employ the following: (1) the teachings of the Bible; (2) the theological reflections and wisdom of our spiritual forefathers, or Christian tradition; (3) our reason (which involves a careful use of secular or non-Christian sources of knowledge); and (4) our spiritual experience.[16] Among these, the important authority must be the Scriptures.

To illustrate how this quadrilateral operates, let us consider the fourth-century Trinitarian controversy. In the early fourth century, Arius, an elder in the Church of Alexandria, began to teach that "there was a time when the Son was not". In other words, the Son of God was a creature, not God, even though he is much loftier than all the other

---

16   W. Gunter, *Wesley and the Quadrilateral: Renewing the Conversation* (Nashville: Abingdon Press, 1997).

creatures in the world. This ignited the Trinitarian controversy where the orthodox Christians fought hard to defend the divinity of the Son and the Holy Spirit against Arius and his sympathisers. Among the defenders was the great pastor-theologian, Basil of Caesarea. Arguing from *biblical texts*, such as John 14:9, Matthew 11:27 and John 17:26, Basil asserted that the Son shares the same knowledge as the Father and is thus equal with the Father.[17] In his defence of the Spirit's divinity, Basil likewise appealed to Scriptures (1 Cor. 12:3), but added that his teachings also conformed to the "unwritten *tradition* of the Fathers". Apart from these, Basil's Trinitarian teachings frequently brought to bear the philosophical and rhetorical *reasoning* that he acquired from his classical education, and his personal *experience* of the Spirit's illumination, all of which brought further clarity to the divinity of the Son and the Spirit.

Since then, similar "quadrilateral" approaches have been employed to defend the theological teachings that we now cherish: the doctrine of justification, the authority of the Scriptures, and so on. The same approach, I believe, can be applied to our dialogue with Chinese medicine. After an inter-disciplinary study of the Western and Chinese medical traditions (that is, the application of reason and experience), we shall bring the teachings of Scripture, and Christian tradition to bear on these findings, focusing particularly on their conceptions of God (if any), cosmology, anthropology and disease. With regards to Christian tradition, we shall draw insights from what is arguably the first Christian attempt at engaging with an indigenous medical tradition. Namely, the experience of the church fathers, who spent much effort reflecting on the value of Greek medicine.

Besides the quadrilateral model, another interpretive paradigm that we shall adopt for our inter-cultural dialogue is the contextualisation model developed by Jackson Wu. In his monograph,

---

17   Stephen M. Hildebrand, *The Trinitarian Theology of Basil of Caesarea: A Synthesis of Greek Thought and Biblical Truth* (Washington, DC: Catholic University of America Press, 2007), 161–62.

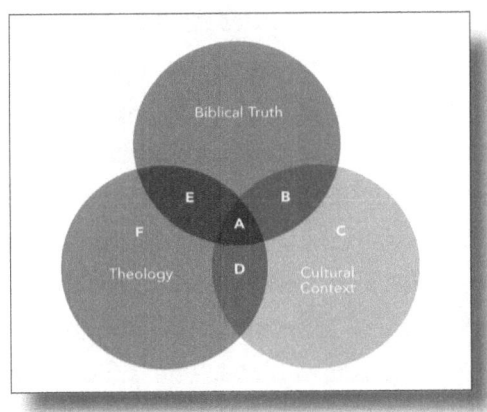

Saving God's Face, Wu proposes that an indigenous cultural or theological idea may be analysed in terms of its relation with biblical truths and its prevailing culture.

According to Wu, some theological or religious ideas are neither compatible with biblical teachings nor have an indigenous cultural context (Area F). Some cultural ideas, on the other hand, are entirely foreign to both theological and biblical teachings (Area C). Then again, there are occasions when "one's theology agrees with the prevailing culture in an unbiblical way" (Area D), such as the popular Christian support for slavery in 18th-century England. Finally, there are theological teachings, such as the doctrine of the Trinity, which cohere with Scriptural truths, but is generally rejected by culture (Area E). What interests us in Wu's model is what he defines as Areas A and B. Area A refers to theological teachings that correspond with those of the Scriptures and an indigenous culture, while Area B represents aspects of an indigenous culture that are compatible with "biblical categories and values" but not regarded as so by prevailing theologies.[18]

How then is Wu's model relevant for our analysis? Basically, it highlights the importance of identifying and attending to medical

---

18   Jackson Wu, *Saving God's Face: A Chinese Contextualization of Salvation through Honor and Shame* (Pasadena, CA: William Carey International University Press, 2012), 51–53.

philosophies or ideas that fall under Areas A or B. Ideas that belong in Area A are, of course, unproblematic, since this underscores the compatibility between a medical idea with Scriptural teachings. Ideas that fall under Area B, however, require more careful attention. This is because they often highlight a question or perspective that could well be Christian or compatible with Scriptural teachings, but is not discussed or explored sufficiently in classical (Western) Christian theology. Typically, such ideas may be foreign to Christians who may then mistake them as unbiblical. The difficulty, of course, is that no ideas ever come with an identity tag, labelled either "Area A" or "Area B". In practice then, the category of Area B reminds us to reflect more critically on a medical idea that is foreign to classical Christian theology, before deciding whether to reject it as unchristian, or accepting it as a valid insight or even a theological contribution from an indigenous culture.[19]

Conclusion

Christian dialogue or engagement with an indigenous medical tradition, such as Chinese medicine, is both an ethical and theological enterprise. Ethical because we are called to love our neighbours and must, therefore, represent them accurately. This, in turn, calls for an inter-disciplinary approach towards understanding Chinese medicine. It is only when we have done so that we can undertake a robust theological analysis of this tradition. To this end, we propose a two-fold approach. The first is to employ the quadrilateral model whereby

---

19   A good example is the Confucian idea of filial piety. In many ways, this teaching coheres well with the Scriptural teachings of honouring one's parents, and thus belongs to Area A. The Confucian emphasis on filial piety, however, also introduces questions that may not be asked by a non-Chinese Christian: for example, whether a newly married couple should live with their in-laws. While this is a non-issue for most Christians in Western societies, this can be a hot potato issue for Chinese Christians. The questions and perspectives that emerge from such complexities then belong to Area B and can contribute to the wealth of spiritual wisdom of the Church.

we subject our study of Chinese medicine to the scrutiny of Scriptural teachings, Christian tradition, reason and experience. With regards to Christian tradition, we shall employ insights from classical Christian theology and the church fathers' experiences in appropriating Greek medicine. Besides this, our analysis will also be supplemented by Jackson Wu's model of contextualisation. Accordingly, particular attention will be paid to Chinese medical ideas that are compatible with Scriptural teachings (Area A), and also those that are less explored by classical Christian theology (Area B).

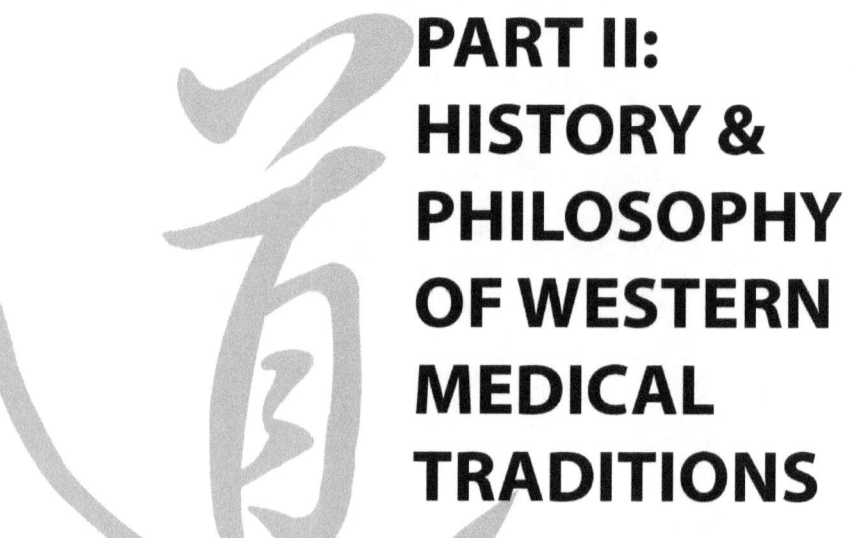

PART II: HISTORY & PHILOSOPHY OF WESTERN MEDICAL TRADITIONS

In Chapter 2, we underscored the ethical imperative in a Christian dialogue with Chinese medicine: we must represent and understand the medical tradition on its own terms. Before that can be done, however, we must recognise, first of all, that we do not enter such a dialogue entirely objective or unbiased. Rather, like the Catholics of Galileo's day, most of us bring into this dialogue a certain set of philosophical and methodological assumptions, and interpret Chinese medicine on these premises. For the most part, these assumptions are none other than the biomedical standards we are more familiar with. For this reason, the next three chapters will see us exploring the history and philosophical basis of Western medicine. We begin with Chapter 3, which will survey the history of Hippocratic medicine—the predecessor of modern medicine—and consider how the early Christians played an important role in the legitimisation and transmission of Hippocratic medicine. For our purposes, much can be learnt here since this was the first Christian attempt at dialoguing with and, eventually, adopting an indigenous medical tradition (in this case, Greek). Chapter 4, or part 2 of our survey of Western medicine, will trace the development of medicine from the Renaissance to the 20th century, when modern medicine came into its full bloom. This historical survey sets the stage for Chapter 5, where we shall unpack the philosophical and methodological assumptions of Hippocratic and modern medicine, both what they share in common, and where they differ. Essentially, the aim here is to shed light on the epistemological assumptions that we may bring to our assessment of Chinese medicine and how these biases may influence our evaluation process.

3

WESTERN MEDICAL TRADITIONS I:

ORIGINS, DEVELOPMENT & CHRISTIAN RECEPTION

Introduction

It has sometimes been suggested that the early Christians attributed all diseases to the demonic and advocated only supernatural forms of healing. Jesus himself undoubtedly healed many people, including some whom eyewitnesses regarded as demon possessed. Nevertheless, it is also evident right from the start that the first Christians had more medical options than just religious healing.[1] Luke the Evangelist, for one, was described fondly by Paul as "the beloved physician" (Col. 4:14). Presumably, this epitaph was earned when the doctor healed the apostle of the many injuries and ills that he suffered during the course of his ministry. Even so, it is not quite clear what kind of medicine Luke or, for that matter the first Christians, employed in the first century. Our knowledge only becomes better in the late fourth century, when Christians began to make references to Greek or, more specifically, Hippocratic medicine with approval.[2] In fact, after the fall

---

1   Gary B. Ferngren, *Medicine & Health Care in Early Christianity* (Baltimore: Johns Hopkins University Press, 2009), 140.

2   Church history and theology usually refer to the first five centuries of the Church as the

of the Western Roman Empire in the fifth century, the Church would play a pivotal role in not only preserving but also transmitting the legacy of Greek medicine through the Middle Ages. How this happened will be the focus of this chapter. More importantly, we will also examine the theological principles involved in the early Christians' evaluation and eventual adoption of Greek medicine, and what these might teach us in our contemporary dialogue with Chinese medicine.

Medicine in the Ancient World

In 1901, a French archaeological team in Susa (present-day Iran) unearthed one of the most important artefacts in Ancient Near Eastern history: the Code of Hammurabi Stele (c. 1754 BC). Biblical scholars have long been intrigued by the parallels between these Babylonian laws and those enshrined in the Torah, such as the demand for one to repay "an eye for an eye".[3] The same code has also fascinated historians of medicine, since it offers a rare glimpse into the state of medical practice in ancient Babylon.

> If a surgeon performs a major operation on a nobleman, with a bronze lancet and caused the death of this man, they shall cut off his hands.

> [The fees for life-saving operations are] ten shekels of silver for a nobleman, five shekels for a poor man and two shekels for a slave.[4]

While these sentences do not reveal much about Babylonian

period of the church fathers or the patristic period (the word, pater, means "father" in Latin). Most Christian traditions, whether Protestant, Catholic, Orthodox, Armenian or Coptic, regard this era as the formative period for Christian doctrine and practice. In this book, we will refer to the church fathers interchangeably with the terms "the fathers" and "the early Christians".

3   See Exodus 21:24.

4   T. Halwani and M. Takrouri, "Medical Laws and Ethics of Babylon as Read in Hammurabi's Code", *The Internet Journal of Law, Healthcare and Ethics*, 4, no. 2 (2006), 3.

medical therapy—beyond the fact that they practiced surgery—it is plain that, as early as the Bronze Age, medical practice was fairly common in Babylon, so much so that their legal responsibilities and fees had to be circumscribed by law. This being said, Mesopotamian medicine, like its Egyptian counterpart, was not quite the secular medicine which we take for granted now. Although the ancients often attributed maladies to natural causes, such as cold, malnutrition or putrefaction, they ascribed even more to the supernatural—sorcery, attacks by demonic spirits, divine punishments and the like. Their healing remedies generally paralleled diverse aetiologies: drug treatments, surgery, prayers, magic, amulets and sacrifices.[5]

Similar sentiments were observed in ancient Greece centuries later. Homer's Iliad (c. 850 BC), for example, took for granted that many injuries and sicknesses could be treated without recourse to supernatural aid.[6] Yet when a plague struck, it was also plain that the gods were involved and a priest should be called for rather than a physician.[7] Things, however, took a different turn during the classical period, when philosophers such as Parmenides (515–450 BC), Heraclitus (c. 500 BC) and Empedocles (c. 460 BC) began to speculate about the nature of reality, human constitution and disease. Out of these reflections emerged a growing conviction that diseases could be accounted for primarily by natural means. Plato (429–347), for example, proposed that all physical reality was constituted by the four elements—earth, water, air and fire—which, in turn, formed the four humours or basic building blocks of the human body—blood, phlegm, bile and black bile. Illnesses therefore occurred whenever

---

5   The word, aetiology, refers to the study of the causation or origins of a disease. Roy Porter, *The Greatest Benefit to Mankind: A Medical History of Humanity from Antiquity to the Present* (London: Fontana, 1999), 44–47.

6   The authorship and dating of Iliad is strongly contested. The Greek ancient historian, Herodotus (484–425 BC), dated it to 850 BC, while modern scholars generally place its composition between the 9th–8th century BC.

7   Vivian Nutton, *Ancient Medicine* (London: Routledge, 2005), 37–39.

the proportion of humours in one's organs was imbalanced.[8] Alcmaeon (c. 510 BC), on the other hand, attributed diseases to either a disharmony between the "forces" in one's body—moist, dry, cold, hot, bitter, sweet and so on—or to external factors like water quality, hardship and local environment. These and other forms of natural aetiologies—that is, natural causes of diseases—found their way eventually into classical and Hellenistic medical treatises, such as the Hippocratic corpus. As we shall see, the latter, in particular, will play an important role in the subsequent evolution of medicine in the West.

From Hippocratic to Galenic Medicine

The Hippocratic corpus is a collection of some 60 or so medical treatises, composed around the late fifth century to the mid-fourth century BC. While some of these could have been written by the historical Hippocrates of Cos (460–370 BC), he is unlikely to be responsible for the whole collection. This can be seen in how these different treatises taught medical theories that sometimes conflicted with one another:[9] for example, the medical treatise, *Breaths*, taught that all diseases were caused by toxic breath or changes in the air quality. *The Nature of Man*, on the other hand, adopted Plato's doctrine of four humours instead and argued that all sicknesses were due to imbalances in one's humours. Nevertheless, a medical "school" did develop around this corpus—Hippocratic dogmatism—which would find itself vying for dominance against other medical approaches, such as Methodism and Empiricism, by the first century AD.[10]

Hippocratism did become mainstream medicine in the West

---

8 *Timaeus* 32, 54–56, 82–86.

9 Owsei Temkin, *Hippocrates in a World of Pagans and Christians* (Baltimore; London: Johns Hopkins University Press, 1991), xi; Nutton, *Ancient Medicine*, xiv, 37–39, 60, 74, 486.

10 Keimpe Algra, *The Cambridge History of Hellenistic Philosophy* (Cambridge: Cambridge University Press, 1999), 604–8.

eventually. This is due, in no small measure, to the teachings and popularity of Galen of Pergamum (129–200). Galen was a one-time physician of Emperor Marcus Aurelius (121–180), a surgeon, and a brilliant philosopher to boot. During his lifetime, he not only composed tomes of medical, psychological and philosophical treatises but also conducted numerous dissections and medical demonstrations. These did much to popularise his vision of Hippocratic medicine—as one based on Plato's humoral doctrine, and also to discredit the teachings of his competitors. While Galen did not live to see his views dominate Roman medicine, his efforts did set this in motion, so much so that two to three centuries later, the mode of medical discourse would shift dramatically from "disputes over alternatives to Galen" to "arguments over the interpretation of Galen".[11]

However, we must not imagine that Galenic medicine enjoyed the kind of ideological dominance that Western biomedicine now takes for granted in most countries. On the contrary, the sick were not above consulting other forms of medical therapies. For some, particularly those living in rural areas, this could be due simply to the fact that they had no access to or could not afford physicians. In such cases then, all they could resort to were folk therapies or religious healings, such the use of talismans, amulets, or prayers to the gods.[12] There were also those patients who saw no conflict between employing secular medicine *and* religious therapies. The orator and hypochondriac, Aelius Aristides (117–191), for instance, had no qualms consulting both his physicians and the priests of Asclepius whenever he fell ill.[13]

This pluralistic approach towards healing, by and large, would persist till the 19th century, when Western medicine experienced a dramatic paradigm shift. This shall be addressed in greater detail

---

11   More will be said about Galenic-Hippocratic medicine shortly. Nutton, *Ancient Medicine*, 292.

12   Ibid., 292.

13   Temkin, *Hippocrates in a World of Pagans and Christians*, 184–85.

in Chapter 4. For now, however, we must turn our attention to the Christian adoption and transmission of Galenic-Hippocratic medicine.

Christian Adoption and Transmission of Galenic Medicine

Like their pagan peers, the majority of the church fathers, such as Origen (c. 184–c. 253), John Chrysostom (347–407), Gregory of Nazianzus (329–390) and Augustine (354–430), concur that medicine is an art and a gift of God, given for the benefit and relief of humankind.[14] Judging by their writings, it appears that they likewise adopted Galenic medicine as the norm from as early as the fourth century onwards.[15] What then is the Hippocratic-Galenic medicine they inherited? Briefly, it is a medical worldview that presupposes the ontological legacy of the Greeks. That is, to perceive all reality primarily in terms of elements, to ask "by which smallest irreducible elements are all things made of?" For Galen, this meant taking on board Plato's doctrine of the four elements and the Hippocratic theory of humours. Accordingly, diseases were due primarily to imbalanced proportions of the four humours in one's organs.[16] Physical healing then called for the correction of these imbalances, either by drugs, dietetics, cautery or surgery.[17]

Unfortunately, the state of medical practice in the Western Roman empire experienced a catastrophic downturn in the fifth

---

14   There are, of course, exceptions to these such as Tatian, Aronobius and Ps-Macarius. The reasons for their objections are quite varied and not an opposition to natural medicine itself. Tatian's opposition to the use of medical material substances, for example, is due to his concerns that the demonic would work through the materials and hold the patient captive. Darrel W. Amundsen, *Medicine, Society, and Faith in the Ancient and Medieval Worlds* (Baltimore; London: Johns Hopkins University Press, 1996), xv, 136–41, 146.

15   See Basil of Caesarea, *Longer Rules* 55; Gregory of Nyssa, *On the Creation of Humanity* and Nemesius of Emesa, *On the Nature of Man*.

16   *Timaeus* 28–29; Nutton, *Ancient Medicine*, 119.

17   Ferngren, *Medicine & Health Care in Early Christianity*, 51–52; Galen and Mark Grant, *Galen: On Food and Diet* (London: Routledge, 2000), 6.

century.[18] In the year 410, the Visigoths shocked the Romans by sacking the eternal city of Rome. This marked the first of a series of barbaric invasions that eventually overran the entire Western empire. By the early sixth century, the city of Rome was in ruins and the rest of the Western empire, which spanned from Italy to the British Isles, Spain and North Africa, was divided up and conquered by different barbaric tribes: the Visigoths in Spain, the Ostrogoths in Italy, the Vandals in North Africa and the Franks in present-day Germany and France. This was a dismal period for Europe as it saw its economies disrupted, urban life withered and its schools all but disappeared. Not surprisingly, Roman culture and education declined rapidly, along with medical practice.[19] It is not surprising, therefore, that scholars sometimes refer to this period between the fifth to tenth centuries as "the Dark Ages".

In spite of this, much learning was still taking place within the Church. Cassidorus (c. 490–585), the "Prime Minister" of the Ostrogoths, and Isidore, the Bishop of Seville, were both polymaths who could compose encyclopaedic tomes that covered virtually every known subject from the liberal arts, medicine, law, history, theology, zoology to architecture.[20] To these, we may add several other Christian intellectuals from the same period, such as Theodore of Tarsus (602–690), the Venerable Bede (672–735) and Alcuin (735–804). The common thread between them was that they were all monks. The fact of the matter is, when the Roman education system broke down, it was preserved by and remained vibrant in the monasteries, particularly those in the British Isles. This, plus the fact that the monasteries were often endowed with libraries full of manuscripts, made these institutions the *de facto* custodians of Roman culture and learning. As

---

18   To better govern its vast territories, the Roman Empire was divided into two halves: the Western and Eastern empires since the late third century.

19   Joseph H. Lynch, *The Medieval Church: A Brief History* (London; New York: Longman, 1992), 85.

20   Ibid.

we shall see, these medieval monks will play a crucial role in not only revitalising intellectual life in European lands, but also reintroducing Hippocratic medicine to these countries.

How then did the monks get involved in the practice and transmission of Greek medicine in the first place? Monasticism, as a movement, began to flourish in the fourth century when numerous Christians from all over the Roman Empire decided to pursue a life dedicated to solitude and holiness for God. Although some monks lived alone or in small groups, many more congregated in monastic communities. Inevitably, some of them fell ill and it soon dawned upon them that they needed to learn and practice medicine in order to care for their sick brothers. Before long, the monks were also extending these services outside the monasteries to serve the poor and the needy.

The first public hospital, the *Basileias*, was established in Caesarea by Basil the Great (329–379).[21] Similar institutions soon followed suit in Constantinople, Rome, Merida (Spain) and other parts of the Empire. [22] By the medieval period, this model of monastic-run hospitals had proliferated and become the norm throughout the continent. Many famous hospitals in Europe date back to this period and their names still testify to their religious origins: St Bartholomew's Hospital in London, Hôtel Dieu in Paris, and St. Maria Nuova in Florence.[23] The same period also saw many priests joining the monks in their medical practice, as a means of ministering to their parishes. This tradition of clerical involvement in medicine would continue even till the 18th century. When John Wesley (1703–1791) became a missionary in Georgia, for example, one of the first things he did was to set up a dispensary to serve his parish. Later on, he even published

---

21   Ferngren, *Medicine & Health Care in Early Christianity*, 124.

22   Gary B. Ferngren, *Medicine and Religion: A Historical Introduction* (Baltimore: Johns Hopkins University Press, 2014), 292, 301.

23   W. F. Bynum, *History of Medicine: A Very Short Introduction* (Oxford; New York: Oxford University Press, 2008), 79.

a medical guide, called the *Primitive Physick*, to educate the laity in basic medical knowledge and therapy.[24]

The monks' "monopoly" over medicine, nevertheless, underwent a significant change in the eighth century. When Charlemagne (742–814) became king of the Franks, he initiated what would be called the Carolingian Renaissance (suitably named after his empire) to reform both the Frankish Church and society. To kick off these reforms, he turned to the aid of the British monks, who not only reorganised the church hierarchy and practices, but also established three distinct schooling systems in the kingdom: the court school, the monastic school and the cathedral school.[25] Roman learning, including medicine, was thus reintroduced into the continent.

Over the next few centuries, education in Europe grew by leaps and bounds, so much so that, by the 13th century, the cathedral schools had evolved into the universities we now recognise—the Universities of Paris, Oxford, Cambridge, Bologna, and others. These medieval universities contributed to the development of medieval medicine in two important ways.

Firstly, they became the institutions by which medicine was taught and propagated as one of their three key disciplines—the other two being law and theology. Secondly, by their emphasis on the role of books and, therefore, libraries in the study of medicine, they reaffirmed Galen's writings as the undisputable authority for medical theory and practice. The significance of their impact cannot be understated since Hippocratic medicine would retain its popularity until as late as the 18th century.[26]

---

24   Clerical practice of medicine is not without controversy. Church authorities were sometimes concerned whether the clergy became too preoccupied with medical practice so much that they neglected their spiritual duties for the sake of the medical fees. Indeed, the Second Lateran Council even attempted to forbid the practice of medicine by the regular (monastic) clergy. This law, however, was never implemented. Ferngren, *Medicine and Religion*, 301, 313–15.

25   F. Donald Logan, *A History of the Church in the Middle Ages* (London; New York: Routledge, 2002), 59–63.

26   The 12th–13th centuries saw renewed Western contact with the Byzantine and Islamic

Christian Reception of Galenic Medicine: An Evaluation

Thus far, we have seen how the Church adopted Hippocratic-Galenic medicine, and even played the crucial role of preserving and re-introducing this tradition back to Europe. In the section that follows, we shall turn our attention to the church fathers' teachings about Greek medicine. Specifically, we look at *why* they regarded this medical tradition as suitable for Christian usage in the first place, and *how* they employed it in their ministry.[27] Our aim here is to elucidate the theological principles they developed in their reflections and consider how these insights may be applicable in our contemporary dialogue with Chinese and other forms of indigenous medicine.

Secular Medicine & Theological Legitimacy

We begin with the observation that Hippocratic medicine was, first and foremost, a form of secular or rational medicine. By this we mean that it does not attribute sicknesses to the whims and fancies of the gods, spirits or dead ancestors, but to predictable natural causes or, more specifically, rational laws that can be described by theories such as Galen's doctrine of the humours. This naturalisation of Greek medicine, I suggest, would have been attractive to the early Christians for two reasons. The first is the fact that it decouples medical practice from the bounds of Graeco-Roman idolatry.[28] The second and more important reason is that this emphasis on natural aetiology would have cohered very well with the Christian doctrine of Creation. If God

---

empires as a result of the Crusades. This introduced new medical texts by Byzantine and Islamic scholars like Rhazes (865–925), Avicenna (9890–1037) and Averroes (1126–1198) into Europe. As most of these treatises were influenced by Galen's ideas, they reinforced the stature of Galen in the medieval medical curriculum. Bynum, *History of Medicine*, 75.

27   For a detailed study of the early Christians' reception of Hippocratic medicine, see Temkin, *Hippocrates in a World of Pagans and Christians*.

28   This is not to say that pagan physicians do not ascribe the gift of medicine to their gods or have abandoned their beliefs in the Graeco-Roman deities. In fact, most still do. Nevertheless, they also held in common with the Christians that "everything, including diseases had its nature, and natural events were neither due to the caprice of gods nor subject to human will". Ibid., 190.

is the God of law and order, He must have, in some way, bestowed the same to His creation. The corollary is that sicknesses are due to the violation of His created order while health is a result of abiding by the same laws.

This brings us to the first principle we can derive from the early Christians' adoption of Greek medicine. Namely, whenever a medical tradition ascribes natural causes to diseases, it conforms to the above theological logic and should therefore be regarded as *theologically legitimate*. Two qualifications are necessary here, however.

First of all, such theological legitimacy should not require an indigenous medicine to conform to the philosophical or scientific frameworks assumed in either Galenic medicine or modern biomedicine. The reason for this is obvious: both forms of Western medicine actually assume rather different epistemic paradigms but are yet regarded as valid forms of rational medicine during their time. Seen from this perspective then, we can certainly count classical Chinese medicine as a kind of secular medicine since it also ascribes natural causes to diseases.[29] The key difference being that its theories are based on a rather different philosophy of *yinyang*, which is unknown to the Greeks, but assumed by virtually all ancient Chinese sciences.

Second, even if an indigenous medicine is *theologically legitimate*, this says nothing about its scientific legitimacy. A good example again is Galenic medicine. Despite its secular and rational emphasis, Galen's theories are now all but abandoned in the West and his aetiology of humours deemed unscientific. The same question of scientific legitimacy has often been raised, of course, about Chinese medicine. This is an important but complex subject and will be taken up later in Chapter 10.

The Role of Philosophy in Medicine
Readers may notice by now that Greek philosophers followed a very

---

29   More will be said about the naturalisation of Chinese medicine in Chapter 6.

distinctive mode of thinking. That is, they often enquired about the fundamental nature (*phusis*) of things or asked which elements (*stoicheia*) constituted basic reality—whether this was air, water, earth, fire, atoms or numbers.[30] The answers they derived, particularly the doctrines of the four elements, eventually became the metaphysical basis for Hippocratic-Galenic medicine. Readers may also notice that the Greeks' preoccupation with "nature" (or to use the technical term, ontology), and the Hippocratic doctrine of humours were actually perspectives and ideas quite foreign to the Scriptures. This is not to imply that these ideas contradicted biblical teachings. Rather, it is to recognise that Scriptures do not have much or, indeed, anything to say either for or against these ideas or modes of thinking. Beyond the fact that God created a good world and bestowed it law and order, the Scriptures have, by and large, left the questions of natural philosophy and metaphysics unanswered.[31] This, I suggest, is probably one reason why the early Christians had little trouble adopting Greek medicine and its metaphysical assumptions. Simply because, as we moderns would put it, it was the "best science" of the day.[32]

This is not to say that the fathers adopted Greek philosophical ideas or approaches uncritically. In fact, they debated much on and critiqued different aspects of Greek philosophy. So, while they were happy to adopt Plato's doctrine of the four elements, for example, the fathers were cautious not to endorse the philosopher's belief that

---

30   Most intriguing, Geoffrey Lloyd has highlighted that such questions about nature have not been the "central preoccupation" of the ancient Chinese. G. E. R. Lloyd, *Adversaries and Authorities: Investigations into Ancient Greek and Chinese Science* (Cambridge: Cambridge University Press, 1996), 6–8.

31   In all likelihood, biblical authors would have abided by the anthropological and medical theories of their day. For example, when Deuteronomy 6:5 called the Israelites to love God, it spoke of them as loving God from their heart (*lēb*) because it regarded the heart as the seat of one's intellect, mind or rationality. Eugene H. Merrill, *Deuteronomy* (Nashville, TN: Broadman & Holman, 1994), 164.

32   The modern equivalent, of course, is Christians' adoption of Western biomedicine. Likewise, the Scriptures have nothing to say about germ theory, antibiotics treatment, evidence-based medicine, DNA, gene therapy and other forms of biomedical knowledge. This, however, has not stopped Christians from regarding the discipline as legitimate medicine.

all matter was eternal. This was because such belief was tantamount to ascribing divinity to matter and, more importantly, erasing the distinction between Creator and creature!

What do all these mean then when it comes to our contemporary dialogue with Chinese medicine? Basically, there are few religious grounds for Christians to reject any form of secular medicine *a priori*. Just because a medical tradition is based on an indigenous philosophy is insufficient reason for disqualifying it. This is the second theological principle we can derive from the fathers' adoption of Greek medicine. This being said, there remains a need for Christians to engage the indigenous ideas critically and to assess their compatibility with Christian teaching. In all likelihood, we will find ourselves affirming some of these ideas while rejecting others. For those familiar with church history, this process is by no means unique, but has taken place every time Christianity encountered a foreign culture, whether this was Greek, Roman, Indian or Chinese.[33]

The Role of Medicine in God's Providence and Salvation
If the fathers did not have much difficulty with the metaphysical premises of Greek medicine, was there anything about the tradition they were more concerned about? Judging from the fathers' writings, it is clear that most of their energies were devoted to the role of Greek medicine in God's providence and salvation.

To begin, the fathers have always understood diseases and illnesses as the unfortunate consequences of Adam's Fall. Seen from this perspective, God's gift of medicine is but one of His providential means of relieving human suffering and can never be an elixir of immortality. On the contrary, sickness and death will always be inevitable facts of life and can only be eradicated at the general

---

33   As discussed in Chapter 2, Christian theologians, on the basis of Scriptures such as Psalm 19:1 and Romans 1:18–20, have long affirmed that God revealed aspects of Himself and His character in nature and all cultures.

resurrection.[34] Scriptural teachings, moreover, also compelled the early Christians to adopt a varied and complex aetiological system that went beyond just humoral imbalances. Illnesses, in other words, could have been due to a whole host of other reasons. Often, diseases and suffering were meted out by God as punishments for misdeeds (Exod. 9:8–12, 2 Kgs. 5:25–27). Sometimes, they were employed by God as means of training His people (2 Cor. 12:7). In some cases, they even functioned as a symbol of God's covenant grace (Gen. 32:25) or became occasions where one participated in God's cosmic duel against Satan (Job 2). In such cases, Basil of Caesarea's advice was more applicable. Healing then called for "assiduous prayers" and repentance, rather than reliance on medical therapy.[35] Regardless of whether one was healed naturally or supernaturally, the fathers were adamant that God was the ultimate healer of all diseases (Deut. 32:39, 2 Chron. 7:13–14), and medicine was but one of His means of healing.

These theological reflections, I believe, remain applicable when we consider other forms of indigenous medicine, such as Chinese or Ayurvedic (Indian) medicine. As long as an indigenous secular medicine brings relief and healing to the sick, it should be regarded likewise as a means of God's providential care. Nevertheless, the fact that death and suffering are etched irretrievably into our cosmic condition should also caution us that no medicine can ever claim to offer perfect health, let alone immortality. Furthermore, we can no longer assume a positive correlation between physical health and spiritual well-being, as was the case in Eden. The former is no longer a reliable indicator of the latter (John 9:1–3). Paradoxically, sicknesses, by God's providence, can actually become the means by which God awakens us from our spiritual stupor or strengthens our spiritual tenacity.

---

34   Jean-Claude Larchet, *The Theology of Illness* (Crestwood, NY: St. Valdimir's Seminary Press, 2002), 26–33.

35   Basil, *Longer Rules* 55 (Translated by Monica Wagner in *Fathers of the Church* Vol. 9, 332).

Medical Metaphors and Christian Teaching

The early Christians' interest in Greek medicine was not confined merely to its theological legitimacy and role. In fact, Hippocratic theories, therapies and practice also provided the church fathers with rich analogies and models for teaching and pastoral ministry. Among these, the most prominent is the figure of the Hippocratic physician. Ever since the classical period, Greek philosophers have often regarded themselves as "physicians of the soul". "The medical art", as Democritus (c. 460–370 BC) put it, "heals diseases of the body, whereas wisdom relieves the soul of passions".[36] In the second century, this motif was taken on board by the Christians and they began to exalt Christ likewise as the "Great Physician" (*Christus medicus*).[37] Before long, the epitaph was also applied to Christian pastors, so much so that, by the fourth century, church fathers, such as John Chrysostom and Augustine, could take for granted that their pastoral counsel was a form of psycho-medical therapy.[38]

Intrinsic to this physician metaphor, of course, is the understanding of human sin as a disease that requires healing. This is what many of the fathers took it to be. John Chrysostom, for example, often described sinners as severely diseased persons who were "very old and crazed", deformed and hideous, or overcome by the leprosy of sin. Relief, as he saw it, could only come from Christ, who could heal and restore them into a pristine spiritual beauty and vibrancy.[39]

As to how such spiritual healings operated in practice, the key Hippocratic therapies—surgery, drugs, dietetic regimen—

---

36   Quoted from Temkin, *Hippocrates in a World of Pagans and Christians*, 8.

37   *Apostolic Constitutions* 33; Amundsen, *Medicine, Society & Faith*, 133.

38   Paul R. Kolbet, *Augustine and the Cure of Souls: Revising a Classical Ideal* (Notre Dame, IN: University of Notre Dame Press, 2010), and Wendy Mayer, "Shaping the Sick Soul: Reshaping the Identity of John Chrysostom", in *Christians Shaping Identity from the Roman Empire to Byzantium: Studies Inspired by Pauline Allen*, ed. Geoffrey D. Dunn (Leiden: Brill, 2015), 150–54.

39   John Chrysostom, *hom. in Rom.* 14; *hom in Tit.* 3:16; *hom. in Col.* 8.

again provided the fathers with much food for thought.[40] When faced with the problem of unrepentant sinners, the author of the *Apostolic Constitutions* took his cue from Hippocratic surgery and recommended that such people be cut off (or excommunicated) like "gangrene". This was because they could potentially corrupt and destroy "the whole body of the church".[41] In his extensive reflection on the relationship between medicine and Christian spirituality, Basil of Caesarea found the doctrine of humoral balance a worthy model of discipleship and commended it heartily to his monastic readers. Just as the flesh must "eliminate foreign elements (or humours) and add whatever is wanting", he explained, so also should one remove whatever vice that damages his soul and increase any virtue that is befitting him as an image of God.[42] In a similar vein, he advised his readers to accept pastoral reproach as they would bitter medicine. For just as the latter brought relief to their bodies, spiritual reproach— though difficult to bear—was also efficacious for healing their souls.[43] At the end of his treatise, Basil went so far as to recommend his readers to take up the medical regimen. The regimen, he explained, "prohibits sensual indulgence, it is opposed to satiety, it forbids as inexpedient an elaborate diet and an exaggerated liking for condiments. In general, it regards want as the mother of health". Consequently, if a monk practised it regularly, he would find himself reaping not only bodily health but, more importantly, spiritual self-control.[44]

The therapeutic use of drugs, surgery and dietetics, is, of course, not unique to Hippocratic medicine. Neither is the idea of healing as a restoration of balance (in this case, of humours) in one's body. As we shall see, such ideas and practices are also common in Chinese medicine. It remains to be seen what spiritual analogies Chinese

---

40   Galen and Grant, *Galen: On Food and Diet*, 6; Basil, *hom. Deus non auct. mal.* 3; Ferngren, *Medicine and Religion*, 95.

41   *Apostolic Constitutions* 2:20, 2:41.

42   Basil, *The Long Rules*, 55.

43   Ibid.

44   Ibid.

medicine may offer for communities familiar with this tradition.[45] Among the above reflections on Hippocratic medicine, the most significant, perhaps, is the patristic notion of sin as a disease that requires therapeutic healing. This is a helpful reminder, particularly for Protestants. In evangelical teaching on Christian salvation, our emphasis has often been on the fact that Christ has died to pay for the penalty of our sins and, through Him, we are forgiven by God. Although this doctrine of penal substitution is entirely right, it is but one important dimension of Christian salvation. This is because we are not only saved *by* Christ but are also saved to *become like Christ*. This is when the patristic view of salvation as medical healing is helpful. By reminding us that our sinful tendencies are still in need of practical and daily healing, it beckons us to die daily to ourselves and be renewed in the Spirit so that we may attain that end which God has purposed for us: Christ-likeness.

Medical Practice as Christian Compassion

Earlier, we mentioned that the fourth-century monks extended their medical services beyond the monasteries to serve both the poor and needy. Seen from their times, such philanthropy was actually a very radical move. "Graeco-Roman paganism", as Ferngren explains, "lacked any religious and philosophical basis for charity that encouraged a personal concern for those in physical need". As the Romans saw it, the sick, disabled and the weak were worthless people and undeserving of their care and concern. In fact, it was commonly assumed that if anyone were poor or sick, he probably deserved it in the first place.[46] Given such sentiments, it is hardly surprising that medical services were only offered to those worth their salt, such as the soldiers or gladiators. The idea that one should

---

45   This, we shall explore, in Chapter 11.

46   Ferngren, *Medicine & Health Care in Early Christianity*, 144; Helen Rhee, *Loving the Poor, Saving the Rich: Wealth, Poverty, and Early Christian Formation* (Grand Rapids, MI: Baker Academic, 2012), 14–19.

provide medical care to the poor and needy was entirely unheard of and, in fact, unfathomable. To put it differently, left to itself, Roman and subsequent Western society would never have bothered with the plight of the poor and ill.

What caused this radical change then, so much so that the entire Western world, till this day, remains a strong advocate for the rights of all humanity and the care of the marginalised? This paradigm shift, I suggest, was motivated largely by two new teachings introduced by the Church. The first was the recognition that God had sent His Son to become a human being, so that He could not only live with, heal and teach us, but also redeem us. God did not owe this to us, of course, but did so out of His infinite love for humanity so that, "while we were yet sinners, Christ died for us" (Rom. 5:8). Second, Christ also taught a significant parable concerning the care of the sick: *The Parable of the Good Samaritan*. By going through the trouble of helping the injured Jew, the Samaritan demonstrated clearly the essence of Christian love: namely, it is a love that is willing to trouble itself, transcend racial prejudices and is ever ready to make sacrifices. When both teachings were taken seriously, the practical outcome was inevitable: all Christians, including the monks, were called to love and care for the poor and sick, the co-bearers of God's image. This then was the impetus for the monks' engagement in medical care, and the reason why charitable institutions sprang up in churches almost right from the beginning of the Christian movement.[47]

With regards to Chinese medicine, this patristic emphasis is instructive. If Chinese medicine turns out to be efficacious, at least for some illnesses, surely it can play a role in Christians' outreach to the sick and the marginalised. This, of course, remains an open question, until we consider properly the clinical efficacy of Chinese medicine in Chapter 10.

---

47   Ferngren, *Medicine & Health Care in Early Christianity*, 144–45.

The Relationship Between Spiritual and Physical Well-Being

Before we conclude our discussions on the fathers' reception of Hippocratic medicine, I would like to make some observations about the influence of Greek anthropology on their views of psychosomatic health. As we shall see in Chapter 5, this will play a crucial role in how we understand and assess the value of Chinese medicine.

Since the classical period, the Greeks have, by and large, adopted a dichotomised view of the human being. That is, human nature comprised two parts: the body (*soma*) and the soul (*psyche*). Philosophers often disagreed on what constituted the soul, whether it was entirely rational, or included spirited and appetitive aspects. Nevertheless, most concurred that the body was material while the soul was made up of very fine, or rarefied material.[48] The body and the soul, moreover, were intimately related. The responsibility of the soul, or its rationality, was to lead the body, so that it might not hinder the soul from attaining a state of happiness or well-being (*eudaimonia*).[49] This dynamic between one's reason and bodily desires was well illustrated in Plato's famous chariot allegory. The soul, as he put it, was "like the natural union of a team of winged horses and their charioteer". If the chariot was to move towards the right direction, the charioteer, or rationality, must restrain and lead the horse of bodily desires.[50] Seen from this perspective, it is hardly surprising that the Greeks always regarded the soul to be superior to the body.

Such a view of human nature had two implications for how the Greeks understood the relation between spiritual and physical well-

---

48   Plato, for example, divides the human soul into three parts: the rational, the spirited and the appetitive. The appetitive governs one's bodily desires (such as thirst, hunger, and sexual desire) while the spirited is the part that gets angry. Other philosophers simply saw the soul as "the seat of divinity within the mortal form". Suffice to say, Plato's tripartite model would become popular by the Graeco-Roman period. John Anthony McGuckin, *Westminster Handbook to Patristic Theology* (Louisville, KY: Westminster John Knox Press, 2005), 317; Gregory A. Smith, "How Thin Is a Demon?", *Journal of Early Christian Studies*, 16, no. 4 (2008): 479–512; *Timaeus* 42–43.

49   *Phaedo* 65d–69c.

50   *Phaedrus* 246a–b.

being. First of all, spiritual well-being was always regarded as more important than bodily health. If one had to choose between the two, the priority had to go to the cultivation of the soul, even if this was detrimental to the body. This being said, it was not uncommon for the Greeks to presume psychic health as having a positive impact on physical well-being.[51] The reverse, however, did not hold true. Generally, the Greeks were less sanguine about the potential benefits of physical health for the soul. The Neo-Platonic philosopher, Plotinus (204–270), it appears, saw no relationship between the two and so refused medical treatment for his intestinal diseases. As for Plato, the two were linked only in the sense that some psychological illnesses, like madness and stupidity, could be due to somatic causes.[52]

In short, the Greeks understood the psychosomatic relationship as *asymmetric*, where the soul was always prioritised over the body. In terms of *bilateral influence* between the two, psychic well-being was often regarded as having a positive impact on the body, while the reverse is true only in the negative sense.[53]

With regard to the early Christians, it was clear that they took on board the above psychosomatic dichotomy and likewise emphasised

---

51   The Hellenistic physician, Erasistratus, for example, attributed Prince Antiochus' illnesses to his infatuation with his young step-mother. In a similar vein, Plotinus believed that his disciple's recovery from gout and weakness in his limbs was due to his retirement from politics and adoption of a philosophic life. Temkin, *Hippocrates in a World of Pagans and Christians*, 15; Porphyry, *Life of Plotinus*, 7.

52   Porphyry, *Life of Plotinus* 1–2; Nutton, *Ancient Medicine*, 117.

53   The reason for this, as G. E. R. Lloyd explains, is to be found in socio-political context of classical Greek society. In his comparative study of ancient Greek and Chinese sciences, Lloyd observes that Greek philosophers and politicians must constantly vie for their ideas (not to mention, prestige and followers) by denying those of their competitors. The net result is that the Greeks tend to conceptualise their ideas dualistically (mine versus theirs) and that their ideas often take on a characteristic bias for one pole over the other (mine is better than theirs). This asymmetric bias is evident not only in matters of ontology, where "becoming depends upon being, but *not* vice versa. Appearance depends upon reality, but *not* vice versa". It is also prevalent in Late Antique society, where it is universally assumed that the enslaved must always be subjected to the free, the female is but a deformed male, and the Greeks are always superior to the barbarians. Lloyd, *Adversaries and Authorities: Investigations into Ancient Greek and Chinese Science*, 121, 128, 130.

the cultivation of the soul. As they saw it, sin arose from the soul, not the body. Indeed, it occurred whenever the soul allowed the flesh to "gain mastery over her charioteer [reason] and exalts itself".[54] This was also the reason why the Christian monks embraced a harsh asceticism: it was to subdue and subordinate their bodily desires to the rational soul in order that they might become virtuous like Christ.

As for the relation between spiritual and bodily health, a similar ambivalence was observed among the early Christians. Antony (251–356), for example, understood Christ's salvation solely as the restoration of one's *psyche* which had little bearing on one's bodily health. Pachomius (292–348), in his *Letters*, likewise assumed that monks would fall sick at one time or another, regardless of their sanctity or ascetic practice. The *Coptic Life of Pachomius* took an even more radical stance. Pachomius, we were told, refused to moderate his ascetic practice or receive medical treatment even when he was ill. This was because sickness had become for him a means of drawing closer to God and therefore a surer mark of his sanctity.[55] In other words, bodily health correlated negatively with spiritual health.

Athanasius of Alexandria (296–373), however, believed that psychic health can be beneficial for the body. This was why his biography of Antony portrayed the monk as enjoying a pristine health and youthfulness, even though he practised a harsh asceticism in a deserted fortress for 20 years.[56] An interesting variant of this view is that given in the *History of the Monks in Egypt*. Here, asceticism did take a toll on several monks, with John of Lycopolis, for example, so worn out that "beard no longer grew on his face".[57] Nevertheless, these Egyptian monks did not pay the price of a premature death for contravening medical norms. Rather, they lived on to ripe old ages,

---

54   John Chrysostom, *hom. in Eph.* 5.
55   Crislip, *Thorns in the Flesh*, 55–56, 140–44, 150, 154.
56   Ibid., 60–68, 72; *Vita Antonii* 14.
57   *Historia monachorum in Aegypto* 1.17.

as was the case for John of Lycopolis (more than 90 years old) and Cronides (110 years old).[58]

Based on the above, it was evident that the fathers, by and large, imbibed the anthropological assumptions of their pagan peers. There was, however, one important difference between the two. Namely, the fathers affirmed that their bodies could contribute positively to the cultivation of divine love and virtues. Ample examples of this can be found in the *Sayings of the Desert Fathers*. Physical labour, for example, was deemed necessary not only for one's livelihood, but also as a safeguard against certain temptations, such as spiritual despondency.[59] Much spiritual insight, moreover, could also be gained by listening to one's bodily experiences. Such was the case for Abba Poemen, who held a pebble in his mouth so that he could develop inner quietude. Likewise, a monk's inability to take hold of the wind then became for him a sober reminder of how we cannot prevent temptations from coming into our minds.[60]

Finally, the body was also understood as the medium by which we expressed God's love and virtues. This was why an old monk was willing to stop fasting and eat, simply because he saw it as more important to show love and hospitality to his visitors.[61]

What then do all these discussions about patristic anthropology have to do with our dialogue with Chinese medicine? The Chinese medical tradition, as we shall see, has also reflected extensively on the relationship between spiritual and physical well-being.

---

58   For example, we are told that Abba Theon ate only "vegetables … that did not need to be cooked" and Abba John of Lycopolis ate "nothing apart from fruit" and avoided "anything that needed to be cooked". These were not curious observations on the part of the author, but most likely his recognition that the monks had contravened Galenic dietetics. According to Galen, cooking was necessary in order to ripen fruits and vegetables and to aid digestion. *hist. monach.* 1.17, 6.4; alim. fac. 2.4, 6.4; Galen and Grant, *Galen: On Food and Diet*, 7.

59   *Sayings of the Desert Fathers*, Antony 1, Silvanus 5 [Benedicta Ward and Anthony Bloom, *The Sayings of the Desert Fathers: The Alphabetical Collection* (Kalamazoo, MI: Cistercian Publications, 1984)], 1, 223.

60   *Sayings*, Agathon, 15; Poemen.

61   *Sayings* 13.10.

These reflections, however, are based on a rather different Chinese anthropology and so beg the question whether they are compatible with Christian teachings. This question will be taken up in Chapter 11, after we have reviewed the history and philosophy of Chinese medicine (Chapters 6–8).[62]

Conclusion

Most ancient societies practised a combination of natural and religious forms of healing. The decoupling of the two approaches began in the fourth century BC, when Greek philosophers began to postulate natural causes to the cosmos, human beings and diseases. This set the stage for the development of secular Greek medicine which became popular during the Roman imperial period. While competition was rife between the different medical schools, Hippocratic-Galenic medicine would become dominant by the fifth century. Its practice, unfortunately, waned during the Dark Ages, when the Western Roman Empire was overrun by barbarians and went into decline. Galen's legacy, however, was preserved by the Church, primarily in its monasteries. The renewal of education and religion during the Carolingian Renaissance saw the monasteries reintroducing Galenic medicine to Western Europe. Eventually, Galen was taught in the medieval universities and regarded as the authoritative figure in medieval medicine.

The early Christians' adoption of Galenic medicine was due, in no small measure, to their continued reflections on the value and role of medicine. For our purposes, these reflections also provide much insight as to how one can engage an indigenous medical tradition theologically. First of all, we observe that Galenic medicine was premised on natural laws and philosophy. Christians would have

---

62   For a comparison of Patristic anthropology with Chinese medical anthropology, see Pak-Wah Lai, "Comparing Patristic and Chinese Medical Anthropologies: Insights for Chinese Contextual Theology", *Studia Patristica* 91, no. 17 (2017): 213–24.

found this compatible with and amenable to their belief that God is a Creator of law and order. Secondly, the church fathers did not think that it was problematic for Galenic medicine to be based primarily on a secular philosophy, i.e., Greek metaphysics. This suggests, quite helpfully, that just because a medical tradition assumes an indigenous philosophy it need not be disqualified from Christian usage *a priori*. Rather, one must engage these indigenous ideas critically before rejecting or adopting them. Thirdly, Hippocratic medicine provided the many rich metaphors for Christian teaching and soul care. Should Chinese medicine be found compatible with Christian beliefs, it could well become another resource for didactic or spiritual metaphors. In a similar vein, the practice of Chinese medicine can also become another avenue for Christians to show compassion to the sick and the needy. Finally, patristic reflections on Christian anthropology have been influenced, quite significantly, by Greek conceptions of spiritual and physical well-being. Chinese anthropology, as we shall see, is quite different from its Greek counterparts. Its value and compatibility with Christian teaching would have to be assessed at a later stage.

4

WESTERN MEDICAL TRADITIONS II:

Scientific Revolution & Rise of Modern Biomedicine

Introduction

When I was studying in England, my family would make weekly trips to the nearby Tesco supermarket for groceries. Whenever we arrived, my four-year-old son would dash through the entrance before making a beeline for the aisles on the right. Meanwhile, my wife would take her time and push her cart in the opposite direction. The reason for this was simple. The toys were on the right while the groceries on the left. More intriguingly, if I were to ask my son what else was available in Tesco, he might not be able to say much, the reason being that all he was concerned about was the toy section. Such behaviour is not unique to juveniles, of course. Most of us, in fact, behave similarly, being more familiar with some quarters of a supermarket, yet entirely clueless about what else it may offer until we start looking for something else. This is because our interests and the questions that we ask—"where are the toys?" or "where is the baking section?"— largely determine what we know and where our blind spots are.

The same can be said about human learning. The questions that we ask about the world, to a great extent, determine the answers we get. Change our perspective or the way we frame our questions and we find ourselves arriving at rather different answers. This is certainly the case for medical practice in the West. In this chapter, we will trace how a paradigm shift in learning eventually transformed European medicine from its esteem for Galen to the biomedicine we are now familiar with. Our journey will explore the contribution of Christianity in this intellectual revolution and take us through the significant moments in the rise of biomedicine. Following this, we shall reflect on the main characteristics and ideological emphases of biomedicine in Chapter 5, and consider how it is, in many ways, still shaped by its Greek legacy. What we gather here will then become our basis for a dialogue between biomedicine and the Chinese medical tradition in the later part of our book.

The Renaissance and the Scientific Revolution

In the previous chapter, we mentioned that intellectual knowledge, as understood in the Middle Ages, was thought to be found in the writings of the great authorities for each discipline: the Bible and the church fathers for theology, Aristotle for philosophy, and Galen for medicine. For the medieval student, the sources for such authorities were available mostly in the form of anthologies or, for the most part, as commentaries by medieval scholars, such as the *Sentences* of Peter Lombard (1096–1160). This was not a problem for them, however, simply because the primary task of learning, as they saw it, was to acquire knowledge systematically and to reconcile any apparent contradictions between these sources. It would not have occurred to the medieval scholars that their sources, which were mostly Latin translations, could be based on spurious or inaccurate manuscripts, or that the teachings of Greek authors, such as Plato, Aristotle or Galen, could differ in some measure when read in their original languages.

These assumptions, however, began to change in the early 15th century. In northern Italy, new and different questions were being asked about learning; questions that demanded alternative answers. Increasingly, scholars were convinced that their studies should not be based on what the medieval masters taught, but on the original sources ("*ad fontes*" in Latin) of each subject. This change in perspective soon gave rise to new modes of learning. Henceforth, one's studies must not only employ the most reliable and accurate manuscripts, but must be conducted also in the original languages of these texts. Thus, the Old Testament must be studied in its original Hebrew and Aramaic, while the New Testament in Greek. Equally important was the belief that texts should always be interpreted in their historical context and not in abstract from the original works. This new paradigm of learning, along with its adoration for all things ancient, would give birth to a new intellectual movement in Europe: the Renaissance.

The Renaissance began initially as the parochial interest of a few lawyers in Padua, northern Italy. It did not take long before it became a significant cultural phenomenon in major Italian city states, such as Florence, Rome and Milan. By the end of the 15th century, this Humanist movement (as it was also known) had reached northern Europe and begun to exert its influence. Cities like Wittenberg, Heidelberg and Frankfurt soon saw their universities abandoning the traditional pedagogy of the medieval scholars (or medieval scholasticism) and adopting the new approaches of the humanists instead.[1] Among the humanists, there were many, such as Erasmus (1466–1536) and Martin Luther (1483–1546), who held up hopes that this new cultural development would do much good in the Catholic Church by reforming its teachings and correcting its many abuses. These aspirations led eventually to the Protestant Reformation, where humanist learning would play an important role in the teachings of the magisterial Reformers such as Luther, Philip Melanchthon (1497–1560) and John Calvin (1509–1564).

These different developments also proved significant for the

---

1   Charles G. Nauert, *Humanism and the Culture of Renaissance Europe* (Cambridge; NY: Cambridge University Press, 1995), 132–36.

birth of modern science. Medieval Europe, through the 12th-century translations of Greek and Arabic works, was already familiar with ancient Greek sciences, such as those taught in Aristotle's *Physics* (4th century BC), Ptolemy's *Almagest* (2nd century AD) and Euclid's *Elements* (c. 300 BC).[2] These, in turn, would have bequeathed to the West a respect for the role of logic and mathematics in the study of the cosmos. This instinct was clearly at play when Nicholas Copernicus (1473–1543) rejected Ptolemy's astronomy. His argument, interestingly, was based not on his own empirical observations but simply on the apparent mathematical inelegance of the Ptolemaic model.[3]

More was at work, however, besides the esteem for mathematics. Early modern astronomers and natural philosophers (this was what they used to call scientists) such as Johannes Kepler (1571–1630), Galileo (1564–1642) and Isaac Newton (1643–1727) also held in common the conviction that the world was created by a good and rational God.[4] As they saw it, God had composed two books: the Book of Revelation—the Bible—and the Book of Nature, the latter of which must be investigated empirically through the language of mathematics. As Kepler put it:

> Why waste words? Geometry existed before the Creation, is co-eternal with the mind of God, is God himself... geometry provided God with a model for the Creation and was implanted into man, together with God's own likeness—and not merely conveyed to his mind through the eyes.[5]

---

2   The 12th century saw a growing economic and intellectual exchange between Western Europe and the East, that is, the Byzantine Empire and the Arabs. It was this that led to the influx of new manuscripts (in Greek and Arabic) into Europe and catalysed the translation movements in cities like Toledo and Paris.

3   Denis Alexander, *Rebuilding the Matrix: Science and Faith in the 21st Century* (Grand Rapids, MI: Zondervan, 2003), 76–79.

4   John Hedley Brooke, *Science and Religion: Some Historical Perspectives* (Cambridge; NY: Cambridge University Press, 1991), 117–51.

5   By postulating geometry as co-eternal with God, Kepler seemed to have erased the

In other words, the Christian doctrine of Creation was instrumental in cultivating both a belief in the possibility of science and also an interest in scientific pursuits. Modern science, concluded A. N. Whitehead,

> must come from the medieval insistence on the rationality of God, conceived as with the personal energy of Jehovah and with the rationality of a Greek philosopher…My explanation is that the faith in the possibility of science, generated antecedently to the development of modern scientific theory, is an unconscious derivative from medieval theology.[6]

It was Francis Bacon (1561–1626), however, who would prove influential in how modern science proceeded subsequently. In his *Novum Organum*, Bacon criticised the teachings of Aristotle and other medieval authorities as "preposterous philosophies which have… led experience captive, and triumphed over the works of God." In their stead, he urged his readers to "commence a total reconstruction of sciences, arts and all human knowledge" through the empirical study of nature.[7] True to his word, Bacon, on one occasion, decided to investigate whether snow could preserve meat. This he did by stopping at the countryside and stuffing a fowl with snow in the midst of a cold, bitter winter. The experiment proved him to be correct. The philosopher, unfortunately, contracted pneumonia and died soon after as an unwitting martyr for his belief!

Notwithstanding this, the empirical approach to knowledge was embraced enthusiastically by many, particularly in England. Robert

distinction between creation (including geometry) and God. Notwithstanding this, it remains clear that Kepler's theism was instrumental in his pursuit of astronomy. Quoted from Alexander, *Rebuilding the Matrix*, 80.

6   Alfred North Whitehead, *Science and the Modern World. Lowell Lectures*, 1925, (New York: Macmillan, 1925), 18.

7   Quoted from Alexander, *Rebuilding the Matrix*, 85–87.

Boyle (1627–1691), for example, spent most of his life engaged in experiments and in so doing, discovered Boyle's Law and pioneered modern chemistry. William Harvey (1578–1657) likewise examined animal anatomy studiously and concluded that blood was pumped around the body by the heart, thus refuting the earlier theories of Galen and Avicenna. Among the English empiricists, the most influential remains Isaac Newton. His laws of classical mechanics would become the scientific basis for the many technological advances that catalysed the 19th-century Industrial Revolution. Philosophically speaking, the elegance and precision of the Newtonian laws also persuaded many that the world was but a mechanical universe that could be understood precisely, particularly through mathematics. Indeed, this belief would inspire many academics to pursue a similar theoretical precision in their own disciplines, whether this was history, theology or even medicine.[8]

Experiments have been and, in many cases, are still a tedious and messy business, involving the setting up of delicate instruments, dissection of animal entrails or human cadavers, and long hours of painstaking measurements. Since ancient times, such manual labour was never welcomed but was, in fact, disdained by the intelligentsia. The mechanical workshop, as Cicero (106–43 BC) declared, "contains nothing fit for a freeborn man."[9] What happened then that persuaded the intellectuals of early modern Europe to change their minds? The answer, once again, lay in Christian theology. Since the beginning of the Church, Christians had long emphasised the value of work in spiritual formation. Christian monks, for example, regulated their ascetic practice through a daily rhythm of prayer *and* work. All prayer and no labour, as they saw it, was detrimental to the soul. Churches and monasteries, moreover, saw it as their duty to care for the poor, the widowed and the sick. This, as we discussed previously,

---

8   W. F. Bynum, *History of Medicine: A Very Short Introduction* (Oxford; NY: Oxford University Press, 2008), 99.

9   Alexander, *Rebuilding the Matrix*, 92.

led to the eventual establishment of public infirmaries as a concrete means of fulfilling Christ's commandment to love our neighbours. This Christian esteem for work would gain yet greater prominence during the Reformation. In his exposition on the priesthood of all believers, Martin Luther declared that all kinds of work, manual or otherwise, were valid expressions of Christian priesthood. Accordingly, mundane labours, such as ploughing, milking the cow or, in our case, conducting tedious experiments were not inferior activities but were as significant as the duties of the priests.[10] Luther's re-conception of work soon gained traction in Europe and would play an important role in the subsequent scientific revolution. By removing the deeply entrenched cultural stigma against manual labour, his teachings made it possible for intellectuals to engage in experimentation as a dignified business. If not for this, it is doubtful whether the modern scientific movement would have attained the momentum and achievements that it had.

Popular thinking has sometimes seen science and religion as being contradictory or, in fact, in conflict with one another. As demonstrated above, Christian theology actually played a positive and remarkably important role in the rise of modern science during the 17th to 18th centuries.[11] As we shall see, the medical world soon felt the impact of the new scientific insights and methodologies discovered in this period. This led eventually to an evolution and, in some ways, an overhaul of Western medicine in the next few centuries. How this happened will be the focus of our next section.

The Evolution of Medicine from the 17th to 18th Centuries

By now, it should be clear to readers that medieval medicine is

---

10   Martin Luther, *The Epistles of St. Peter and St. Jude: Preached and Explained* (NY: Anson D. F. Randolph, 1859), 106.

11   Gary B. Ferngren, *Science and Religion: A Historical Introduction* (Baltimore, MD: Johns Hopkins University Press, 2002), ix.

not quite the same as its contemporary counterpart. Our General Practitioners no longer speak of humoral imbalances, but rather of bacterial infections, viruses, cancer or genetic defects as the causes of our illnesses. This being said, both medical traditions still share and esteem a common foundational discipline: anatomy.

That the human body may be dissected for investigation was an idea unheard of and, in fact, sacrilegious in classical Greece. Such practice only became acceptable, albeit for a short while, during the Hellenistic period, when the Alexandrian physicians, Herophilus of Chalcedon (c. 335 BC) and Erasistratus of Julis (300–240 BC) received imperial permission to dissect dead criminals.[12] After a hiatus of more than three centuries, Graeco-Roman interest in anatomy revived in the second century AD, with Galen of Pergamum as its best spokesman.[13] Indeed, Galen's *On the Usefulness of the Parts* is the most detailed and complete account of human anatomy from this period. When his teachings became dominant subsequently, this treatise and other Galenic writings became pretty much the gold standard for anatomy during the Middle Ages. As for Galen himself, he was widely esteemed as an inspiration for those keen to develop his anatomical legacy.

The first medieval public human dissection took place in Bologna (1315). Anatomical interest soon became widespread, with more dissections conducted and many books written about the subject, most notably Andreas Vesalius' *De humani corporis fabrica* (*On the Fabric of the Human Body*, 1543). Indeed, the next three centuries would see anatomical studies becoming "the queen of the medical science"[14] and making significant discoveries, the most influential, perhaps, being William Harvey's discovery (1628) that the heart was responsible for pumping blood through the body. This medical

---

12   Heinrich Von Staden, "The Discovery of the Body: Human Dissection and Its Cultural Contexts in Ancient Greece", *Yale Journal of Biology and Medicine*, 65 (1992): 223–41.

13   Vivian Nutton, *Ancient Medicine* (London: Routledge, 2005), 213.

14   Bynum, *History of Medicine*, 88–91.

insight would prove valuable 300 years later, when the first open-heart surgeries were successfully performed in the 1950s.[15]

The discrepancies between these new discoveries and Galen's anatomical theories did not go unnoticed. In line with the spirit of the Renaissance and scientific empiricism, doubts were soon cast upon Galen's teachings so much so that by the early 17th century, his influence had more or less waned. His hero, Hippocrates, did not suffer a similar fate, however.[16] The fact of the matter is, early modern medicine knew far more anatomy than its physicians could use and what was discovered had little impact on medical therapeutics. Consequently, Hippocratic therapies, such as "bloodletting, emetics (to invoke vomiting), cathartics (to induce purging), and the gamut of remedies associated with humoralism continued as the mainstay of doctors".[17] Indeed, the Hippocratic orientation towards patients, that is, to rely on the "patients' accounts of their own feelings and symptoms to make their diagnoses", continued to define medical encounters right until the 1920s.[18]

Two further developments in 16th- to 17th-century medicine were noteworthy. The first was Paracelsus' (1493–1541) "emphasis on chemistry, as a way of understanding the way the human body works, and as a source of drugs to treat disease." This paved the way for the use of metals, such as mercury and arsenic, and traditional botanicals to treat diseases.[19] The second had more far-reaching consequences. During his clinical practice, Thomas Sydenham (1624–89) observed that the Peruvian bark (quinine) was efficacious for curing malaria in *all* kinds of patients. This led him to conclude that "diseases should be reduced to definite and certain *Species* … with the same care which we see exhibited by Botanick Writers in their Phytologies". Accordingly,

---

15   James Le Fanu, *The Rise & Fall of Modern Medicine* (London: Abacus, 2014), 95.

16   Roy Porter, *Medicine: A History of Healing* (London: Michael O'Mara, 1997), 229.

17   Bynum, *History of Medicine*, 95, 103.

18   Ibid., 110; Le Fanu, *Rise & Fall of Modern Medicine*, 235.

19   Bynum, *History of Medicine*, 97–98.

Nature, in the production of diseases, is uniform and consistent ... and the selfsame phenomena that you would observe in the sickness of a Socrates you would observe in the sickness of a simpleton. Just so the universal characters of a plant are extended to every individual of the species.[20]

To be sure, Sydenham did not apply his conclusion to all diseases across the board. At least in the case of chronic illnesses, he continued to attribute these to humoral causes. Nevertheless, his reflection, explains Bynum,

can be seen as a kind of turning point in clinical thinking. It encouraged doctors in the generations that followed to classify diseases; more significantly, it began the modern process of teasing out the difference between the disease and the person suffering from the disease, and of identifying those universal features of each kind of disease that could make a specific therapy rational.[21]

Henceforth, disease gained an ontological status and was to be distinguished from the diseased. More importantly, it was now the focus of diagnosis and therapy. As we shall see, this notion of disease as a distinct and separate entity would gain greater specificity in the 19th century, with the development of germ theory.

The Birth of Biomedicine in the 19th Century

The birth of modern biomedicine proper is usually attributed to the 19th century. During this period, several influential developments took place, the most important being the evolution of the hospital into a modern institute of medical training and research, the invention of

---

20   Quote from Roy Porter, *The Greatest Benefit to Mankind: A Medical History of Humanity from Antiquity to the Present* (London: Fontana, 1999), 230.

21   Bynum, *History of Medicine*, 105.

new medical technologies, the discoveries of new medical paradigms (particularly cell and germ theories), public healthcare reforms and advancements in surgery.

Ever since the Middle Ages, hospitals had been regarded as religious institutions where the poor, the pilgrims and the infirm could receive refuge and hospitality.[22] For the most part, they were not known for their ability to heal or as curative centres, but rather as places where the ill could receive care, much like the hospices of today.[23] In the aftermath of the French Revolution (1789), however, a new medical model was introduced in Paris: hospital medicine. Under this scheme, three new aspects of medical education were emphasised. Firstly, the student's training ought to be intensely practical, where he read little, saw much and did much. Secondly, this practical training was to take place within the hospital. Thirdly, all medical students were to be trained in *both* medicine and surgery. It did not take long before hospital medicine gained popularity and was duplicated throughout Europe and eventually in the United States. Till this day, it remains the primary model of training for aspiring physicians.[24]

As may be expected, this new method of learning redefined modern medicine in several ways. It systematised physical diagnosis into the four cardinal dimensions that are still taught today: inspection (looking at the patient), palpation (examining the body by touch), percussion (tapping the chest or abdomen) and auscultation (listening to the heart or chest) by means of the stethoscope (then newly invented, in 1816). Like their Hippocratic predecessors, the French physicians continued to keep careful clinical records during their diagnostic encounters. Where they differed was that they also conducted autopsies to compare their clinical observations with what

22   Ibid., 78.

23   Gary B. Ferngren, *Medicine and Religion: A Historical Introduction* (Baltimore: Johns Hopkins University Press, 2014), 320.

24   Bynum, *History of Medicine*, 118, 153.

may be discovered about their patients, post-mortem. What they would be looking out for were "pathological changes produced by the disease", characterised by lesions on the affected organs. This search for clinico-pathological correlations was again a result of the new paradigm of hospital medicine. By emphasising both medical and surgical training, the French model inadvertently imported "surgical thinking into medicine proper." Traditionally, medical doctors were "concerned with the whole body, with humours … or other generalist conceptions of disease". Surgeons, on the other hand, were always confronted by the local: broken bones, organic abnormalities and the like. When the two disciplines were brought together, physicians began to see pathology through surgical eyes. Henceforth, "the lesion acquired medical significance" as the embodiment of pathological changes induced by a disease. [25]

Alongside these changes were rapid advances in diagnostic technologies. These included the invention of the stethoscope mentioned earlier, the ophthalmoscope (1851) used in eye examinations, and the kymograph (1840s), which records changes in the blood pressure.[26] The same century also saw extensive applications of the microscope, invented earlier in the 17th century. Indeed, two new and significant medical paradigms would not have been possible if not for the microscope: cell theory and germ theory.

Cell Theory

Between the 16th to 19th centuries, the "basic unit of medical understanding of disease" was evolving rapidly. Galenic physicians had long assumed the "basic unit" to be the humours of one's body and thus focused their therapeutic concerns on the whole body. The anatomical studies of Giovanni Battista Morgagni (1682–1771), Xavier Bichat (1771–1802) and others gradually shifted the focus to the organs and some 21 types of tissues found in the body, including the ner-

---

25   Ibid., 119, 137, 215–231.
26   Ibid., 255–256.

vous, osseous, fibrous and mucous.[27] It was the Germans, however, who first argued that pathologists should focus their attention on the cells instead. First introduced by Theodor Schwann (1810–82), cell theory soon became popular under the auspices of Rudolf Virchow (1821–1902) who convinced the medical community that cells not only grew by division but were also

> the fundamental units of physiological and pathological activity, and that routine clinical events, such as acute and chronic inflammation, cancer growth and spread, and bodily reactions to external stimulation such as irritation or pressure, could be fruitfully conceptualised in cellular terms.[28]

As we shall see, this pursuit of the "basic unit of medical understanding" did not stop at the cellular level. In the 20th century, it would dive deeper into the depths of the human body and emerge with a greater discovery: that our genes and DNA play an even greater role in our health and well-being.

Germ Theory

When smallpox inoculation became popular in late-18th-century England, the idea that diseases were caused by micro-organisms, such as bacteria or viruses, was still unheard of. By the 1890s, germ theory was not only established, but integrated and taught in all medical textbooks. This paradigm shift is due in no small measure to two important pioneers in this field: Louis Pasteur (1822–1895) and Robert Koch (1843–1910).

Pasteur's initial research was on the role that micro-organisms played in the distortion of crystal optics and in fermentation. After investigating a silkworm plague in the French silk factories,

---

27   Ibid., 139, 213.
28   Ibid., 219–20.

it dawned upon him that bacteria could also cause diseases and he thus spoke increasingly of a "germ theory of disease". Pasteur's claim to fame, however, remained his work on anthrax and rabies, where he concluded that these were caused by germ-like organisms (the first by the *Bacillus anthracis* and the second, as subsequent research showed, by a virus). More importantly, he also developed vaccines that successfully inoculated patients infected by these diseases.[29]

Pasteur's germ theory was further validated by a younger German physician, Robert Koch. Koch's first significant work was also on anthrax, where he managed to map out the complex life cycle of the bacterium and demonstrated how it could lie dormant in the soil for many years. His crowning achievements, however, remained his identification of the bacteria responsible for the two most dreaded diseases in 19th century: tuberculosis (1882) and cholera (1884).[30]

By identifying germs as the cause of diseases and distinguishing them from the patient's body, germ theory further legitimated Sydenham's model of disease. Practically speaking, it also brought clarity and specificity to the diagnostic process. Objective diagnostic criteria could now be developed to identify these menacing micro-organisms. Diseases that used to fall into broad categories, such as "filth disease", could now be differentiated according to their bacterial causes, as typhoid, cholera, scarlet fever or typhus. Fevers, on the other hand, were no longer regarded as diseases but relegated to mere symptoms instead.[31]

Koch and his fellow scientists' preoccupation with cholera were hardly surprising. The 19th century alone saw the outbreak of six cholera pandemics in Asia, Europe and the United States. In Great Britain, the plague struck twice. In the 1830s, it claimed 6,536 victims in London. In 1854, it took another 23,000 lives across the British Isles. It was during this second epidemic that John Snow (1813–

---

29   Ibid., 223–31.
30   Ibid., 234–37.
31   Ibid., 241–42.

1854) began to investigate the cause of the disease. One experiment he conducted was to compare two groups of people: the first who used Thames water from its upstream, and the second who used unfiltered water downstream, after "the sewers of London had emptied into it." As it turned out, the latter group was 13 times more likely than the former to contract cholera, thus providing strong evidence that cholera was transmitted through contaminated water.[32]

Snow's experiment exemplified two further aspects of 19th-century modern medicine. The first was the growing tendency among medical physicians and scientists to employ mathematics or, more specifically, statistics to validate their medical hypotheses, whether this was quantifying clinical observations, post-mortem autopsies or experiments like that of Snow's.[33] The second was the recognition that effective medical care was not merely the business of individual physicians or hospitals, but also a legitimate concern for governments and public institutions. The Industrial Revolution had seen an unprecedented migration of workers into English cities, leading to a rapid deterioration in urban hygiene standards. This, coupled with the lack of proper provision of clean water and sewage disposal, meant that cities like London and Manchester were prime breeding grounds for all sorts of diseases, including cholera.[34] Recognising the huge social costs of poor urban sanitation and hygiene, the British government enacted the first Public Health Act in 1848, legislating town councils to be responsible for sanitary supervision and inspection, drainage, water and gas supplies. Further laws were introduced between 1854–58 to tackle waste and refuse disposal, water pollution, and other sanitation problems. As Thomas McKeown (1912–1988) argued, these public measures, along with improvements in nutrition, would prove crucial in reducing mortality rates in the 19th century.[35]

32   W. F. Bynum, *Science and the Practice of Medicine in the Nineteenth Century* (Cambridge [England]; New York: Cambridge University Press, 1994), 79.
33   Ibid., 42–44.
34   Porter, *Greatest Benefit to Mankind*, 397–427.
35   Although much of McKeown's thesis have been discredited, this part of his theory

Before we turn the page on 19th-century medicine, two significant developments in surgery are noteworthy. This was due largely to the discovery and application of anaesthesia and antisepsis.[36] Prior to the use of anaesthesia, surgery was restricted to the superficial parts of the body—the limbs, the joints or external wounds. The use of ether and chloroform in the 1840s, however, enabled surgeons to control pain better and thus gave them more time to operate. This, of course, dramatically enlarged the range of operations that surgeons could perform. These changes, nevertheless, did not necessarily improve a patient's chances of surviving a surgery. This was because the more invasive a procedure, the greater the chance of post-operative infection and, therefore, death. Clearly, if surgery was to develop successfully, an effective means of controlling and eradicating infections was needed. This was first attempted in the 1860s, when Joseph Lister (1827–1912) began to use antiseptic carbolic (phenol) dressings on surgical wounds. Later, with the establishment of germ theory, surgeons began to adopt aseptic measures as well. Henceforth, surgical equipment, instruments, dressings, the surgeon's hands and the patient's skin were sterilised as thoroughly as possible to exclude germs right from the onset. Not surprisingly, the incidence of infections fell dramatically and patients recovered at a much faster rate.[37]

Biomedicine: Its Golden Age and Beyond

When a newly qualified doctor set up practice in the 1930s, noted Le Fanu, he had only

---

still holds. In addition, most historians concur with his claims that "curative medical measures played little role in mortality decline prior to the mid-20th century." "The McKeown Thesis—The Lancet", accessed 11 February 2016, http://www.thelancet.com/journals/lancet/article/PIIS0140-6736(08)60292-5/fulltext.

36   Porter, *Greatest Benefit to Mankind*, 597–99.
37   Bynum, *History of Medicine*, 245–50.

a dozen or so proven remedies with which to treat the multiplicity of different diseases he encountered every day: aspirin for rheumatic fever, digoxin for heart failure, the hormones thyroxine and insulin for an underactive thyroid and diabetes respectively, salvarsan for syphilis, bromides for those who needed a sedative, barbiturates for epilepsy, and morphine for pain.[38]

The fact of the matter was, even though clinical diagnosis had improved dramatically by the early 20th century, there was still little that a physician could offer, therapeutically speaking.[39] It was no wonder then that William Osler (1849–1919), Regius Professor of Medicine at Oxford, saw it unrealistic to regard the physician's role as making people better. Rather, it was merely to care for the patient, provide a correct diagnosis of her disease, give a prognosis for the likely outcome, and do what was best to relieve her sufferings.[40] What Osler and his peers would not have imagined was that biomedicine would enter a Golden Age from the 1930s to 1960s, when new potent drugs were discovered, surgical techniques developed, medical technologies invented, and therapeutic paradigms redefined, so much so that mortality rates would drop drastically, especially in developed countries.

How did this Golden Age emerge? We begin our story with the new drug discoveries. Germ theory, as mentioned earlier, had identified bacteria as the cause of many infectious diseases and, therefore, the target of rational therapy. For a long time, however, there was no effective means of treating such bacterial infections. In 1928, Alexander Fleming (1881–1955) made a fortuitous discovery

---

38   Le Fanu, *Rise & Fall of Modern Medicine*, 403–4.

39   Porter, *Greatest Benefit to Mankind*, 674–78.

40   William Paton, "The Evolution of Therapeutics: Osler's Therapeutic Nihilism and the Changing Pharmacopoeia", *Journal of the Royal College of Physicians* 13 (1979): 74; Le Fanu, *Rise & Fall of Modern Medicine*, 405–6.

that penicillin mould could inhibit the growth of *staphylococcus* bacteria. His research was picked up a decade later by Howard Florey (1898–1968) and Ernst Chain (1906–1979), who produced enough penicillin to treat a policeman, Albert Alexander. Alexander died, unfortunately, when the supplies of penicillin ran out. His initial recovery, nonetheless, confirmed the efficacy of the mould and set the stage for the production of the first antibiotic. More importantly, Florey and Chain's research clarified "the principles by which *all* antibiotics were subsequently to be discovered." Since then, nine major types of antibiotics, amounting to hundreds of varieties, have been discovered.[41] These are now used to treat all sorts of infections, ranging from the trivial sore throat to the lethal meningitis.[42]

The second game-changing drug, cortisone (or steroids), was discovered, again fortuitously, in the 1940s. Cortisone was used initially to treat inflammations arising from rheumatoid arthritis. While this proved ineffective, cortisone turned out to be a wonder drug of sorts, highly efficacious for treating a host of other illnesses whose causes were yet unknown and for which there were no effective therapies. These included

> [A]llergy (anaphylactic shock, asthma, rhinitis, conjunctivitis and eczema); autoimmune disorders (the connective tissue disorders, haemolytic anaemia, ... and myasthenia gravis); ... acute inflammatory disorders (polymyalgia, optic neuritis, psoriasis) and potentially lethal swelling of the brain and spinal cord following injury.[43]

Penicillin and cortisone were just two of the over 2,000 new

41   Le Fanu, *Rise & Fall of Modern Medicine*, 57–58.
42   "Antibiotics. Side Effects & Types of Antibiotics", *Patient*, accessed 3 March 2016, http://patient.info/health/antibiotics–leaflet.
43   Le Fanu, *Rise & Fall of Modern Medicine*, 77–79.

drugs introduced from the 1930s to the 1960s. Others included antihistamines, synthetic steroids, hormone preparations, anti-epileptic drugs, new analgesics, sedatives and cytotoxic or immunosuppressive agents.[44] Since then, the physician's therapeutic arsenal has more than doubled, with 4,000 approved drugs, another 338 biotech drugs and 5,024 drugs still under experimentation.[45] The significance of this development cannot be understated. There has never been a time in the history of Western medicine as it is now, when a doctor has, at his disposal, such a wide range of drugs to treat the diverse diseases he encounters. More importantly, this abundance of drug therapies has also forged, in popular imagination, an optimistic belief that there can be "a pill for every ill".

While the introduction of anaesthesia and antisepsis widened the range of surgical options available by the early 20th century, there remained several frontiers difficult to overcome. The decades that followed, however, saw many of these challenges resolved through the development of new drugs and medical technologies. Kidney transplantation is a good example. Surgically speaking, it is a relatively straight forward procedure, involving "little more than connecting the blood supply of the donated kidney to that of the recipient." Nevertheless, it was an idea doomed to fail because the recipient's immune system would always identify the donor's organ as a foreign body, much like viruses and bacteria, and reject it. This obstacle was finally overcome when immunosuppressive drugs, such as *azathioprine*, were developed to improve patients' tolerance of donor organs.[46] Likewise, despite several attempts at open heart surgery, no patients ever survived since there was no robust means of taking over the heart's function while it was being operated upon. This problem was resolved in the 1950s when the heart-lung bypass

---

44   Ibid., 405.

45   "DrugBank: Statistics", accessed 1 March 2016, http://www.drugbank.ca/stats.

46   This comes at the price of weakening the patients' immune system. Le Fanu, *Rise & Fall of Modern Medicine*, 237.

machine, or pump-oxygenator, was invented.[47] Our list could go on much longer, with technological innovations transforming surgical possibilities. For example, the invention of the Charnley hip in the 1960s has made hip replacements a routine operation nowadays, and the invention of the laparoscope has made keyhole surgeries possible, thus mitigating the risks of surgery and making surgical interventions possible for those previously deemed too old to be operated on.[48]

Medical technologies offered much more than just new surgical innovations or possibilities. They also extended the physicians' medical gaze, that is, their ability to visualise their patients' diseases. X-rays were discovered in 1895 and soon put into good use for diagnosing fractures and locating other foreign objects in the body. The invention of the Computerised Axial Tomography (CAT) Scan and Magnetic Resonance Imaging (MRI) brought the physician's gaze to yet greater heights by providing detailed three-dimensional images of patients' organs and musculoskeletal structures.[49]

Meanwhile, the search for the "basic unit of medical understanding" had also progressed beyond cell theory. In 1869, the presence of "nucleic acid" in the nucleus of every living tissue cell was discovered by Friedrich Miescher (1844–1895). By the 1920s, two forms of this nucleic acid had been identified: the DNA (deoxyribonucleic acid) and RNA (ribonucleic acid). Initial views that the DNA structure was simple were soon disproved by Francis Crick and James Watson who demonstrated in 1953 that the DNA had a double helix structure and contained a complicated code. This ushered in a new field of research—genetics—the most well-known being, perhaps, the Human Genome Project, which successfully sequenced the human genome within a short span of 13 years (1990–2003).[50] This new genetic science introduced yet another

---

47   Ibid., 95–119.
48   Ibid., 220, 447–452.
49   Porter, *Greatest Benefit to Mankind*, 605–10.
50   The project sequenced only the euchromatic regions, or 90 percent of the human

new paradigm to our understanding of disease. Diseases were now due not only to enemies *out there* (viruses and bacteria) but also to enemies *within* (genetic defects). Since then, a number of diseases, such as sickle-cell anaemia, Down's syndrome, cystic fibrosis, and some forms of Alzheimer's disease, have been identified as hereditary. More significantly, these discoveries have encouraged both public and private institutions to invest billions of dollars in genetic research, in the hope that gene therapies can be developed eventually to treat not only genetic defects, but also common illnesses as well, such as arthritis, diabetes and cancer.[51] The latter focus is particularly important since hereditary diseases afflict only a minority and will not benefit the masses, let alone deliver the economic successes desired by its investors.[52] To date, a few genetic therapies are already in use, while many more are undergoing clinical trials.[53] In the short term, however, the "blockbuster" drugs that pharmaceutical companies are hoping for are unlikely to appear.[54] This is due largely to the extraordinary difficulties involved in understanding how the 20,000

---

genome. The other regions, the heterochromatic were not sequenced under the project. International Human Genome Sequencing Consortium, "Finishing the Euchromatic Sequence of the Human Genome", *Nature* 431, no. 7011 (21 October 2004):931–45, doi:10.1038/nature03001.

51   These "common illnesses" are not due to specific genetic defects. Nonetheless, genetics and environment can play a role in their formation. The question, therefore, is how may gene therapy be applied to these diseases, despite their less straight forward links to the genetics.

52   For example, two breast cancer genes, BRCA1 and BRCA2, are responsible for almost all hereditary forms of breast cancer. Hereditary breast cancers, however, account for only 5 percent of all breast cancers. This discovery (and any form of gene therapy developed against these defects) will have no therapeutic benefit for the remaining 95 percent of breast cancer patients. Le Fanu, *Rise & Fall of Modern Medicine*, 336–37.

53   More will be said shortly about the application of targeted (genetic) therapies in oncology.

54   A blockbuster drug refers to one which enjoys global sales of more than US$1 billion annually. Examples include *atorvastatin*, which is used to prevent cardiovascular diseases, and *etanercept*, which is prescribed for treating autoimmune diseases. Blockbuster drugs account for 60 percent of the US$245 billion sales of the 10 leading pharmaceutical companies. "Has the Era of Blockbuster Drugs Come to an End? | BioPharm International", accessed 29 February 2016, http://www.biopharminternational.com/has-era-blockbuster-drugs-come-end.

human genes operate and interact with one another.[55] Indeed, some, like Le Fanu, even doubt whether we can ever work out the specific relationships between genes and common illnesses, let alone design the gene-based drugs needed to cure such diseases.[56]

In the field of oncology, the successful cure of Acute Lymphoblastic Leukaemia (ALL) in the 1970s encouraged much optimism that all kinds of cancers could be similarly cured. In the US, campaigns were launched against common cancers, with vast amounts of funds channelled to the search for cures. The results to date have been mixed, however.[57] While chemotherapy proved effective for curing 90 percent of childhood cancers and some forms of leukaemia, it has enjoyed less success against the common types of cancers. A 2004 study of the efficacy of chemotherapy, for example, observed only a modest improvement of 2–3 percent in 5-year survival rates.[58] The reason for this stark difference lies in the biological difference between ALL and the common types of cancers. The latter are mostly "solid" tumours which arise from solid organs (like the breasts, lungs, stomach and the colon) before metastasising throughout the body. These solid organs, which have contact with the external environment through various ways, are endowed with the ability to eliminate or nullify the effects of environmental toxins, including chemotherapy drugs. It is hardly surprising, therefore, that

---

55   Robin McKie, "Stunning Gene Therapy Breakthrough Driven by Great Dedication and Graft | Robin McKie", *The Observer*, 17 December 2017. Science, accessed 17 December 2017, http://www.theguardian.com/science/2017/dec/17/stunning-gene-therapy-breakthrough-riposte-to-truth-tarnished-times.

56   Le Fanu, *Rise & Fall of Modern Medicine*, 459–60.

57   New cancer therapies have seen very low success trials, most of which did not even pass the pre-clinical trial stages. "Lab Mice Can't Help Us in the Fight against Cancer | Comment | Voices | The Independent", accessed 4 March 2016, http://www.independent.co.uk/voices/comment/lab-mice-cant-help-us-in-the-fight-against-cancer-8316756.html.

58   Or to put it plainly, the majority of chemotherapy patients will incur a huge financial cost and suffer severe side effects needlessly, as their treatments would have no effect on their 5-year survival rates. Graeme Morgan, Robyn Wardy, and Michael Barton, "The Contribution of Cytotoxic Chemotherapy to 5-Year Survival in Adult Malignancies", *Clinical Oncology*, 16 (2004): 549–60.

chemo drugs have been found to be less efficacious in controlling the growth of solid tumours.[59] This being said, there is evidence that a combination of traditional (surgery, chemotherapy, radiotherapy) and targeted therapies can be helpful for some cancer patients. For instance, the use of Anaplastic Lymphoma Kinase [ALK] inhibitors has proven beneficial against ALK-positive metastatic non-small-cell lung cancer.[60]

The mid-20th century also saw the emergence of another new medical paradigm, that is, preventive treatment against serious or fatal diseases. In 1967, a study was conducted with 140 US veterans, where some were given drugs to lower their blood pressure while others a placebo. As it turned out, 27 veterans in the control group went on to suffer strokes, while only two in the treated group were afflicted. Clearly, the hypertension drug regimen had contributed significantly to stroke prevention. Since this discovery, millions around the world have been placed on hypertension drug regimens to lower their blood pressure. In 1996, this amounted to more than one in three Americans between the ages of 35 and 74.

In the 1990s, a similar argument was made about lowering cholesterol levels to reduce the risks of heart disease. This advice likewise put millions on cholesterol-lowering drug regimens worldwide.[61] Interestingly, a similar culture of prevention has also become prevalent in the area of medical diagnosis. With the widespread availability of diagnostic technologies, far more patients are now being subjected to routine diagnostics, like endoscopy, CT scans or MRIs, than before the 1970s.

Such preventive approaches are not without controversy. When

---

59   Porter, *Greatest Benefit to Mankind*, 595; Le Fanu, *Rise & Fall of Modern Medicine*, 155, 310–15, 803–4.

60   ALK-positive metastatic non-small-cell lung cancers amount to 3–7 percent of all lung cancers. *A Decade in Medicine*, Nature Reviews (Macmillan, 2015)., 16; Mark M. Awad and Alice T. Shaw, "ALK Inhibitors in Non–Small Cell Lung Cancer: Crizotinib and Beyond", *Clinical Advances in Hematology & Oncology: H&O* 12, no. 7 (July 2014): 429–39.

61   Le Fanu, *Rise & Fall of Modern Medicine*, 148–55.

otherwise healthy people are advised to take long-term prescription drugs, the boundary between the sick and the healthy is inadvertently redefined. Moreover, such drugs are not without side effects, such as lethargy, dizziness and headache, and are costly in the long run.[62] All these raise the question of at what point is the project of preventing strokes or other diseases too costly in terms of patient side effects and the spiralling medical costs that are challenging public healthcare systems across the world?

In the area of diagnostics, it is also not entirely clear to what extent a patient should be subjected to routine diagnostics. This problem is further complicated by the fact that, in some countries like the US, routine diagnostics, such as endoscopy, contribute significantly to a private physician's revenue—a clear conflict of interest.[63] Likewise, if shifting the boundary between the healthy and the sick leads to more demand for drugs, would not pharmaceutical companies be inclined to do so in the long term?[64]

More importantly, the constant redefinition of what it means to be sick or healthy has in recent years given rise to a "doing better, feeling worse" syndrome, where more people nowadays perceive themselves as suffering from some form of chronic disorders (whether physical or psychological) and are quite happy to be prescribed drugs for these ailments.[65] This is despite the fact that many of them would have been regarded as healthy by past medical standards. Some of these patients, unfortunately, have gone on to become addicted to medication, such

---

62   In 2013, drugs costs in hospitals and the community in England amounted to 15 percent of the total NHS budget. "A Pill for Every Ill? — BBC News", accessed 1 March 2016, http://www.bbc.com/news/health-30418580.

63   In the US, for example, endoscopy and "catheter lab" can generate up to 80 percent of a specialist's income. Le Fanu, *Rise & Fall of Modern Medicine*, 489–99.

64   Through a series of astute marketing and medical campaigns, Glaxo managed to redefine heart-burn as Gastro-Oesophageal Reflux Disease (GORD) and, in so doing, generated significant sales for its acid suppressant drug, Zantac. Ibid., 770–71.

65   A physician friend of mine laments that the opposite can also be true. He had far too many patients who ignored his advice to take their medication regularly until it was too late!

as sedatives, anti-psychotic drugs, or even cough mixture.[66]

We conclude by surveying briefly the evolution of clinical research in the 20th century. Subsequent to Snow's statistical study of cholera plagues in London, statistical-empirical medical research began to dominate or, indeed, define the medical industry from the 1950–60s onwards, particularly with the invention of the double-blind Randomised Controlled Trials (RCTs). The 1980s would see a further development in this trend with the advent of Evidence-based Medicine, where available drugs' RCTs are meta-analysed and reviewed systematically to help regulators, insurance companies and physicians decide which drugs are most suitable and affordable for patients.[67] Despite the efforts of serious and well-meaning clinical scientists, the way clinical trials are conducted has not always been as objective as what people imagined. Publication bias remains quite prevalent, even in academic journals, with positive results being published much more frequently than negative findings, and primary outcomes being switched not infrequently with secondary outcomes, in order to exaggerate the benefits of drugs under trial.[68] It does not take much to guess that the pharmaceutical companies, which sponsor the majority of these trials, are the key culprits of such bias. All these are only complicated by the fact that pharmaceutical companies spend considerable amounts marketing and lobbying for their drugs, so much so that popular and even political sentiments

---

66   "A Pill for Every Ill: Two Million Brits Have Become Addicted to Prescription Drugs | Features | Lifestyle | The Independent", accessed 26 February 2016, http://www.independent. co.uk/life-style/health-and-families/features/a-pill-for-every-ill-two-million-brits-have-become-addicted-to-prescription-drugs-1764497.html.; Porter, *Greatest Benefit to Mankind*, 685.

67   The history and evolution of the RCT, along with its methodological limitations and challenges in practice, will be explained in greater detail in Chapter 10. *The Cochrane Library* is one such depository of RCT reviews. Established by the UK government since 1992, the database is available freely to the UK public. "Ebm.pdf", accessed 3 March 2016, http://www. medicine.ox.ac.uk/bandolier/painres/download/whatis/ebm.pdf.

68   For example, a 2010 study of publication bias concluded that positive trials are 1.6–2.4 times more likely to be published than negative trials. Ben Goldacre, *Bad Pharma: How Drug Companies Mislead Doctors and Harm Patients*, Kindle (Harper Collins UK, 2013), Kindle Location 256, 521, 3021–48.

have been skewed significantly, quite apart from the clinical efficacy of a drug.[69] More will be said about these issues in Chapter 10, when we evaluate the history, assumptions and limitations of RCTs and how clinical research is currently conducted.

Conclusion

The last 500 years have seen a radical transformation of medicine in the West, from one based on the authority of the ancients to a discipline validated by the norms of empirical science. In this process, new paradigms of human physiology and disease have been conceived, lethal maladies cured, and insurmountable surgical obstacles overcome. Many of these achievements have been due to the technologies developed both within and without the medical world. Indeed, apart from them, humankind could never have imagined peering beyond what our plain eyes can see, let alone, develop the drug and surgical therapies that would usher in the Golden Age of medicine. Since the 1980s, however, the progress of biomedicine appears to have slowed down. This being said, clinical research in diverse medical fields continues unabated, with billions of dollars poured into them. All these could well give rise to new promising drugs and therapies and, perhaps, usher in a new Golden Age of medicine.

Despite its decisive break from the past, modern biomedicine

---

69   It is estimated that the marketing spend of pharmaceutical companies is twice the amount of their research and development budget. A good example of the influence of pharmaceutical marketing and PR can be seen in the drug, Herceptin. In 2005, a sudden media frenzy was generated around the breast cancer drug so much so that the British populace, patient groups and even the Health minister called for the drug's immediate approval. All this was quite bizarre since the manufacturer, Roche, had not even submitted its licence application! As it turned out, the patients who were successfully treated with Herceptin, as the media articles claimed, were introduced to the press by a PR company under the payroll of Roche. Clearly then, the public clamour was but a result of Roche's clever PR tactics. More seriously, Herceptin not only costs a patient tens of thousands of pounds, but has also proven to be marginally effective (4–5%) against some breast cancers. When this benefit is weighed against the finding that a similar percentage of Heceptin users will suffer from cardiac side effects, it is doubtful whether Herceptin is a viable drug to begin with. Ibid., Kindle Location 3719–53.

remains, in many ways, a child of its Greek heritage. As we shall see in the next chapter, biomedicine continues to share several philosophical and epistemic assumptions with Hippocratic medicine, particularly in the way they conceive of human physiology and disease, and the way they justify knowledge. These assumptions, as I will argue later in Chapters 5 and 8, are usually brought to bear whenever biomedicine encounters and evaluates Chinese medicine. It is pertinent, therefore, to have a proper grasp of them in order to appreciate the dynamics and complexities involved in a dialogue between biomedicine and its Chinese counterpart.

5

SEEING MEDICINE FROM
A GREEK PERSPECTIVE

Cultural Paradigms & Tacit Beliefs

It is tough being a Singaporean. When we travel overseas, we are often asked "which part of China do you come from?" Every so often, we are mistaken for Koreans, Japanese or Mainland Chinese. For those who have actually heard of the country, Singapore sometimes conjures up the image of an authoritarian regime well known for its ban on chewing gum. But if there is anything that truly characterises Singaporeans, my guess is that we are some of the most obsessive-compulsive planners in the world. Events at our civil service are often planned up to the minute—what we call "minute-by-minute" scheduling. Ever since the SARS scare, all state schools regularly monitor the body temperatures of their students, just in case someone brings in an unexpected bug.[1] This preoccupation with planning and control is also why chewing gum was banned in the first place. It was not intended to be a killjoy, but to prevent gum from jamming our subway doors and, in so doing,

---

1   SARS refers to severe acute respiratory syndrome, an atypical pneumonia that broke out worldwide from late 2002 to early 2003. SARs affected 8,096 people in total. In Singapore, 238 people fell ill and 33 died from the disease. The more recent Ebola and MERS (Middle Eastern Respiratory Syndrome) outbreaks have, of course, further legitimised such precautions. "Sars in Singapore: Timeline, Singapore News & Top Stories—*The Straits Times*", accessed 21 March 2016, http://www.straitstimes.com/singapore/sars-in-singapore-timeline.

paralysing the entire subway system.[2] How did such obsession with planning arise, one may ask? Well, simply because of Singapore's fragile socio-economic and political situation: we are a young nation with negligible natural resources, and are often vulnerable to geopolitical instabilities from without. Moreover, as a miniscule island state that is even smaller than New York City, we do not have much room to manoeuvre should anything go wrong. For this reason, Singaporeans plan and do so aggressively.

The places we live in and the challenges we face there often determine the questions we ask about the world and the problems that preoccupy us.[3] These, in turn, powerfully shape the way we approach problem solving, our epistemology, our metaphysics, and, ultimately, the way we understand the world.[4] More importantly, as the theories or practices we develop "come to be accepted and to be believed to prove its worth," a "momentum effect", as Geoffrey Lloyd coins it, kicks in. We soon find ourselves assuming these paradigms in our intellectual pursuits and devoting "very considerable efforts" to elaborating and justifying them.[5] The more entrenched these paradigms or tacit beliefs are, the less aware we shall be of them and of how they actually shape the way we perceive the world.[6] It is imperative to recognise that this principle was at play during the evolution of both the Western and Chinese medical traditions. That is, the two asked very different questions about the world and psychosomatic

---

2   Elle Metz BBC News Magazine, "Why Singapore Banned Chewing Gum", *BBC News*, accessed 21 March 2016, http://www.bbc.com/news/magazine-32090420.

3   Jared Diamond argues, quite persuasively, that environmental factors play a crucial role in the rate of development of societies, and how this contributes to the political, cultural and technological differences between different peoples and nations. Jared Diamond, *Guns, Germs, and Steel: The Fates of Human Societies* (New York: W.W. Norton & Co, 1997).

4   G. E. R. Lloyd, *Adversaries and Authorities: Investigations into Ancient Greek and Chinese Science* (Cambridge: Cambridge University Press, 1996), 9.

5   G. E. R. Lloyd, *Disciplines in the Making: Cross-Cultural Perspectives on Elites, Learning, and Innovation* (Oxford: Oxford University Press, 2009), 85.

6   Denis Alexander, *Rebuilding the Matrix: Science and Faith in the 21st Century* (Grand Rapids, MI: Zondervan, 2003), 14.

well-being, and were led to rather different conceptions of health and disease. Should we fail to grasp this, any attempt to bring the two traditions into dialogue will be a futile exercise, a case of "the chicken trying to talk to the duck", as a Chinese saying goes.

In the last two chapters, we surveyed the development of Western medicine from its Greek roots to its modern biomedical expressions. Our intent, however, was not merely historiographical, but to set the stage for our present reflection, which is to evaluate the ideological paradigms intrinsic to Galenic medicine and how these emphases still influence and shape modern biomedicine. As we shall see, the Greek intellectual legacy bequeathed to modern biomedicine three important epistemic assumptions: the medical significance of anatomy; an ontological perspective of disease; and the esteem for mathematics as the means for securing epistemic certainty. To students of modern science, these emphases may come across as self-evident rather than perspectives unique to the West. To remind us that things need not always be how they are perceived, occasional references will be made to Chinese philosophy and medicine. These, however, will be kept to a minimum as more will be said about the history of Chinese medicine, its theories and practices in Chapters 6 to 8.

The Greek Pursuit of Teleology and the Medicalistion of Anatomy

We begin with anatomy. The discipline has been a longstanding feature in Western medical history and is regarded generally as the backbone of modern medicine. It is curious, however, that anatomical studies have had little bearing on medical practice from the classical to Late Antique periods. Indeed, for the most part, Graeco-Roman physicians knew more anatomy than they can actually use.7 What is more intriguing is the fact that when the classical Greeks first examined

---

7   Shigehisa Kuriyama, *The Expressiveness of the Body and the Divergence of Greek and Chinese Medicine* (New York: Zone Books, 1999), 122.

animal entrails, what they were looking out for were not insights for medicine, but rather, signs of divination. This, coupled with the fact that many other medical traditions (such as Ayurvedic and Chinese) had flourished without a need for serious anatomical inquiry, suggests strongly that it was not quite self-evident why anatomy should be associated with, let alone necessary for Greek medicine. All these beg the question why physicians came to be enamoured with anatomy and prized it so highly.

It has been observed that "a great number of (classical Greek) words relating to cognition appeal to the experience of sight." The word, *noein*, for example, means acquiring a clear mental image of something, while the word, idea, is basically derived from the verb *ideō*, meaning "I see".8 The Greeks have often differed, however, as to the specific relationship between what we see and what we know.

On the one hand, we have Plato who cautioned his readers not to be beguiled by appearances, or the particular things that we encounter, but to apply reason in such a way that we may see beyond these shadowy appearances and grasp the true Archetypal Forms (or Ideas) that underlie all things.9 As he famously put it, although there are many beds in the world, they take their form after an archetypal bed, without which the particular beds cannot be recognised or built.[10]

On the other hand, we have Aristotle, who not only rejected Plato's theory of Forms but argued that true knowledge can only be found in a careful study of the particulars. In other words, we only know what a bed is by studying a particular bed in detail. There is really no point speculating about the existence of an archetypal idea of a bed. The significance of this epistemic turn cannot be understated. Aristotle went on to apply this principle to a systematic and empirical study of animals, both by observation and dissection. His writings

---

8 Ibid., 120–22.
9 *Republic* 517a–c.
10 Ibid., 596–599.

on zoology, such as the *History of Animals* and *On the Parts of the Animals*, eventually came up to a quarter of his extant writings and would establish him as the undisputed father of Western science and biology. His authority remained unchallenged throughout the Middle Ages until the advent of the modern Scientific Revolution.

This being said, just because one should learn from one's empirical experience need not imply that one should dissect an animal. Chinese physicians, for example, also valued the empirical observation of their patients' looks, bodily smells and meridian pulses as part of their diagnostic process. Yet, they never saw a need for anatomical investigations.[11] Furthermore, what does one encounter when he dissects an animal? For most people, it is just messy entrails and repugnant smells, which hardly lend themselves to useful knowledge. To Aristotle, however, the dissection of animals could be immensely instructive if we recognised beforehand that there was a cause, a purpose and a good to be found among these entrails.[12] To put it differently, dissection was essentially an exercise in teleological gazing, where we attempted to peer beyond the blood, flesh, and bones to contemplate the wondrous design we believed was intrinsic to each animal's anatomy.[13] As we saw in the previous chapter, this logic of the anatomical gaze eventually took root in the Graeco-Roman world, convincing Galen and his peers that anatomy was not only an important means of knowing how "Nature shaped each (anatomical) part perfectly for its end (and use)", but was also an essential part of medical practice.[14]

In subsequent centuries, the dominance of Galenic medicine meant that the medical significance of anatomy came to be taken

---

11   Chinese medical diagnosis commonly involves four procedures: looking, smelling, enquiring (from the patient) and meridian pulse diagnosis (*wang wen wen qie*, 望、闻、问、切).

12   *Parts of Animals* I.5, 645a4–36.

13   Teleology is a philosophical study of nature whereby one attempts to describe things in terms of how they are designed for a specific end, purpose or goal (*telos*).

14   Kuriyama, *Expressiveness of the Body*, 123.

for granted. During the medieval period, the Christian God, quite understandably, replaced Plato's Divine Craftsman (Demiurge) or Aristotle's Unmoved Mover as the Creator and Designer of all things, including anatomy. The advent of the scientific revolution did see a gradual repudiation of Aristotle's zoological theories. Nevertheless, his logic of the anatomical gaze remained unabated, and continued to inspire new generations of anatomists to gaze into the body's mystery and to discern its design. In the last two centuries, beliefs in a Designer and the value of teleology have waned, if not disappeared altogether in biomedicine. This, however, did not diminish the value of anatomy one bit. Instead, anatomical studies went on to play an influential role in the evolution of modern medicine. When French hospital medicine incorporated surgery into medical training during the early 19th century, the surgical bias for anatomy gradually reconceptualised how physicians perceived diseases.

Over time, it came to be understood that the progress of disease was best characterised by the extent of lesions found on a patient's organs. Not surprisingly, this anatomical emphasis motivated scientists, both within and without the medical world, to pursue new ways of visualising the anatomy and its lesions. Out of this, new diagnostic technologies, such as X-rays, CT scans, MRIs, ultrasound scans and laparoscopy, were invented, thereby improving dramatically the physicians' ability to examine their patients' bodies visually. By justifying and elaborating on the medical significance of anatomy, these medical and technological developments did much to establish the discipline as one of the key pillars of biomedicine. More important for our purposes, they also legitimated anatomy as a benchmark for assessing the credibility of other types of medical traditions, including Chinese medicine.[15]

---

15   Ted J. Kaptchuk, *Chinese Medicine: The Web That Has No Weaver* (London: Rider, 2000), 76.

The Importance of Ontology in Greek and Modern Medicine

Teleological design, however, was not the only thing the Greeks looked out for when they observed their world. Another longstanding question that they grappled with, ever since the Pre-Socratic period (6th century BC), was ontology. That is, to enquire what was the nature or the essence of all things? What were they made of? For some pre-Socratic philosophers, the fundamental building block of the cosmos was earth. For others, it was fire. Yet others, it was air, water, atoms, a combination of the four elements, or even numbers. Despite their differences, the Greek philosophers generally agreed that the cosmos ought to be made up of one or more fundamental elements, whose nature can be explored.

Again, Aristotle played a pivotal role in the development of Greek ontological thinking. In his *Categories*, he classified all types of beings into universals or particulars, both of which could be either accidental or non-accidental. A four-fold system thus subsisted: (1) accidental universals; (2) essential universals; (3) accidental particulars; (4) non-accidental particulars (also known as primary substances).[16] To illustrate, let us take Socrates as an example. As an individual, he is a non-accidental particular. He is one of a kind, never to appear again. The whiteness of his skin, however, is an accidental particular. It is particular because it can be distinguished from the whiteness of, say, Plato's skin. It is accidental, however, because the whiteness does not define Socrates as an individual. Whiteness, in itself, can characterise all sorts of things—human beings, horses, cats, and so on—and yet not change them essentially. So, the fact that a horse shares the same colour as a cat does not change it into a cat. Therefore, the colour white is regarded as an accidental universal. Finally, the category of man is a non-accidental universal because it defines all men across the board, whether they are Socrates, Plato or Aristotle.

---

16   *Categories* 1a–2a.

Besides these distinctions, Aristotle also categorised things into "classes of increasing generality".[17] A maple tree, for example, belonged to the same class as other maple trees. Nonetheless, all maples also belonged to a broader class, namely, the class of trees. This distinction can be applied, of course, to all sorts of things, from music, metals and ethnic races, to plants and animals. It is Aristotle, therefore, whom we are indebted to for the distinction between *genus* and *species* that is now taken for granted in botany, biology and medicine.[18]

More importantly, Aristotle's ontological frameworks also permanently shaped how the West (and those influenced by them) perceives reality. In his comparative study of Asian and Western patterns of thinking, Richard Nisbett notes that modern Westerners

(a) have a greater tendency to categorise objects than would Easterners; (b) find it easier to learn new categories by applying rules about properties to particular cases; and (c) make more inductive use of categories, that is, generalise from particular instances of a category to other instances or to the category as a whole.[19]

In comparison, Easterners, particularly those influenced by ancient Chinese thought, often show less interest "in classes of objects sharing the same properties" but are more concerned about the relationships between objects, that is, how does the part relate to the whole. This difference has been validated in several social

---

17   Paul Studtmann, "Aristotle's Categories", in *The Stanford Encyclopedia of Philosophy*, ed. Edward N. Zalta, Summer 2014 , http://plato.stanford.edu/archives/sum2014/entries/aristotle-categories/.

18   The Latin word, *genus*, means type, race or group. The usage of genus and species was popularised by Carl Linnaeus (1707–1778) in his *Species Planatarum* (1753). As mentioned in Chapter 4, he and his fellow botanists played an influential role in Sydenham's development of his disease model.

19   Nisbett defines Easterners as those influenced by ancient Chinese thought, namely, the Chinese, Koreans and Japanese. Richard E. Nisbett, *The Geography of Thought: How Asians and Westerners Think Differently — And Why* (New York: Free, 2003), 139–40.

psychological studies: for example, when triplets of pictures, such as a chicken, a cow and grass, are shown to American and Chinese children, the American children tended to associate these objects according to their taxonomy, while the Chinese on the basis of relationships. Thus, in our example, more Americans would group the chicken with the cow because they shared the common attributes of being animals, while more Chinese would group the grass and the cow together because the former was related to the latter as its food.[20]

How then do these ontological perspectives influence Greek and modern medicine? The earliest introduction of Greek ontology into medical theory is probably Plato's *Timaeus*. According to the philosopher, all material reality is constituted by the four elements of air, water, fire and earth.[21] A combination of these elements, in turn, gives us the four humours—blood, phlegm, bile and black bile—that make up the different organs in our bodies.[22] We fall ill whenever our humours are imbalanced or misproportioned in our organs. Plato's doctrine of humours eventually found its way into the Hippocratic text, *On the Nature of Man*, and was enshrined in Galen's teachings as the *de facto* interpretation of Hippocratic medicine.[23] Under the auspices of Galenic medicine, humoral theory went on to become the dominant pathological and aetiological paradigm in much of European medical history. Although the theory was eventually abandoned in the 19th century, the ontological logic that underlay it persisted. Instead of the humours, the body's organs (and its lesions) became the focal point of aetiological studies—due in no small measure to the prominence of anatomy in the 18th to 19th centuries.[24] As we have seen in Chapter

---

20   Ibid., 138–40.

21   *Timaeus* 53c–d.

22   Owsei Temkin, *Hippocrates in a World of Pagans and Christians* (Baltimore; London: Johns Hopkins University Press, 1991), 12.

23   It is debatable, of course, whether Plato influenced *The Nature of Man* or shared a common ontology with the Hippocratic text.

24   W. F. Bynum, *History of Medicine: A Very Short Introduction* (Oxford; NY: Oxford University Press, 2008), 140.

4, this focus on anatomy was just another step in biomedicine's search for the "basic unit of medical understanding of disease."[25] The next century saw this concept further refined, or redefined, by the advent of cell theory and, later on, genetics. This shift in ontological focus, of course, gave rise to new aetiological frameworks. Abnormal cellular growth is now understood as the cause of cancer, while genetic defects are the reasons for a whole host of other diseases. Yet, whether it is the humours, organs, cells or genes, the same ontological logic remains—the problem and disease lay in the "dot" or the most fundamental "building block" of the human body.

The above, however, is not the whole story of how Greek ontology influenced the evolution of biomedicine. Besides drawing attention to potential ontological deficiencies in the human being, the same perspective also persuaded physicians to invest ontological status to some diseases. By this we mean the germs that attack our bodies. As mentioned in our history of biomedicine, it was Thomas Sydenham who first observed that the Peruvian bark could cure malaria, whether it occurred in a Socrates or a simpleton. This suggested to him that a disease could be common to and yet ontologically distinct from individual patients. In the 19th century, Sydenham's model gained greater specificity with the advent of germ theory. Henceforth, external pathogens, such as bacteria and viruses, were regarded as ontological entities—to be distinguished from the patients—and the proper targets for medical therapy. Sydenham's disease model, of course, owed much to Aristotle's *Categories*. If it were not for the philosopher's distinctions between the universals and particulars, and the *genus* and *species*, biomedicine would never have had the language to describe the ontology of germs to begin with.

In his comparative study of ancient Greek and Chinese sciences, Geoffrey Lloyd observed that the Chinese, quite unlike the Greeks, were not concerned with the question of ontology. To be sure, a vari-

---

25   Ibid., 213.

ety of terms have been used to translate the word nature or *phusis* (in Greek) into Chinese, such as *tian* (天, heaven), *ziran* (自然, spontaneity) or *dao* (道, the way). Nonetheless, it is also apparent that the Chinese did not have a concept of nature to begin with. In fact, they actually "got along [well] without any such central preoccupation".[26] Rather, the focus of their philosophical reflections was elsewhere, or as Nisbett put it earlier, on the relationships or correlations between the parts and the whole, best exemplified by the theory of *yinyang*. More will be said about the development of *yinyang* philosophy and its impact on Chinese medicine in Chapters 6 and 7. For our present purposes, it is important to consider what this philosophical difference may mean for any dialogue between the Western and Chinese medical traditions.

To illustrate the difference between the two traditions, I return again to our earlier analogy. That is, biomedicine's conviction that a disease is to be found in the "dot", whether this is a germ, a cell or a gene. According to this logic, once the problematic "dot" has been identified, the next logical step is to solve the problem, whether it is the use of antibiotics against bacteria, or the design of a gene therapy to correct a genetic defect. When we look at the *yinyang* theory that underlies Chinese medicine, it is clear that a radically different perspective is at work. In contrast to Greek ontology, truth and reality for the Chinese are to be found in the relationships between two or more "dots" or entities. When applied to Chinese medical theory, it means that a person falls ill whenever the systemic relationships between his organs are imbalanced, or there is an adverse environmental impact on his body, or both. By this logic, to suppose, as biomedicine does, that a disease is due primarily to defects in a specific organ or an attack by specific germs is simply inadequate or unsound. Failure to grasp this epistemic difference is, of course, a recipe for miscommunication. Unfortunately, this is

---

26   Lloyd, *Adversaries and Authorities*, 6–7.

exactly what happens whenever the two medical traditions encounter each other. The consequence of this is that biomedical doctors are not only bewildered by Chinese medical theories, but often go so far as to belittle the tradition. Herein then is the first challenge that Greek ontology poses to any dialogue between the two medical traditions.

The second challenge is how this ontological bias not only operates as a critique of Chinese medicine from without, but also from within. As I explained in Chapter 1, modern Chinese medicine, or TCM, is the direct result of Chinese communist policies which mandated the modernisation of Chinese medicine through its integration with its Western counterpart. The net result is the incorporation of biomedical thinking, including anatomy, into the ancient discipline. To be sure, medical traditions have always benefitted from responding to external challenges and encounters with other forms of medicine. As we shall see in Chapters 6 and 7, Chinese medicine also evolved through such interactions. This being said, some of the changes introduced by the Communist regime since the 1960s have caused concerns for many Chinese medical practitioners.

A good case in point is the TCM diagnostic method, *Bianzheng Lunzhi* (辩证论治, to differentiate, identify, discuss and treat). *Bianzheng Lunzhi* was first introduced by the communist authorities in the 1960s as a means of replacing what they perceived as superstitious and outdated theories,[27] that is, the theories of *yinyang* and *wuxing* (five phases) that have long been presumed in Chinese medical theory and practice. Enshrined as official medical dogma in the 1980s, *Bianzheng Lunzhi* is based on the recognition and understanding of "pathological and physiological movements of the body." Therapeutically speaking, it aims to

adjust or support such pathological and physiological

---

27   *Bianzheng Lunzhi* is based primarily on one of the most popular Chinese medical diagnostic methods, *Bagang Bianzheng* (八纲辨证). More will be said about this and other forms of diagnostic methods in Chapter 9.

functions to enable the recovery of the internal *balance*; to enable the excretion and weakening the effect of *pathogen stimulants*; or encourage the potential ability [of the body] to *tolerate attacks by pathogens* and wait for new disease-resistance mechanisms to appear. (*emphasis mine*)

While the allusion to the notion of balance seems to presume the theory of *yinyang*, *Bianzheng Lunzhi* is, in effect, a paradigm based on biomedical premises. What gives this away is its emphasis on overcoming the "pathogen stimulants" and "pathogens", which, quite obviously, involve an ontological view of disease. In other words, Greek ontology has supplanted *yinyang* theory as the new metaphysic for Chinese medicine. What harm might this have, one may ask? Practically speaking, B*ianzheng Lunzhi* trains physicians to identify specific medical syndromes (or "pathological and physiological movements") and to match them with those recorded in the medical classics. This, in turn, enables them to identify the medical therapies relevant for such syndromes. By and large, this works well whenever the syndromes are matched. Yet, there have also been cases where an illness was esoteric and no clear match was found. Whenever this happened in the past, a Chinese physician would seek recourse to *yinyang* theory as a means of working out an alternative diagnosis and therapy. For those trained solely in *Bianzheng Lunzhi*, however, they will find themselves at a loss, not knowing how to proceed with their diagnosis, let alone treat the patient.[28]

Apart from these difficulties, this ontological bias has also made biomedicine more susceptible to narrower views of medical therapy and, sometimes, a more reductionist understanding of disease and the human being.[29] Such biases have played out in at least two

---

28 Rhonda Chang, "Making Theoretical Principles for New Chinese Medicine", *Australian and New Zealand Society of the History of Medicine, Health and History*, 16, no. 1 (2014):66–86.

29 Sean Sanders, ed., "The Art and Science of Traditional Medicine Part 1: TCM Today — A Case for Integration", *Science* 346, no. Suppl (2014):S4–25.

ways. Firstly, by prioritising the disease as focal point of therapeutic research, biomedicine has sometimes leaned too much on the logic of seeking a specific drug to treat a disease, or "a pill for every ill". Often, this leads to a bias for drug therapy over and against other forms of therapeutics that were previously practised in Hippocratic medicine, and are still employed in Chinese and Ayurvedic medicine, such as dietary regimens and therapeutic massage.[30] Consequently, when a biomedical physician hears that an ailment was healed by a non-drug therapy, say, by massage or pure dietetics, he is likely to be bewildered or sceptical about the results.[31] Furthermore, the same logic often compels biomedical therapy to prioritise the eradication of the disease over the well-being of its patients.[32] The net result of this are the side effects that patients experience regularly, but must patiently endure as the necessary trade-off for getting rid of, or controlling their diseases.[33] For example, Paroxetine is a drug commonly used to treat depressive disorders. Patients, however, may experience a wide variety of possible side-effects, ranging from those which are minor (such as drowsiness, dry mouth, loss of appetite, sweating and trouble

---

30   When treating an ailment, a TCM physician generally employs several forms of treatment, in addition to drug therapy. In practice, the extent to which this is possible depends largely on the physician's financial resources and infrastructure support. A private clinic may offer acupuncture and moxibustion treatments, while a state-run TCM hospital in China may offer much more, including therapeutic massage (*tuina*, 推拿), a variety of moxibustion therapies, cupping, acupuncture point injections and electrical needling. These therapies will be explained in greater detail in Chapter 9.

31   In Chapter 9, we will discuss how non-drug therapies often play a prominent or, sometimes, the primary role in TCM therapies.

32   To be sure, the World Health Organisation (WHO), as early as 1948, had already defined health as "a state of complete physical, mental and social well-being and *not merely the absence of disease or infirmity.*" In practice, however, most biomedical physicians take for granted that side-effects are necessary costs that a patient has to pay. This has sometimes led to quite fatal results. World Health Organisation, "WHO Definition of Health', *WHO Definition of Health*, accessed 15 August 2016, http://www.who.int/about/definition/en/print.html.

33   This is in stark contrast to TCM drug formulas. Typically, a Chinese drug formula contains four categories of drugs, including the primary ingredients that treat the ailments, and secondary drugs that offsets any potential side effects. For this reason, managing side-effects are rarely a concern for TCM physicians.

sleeping) to the more serious (such as increased risk of birth defects and even suicidal thinking in children and adolescents).[34] A 2015 study of chemotherapy treatments for advanced cancer patients has actually cautioned against the use of chemotherapy for such patients in view of the fact that the side effects have often turned out to be more detrimental than the cancer itself.[35]

Secondly, in its pursuit of the most "basic unit of medical understanding of disease", the biomedical industry has invested significant financial and human resources into genetic research and therapy. The underlying premise is that once we understand how our genes operate, we would be much closer to finding a treatment for all kinds of diseases. To date, we have progressed much in our knowledge of genetics. Some gene therapies have even been introduced with promising results, such as the use of ALK inhibitors against non-small-cell lung cancers that harbour ALK fusions. Nevertheless, we have yet to see the advent of ground-breaking drugs that match the therapeutic (and commercial) successes of those discovered during

---

34   In the case of Paroxetine, the problem was magnified by the unethical behaviour of the manufacturer, GlaxoSmithKline (GSK). The company had first received marketing authorisation to provide the drugs to adult patients in 1992. During this period, many physicians also prescribed the drug to children "off label" (that is, to use it beyond what the authorisation covered). This was common practice since most drug companies would not conduct trials for children as this was a small and not so lucrative market. It was estimated up to 32,000 children were prescribed the drug annually in UK alone. When Paroxetine's patent was expiring, GSK took advantage of a regulatory incentive that promised pharmaceutical companies a patent extension of 6 months if they extend the use of their drugs to all users, including children (supported by clinical evidence). When GSK applied for a marketing authorisation for children patients, it came to light that the company had conducted nine trials on children between 1994 to 2002, all of which concluded that the drug was ineffective. What was worse is that the drug seemed to have increased suicidal thoughts and behaviour among adolescents. Yet clearly, GSK did not disclose to the public of its findings and allowed the drug to prescribed to children for several years more. For such behaviour, GSK was eventually fined US$3 billion by US Department of Justice. Ben Goldacre, *Bad Pharma: How Drug Companies Mislead Doctors and Harm Patients*, Kindle (Harper Collins UK, 2013), Kindle Location 968–1026.

35   Prigerson et al. have demonstrated that chemotherapy treatment for end-stage cancer patients actually worsen rather than improve their Quality of Life near Death. "JAMA Network | JAMA Oncology | Chemotherapy Use, Performance Status, and Quality of Life at the End of Life', accessed 21 March 2016, http://oncology.jamanetwork.com/article.aspx?articleid=2398177.

the Golden Age of the 1930s to 1960s.[36] It would seem that we have reverted to the problem of Galen and his peers, where, like them, we know much more about genetics than we can actually use. Why has this happened? Increasingly, physiologists are recognising that biological reductionism, or the pursuit of the most basic unit of the human body, does not dramatically improve our understanding of human physiology.[37] Contrary to popular belief, genes alone do not determine "an organism and its functions." Rather, several biological systems actually operate concurrently within an organism, at the cellular, protein and genetic levels, all interacting with one another and also the environment. In other words, multiple physiological causes, not the genes alone, are responsible for the onset of diseases. As long as we do not abandon the idea of genetic determinism and focus on the intricate systemic relationships in our bodies instead, it would be difficult for us to develop the next significant or blockbuster drug in the short term.[38]

Having said all this, there has been growing recognition since the late 1970s that diseases may not be due only to biological but also to psychological and social factors.[39] This biopsychosocial (BPS) model of disease has now been applied successfully in several areas. The study of Type II diabetes is a good example. An approximate 20 million Americans are estimated to suffer from diabetes, of which 90 percent to 95 percent are considered Type II. As a result of the BPS approach, we now know that the high incidence of Type II diabetes is due primarily to the prevalence of obesity and physical inactivity

---

36   Mark M. Awad and Alice T. Shaw, "ALK Inhibitors in Non–Small Cell Lung Cancer: Crizotinib and Beyond", *Clinical Advances in Hematology & Oncology: H&O* 12, no. 7 (July 2014): 429–39.

37   Uwe Sauer, Matthias Heinemann, and Nicola Zamboni, "Getting Closer to the Whole Picture", *Science* 316, no. 5824 (2007): 550–51.

38   Denis Noble, *The Music of Life: Biology beyond Genes* (Oxford; New York: Oxford University Press, 2008), 4.

39   Francesc Borrell-Carrió, Anthony L. Suchman, and Ronald M. Epstein, "The Biopsychosocial Model 25 Years Later: Principles, Practice, and Scientific Inquiry", *Annals of Family Medicine* 2, no. 6 (November 2004):576–82.

among Americans. In other words, in the combat against Type II diabetes, encouraging changes in lifestyle is at least as important, if not more, than developing drugs against the malaise.[40]

Mathematical Medicine

We turn, finally, to the role of mathematics in Greek and modern medicine. Since antiquity, the Greeks have commonly held geometry to be the "surest knowledge accessible to mortal men".[41] Judging by Euclid's (323–283 BC) *Elements*, Greek geometry operates on the premise that there exist several self-evident (but yet undemonstrable) axioms.[42] For example, "if equals are taken from equals, equals remain", "all right angles are equal to one another", or "the whole is greater than the sum of the parts". Once these axioms are established, they then become the basis for deducing other geometric propositions and theorems, such as Pythagoras' and Thales' theorems. The fact that this axiomatic-deductive approach could offer such exact and certain knowledge proved inspirational for the Greeks. When Aristotle laid out the conditions and procedures for demonstrative sciences in his *Posterior Analytics*, he took this as a model, arguing that axioms or first principles can also be found and used for deducing or demonstrating scientific theories. A good example of this would be his teleological assumption, where he presumed that "nature does nothing in vain".[43] When Archimedes (287–212 BC) investigated the phenomenon of flotation, he similarly postulated that fluids were

---

40   S. Wild et al., "Global Prevalence of Diabetes: Estimates for the Year 2000 and Projections for 2030", *Diabetes Care* 27, no. 5 (1 May 2004): 1047–53.

41   Hardy Grant, "Geometry and Medicine: Mathematics in the Thought of Galen of Pergamum 4", *Philosophia Mathematica*, s2–4, no. 1 (1989): 29–34.

42   Euclid's *Elements* is the most substantive extant text on Greek geometry. Lloyd, *Disciplines in the Making*, 35.

43   Aristotle, of course, predates Euclid and it is an open question whether his axiomatic–deductive approach played an influential role in Euclidean mathematics. G. E. R. Lloyd and Nathan Sivin, *The Way and the Word: Science and Medicine in Early China and Greece* (New Haven, CN; London: Yale University Press, 2002), 165–66.

perfectly homogeneous and totally inelastic. In so doing, he worked out his famous theory of flotation, Archimedes' principle.[44] As we mentioned earlier, Galen was clearly inspired by Aristotle's axiom—that nothing is done and vain—and employed it extensively in his anatomical investigations.[45] In addition, he also introduced more axioms of his own, such as "nothing comes without a cause" and "opposites are cured by opposites".[46]

While not all Greek sciences employed this axiomatic-deductive approach, most sought to mathematise their disciplines in order that they may attain, as it were, the certainty intrinsic to Greek geometry. Not content with his idea that all physical reality was made up of the four elements, Plato further proposed a geometric basis for these elements by suggesting that they were constituted by small triangles.[47] When Praxagoras of Cos (300 BC) and his student, Herophilus (c. 325–255 BC), developed their pulse theory, they turned to music (and therefore harmonic theory) as the analogy for the arterial dilations and contractions that they apparently detected in the pulses.[48] Most intriguingly, a recent study of Galen's writings indicates that his medical teachings and practice were very much informed by a rudimentary statistical instinct. This can be seen in how well aware he was of the value of a large sample size, the need to repeat an experiment to derive a reliable scientific conclusion, and the idea of population distribution.[49]

At this juncture, the question may be asked: "Why were the

---

44   Archimedes asserts that the upward buoyant force exerted on a body immersed in a fluid, whether fully or partially submerged, is equal to the weight of the fluid that the body displaces and that this acts in the upward direction at the centre of mass of the displaced fluid.

45   R. J. Hankinson, *The Cambridge Companion to Galen* (Cambridge; NY: Cambridge University Press, 2008), 51–58.

46   Ibid., 61.

47   *Timaeus* 54–56.

48   Lloyd and Sivin, *The Way and the Word*, 168.

49   Athanasios A. Diamandopoulos, Goudas C. Pavlos, and Kassimatis I. Theodoro, "Early Evidence-Based Medicine: Clues on Statistical Analysis in Medicine from Galen's Writings", *Taylor & Francis*, The American Statistician, 61, no. 2 (2007): 154–58.

Greeks so bent on deriving an exact, certain and, inadvertently, mathematical understanding of science?" Besides a desire for "the highest possible standards of rigour", this pursuit of certainty, Lloyd suggested, also stemmed from the competitive spirit that characterised Greek civic and intellectual life.[50] Greek intellectuals, explained Lloyd, mostly lived

> in one or other of the more or less democratic, or more or less oligarchic, city states, whether their own, as citizens, or in others, as metics or resident aliens, or simply as visitors.... Throughout the classical and early Hellenistic periods, they were mainly self-supporting, relying on the wealth of their members and (as much and sometimes even more) on fee-paying pupils.[51]

Operating in this context, competition between Greek philosophers was understandably rife, since they had to vie against each other for not only more prestige but also additional members and students. Such competition was usually expressed in the philosophers' dialectical debates with one another, where they sought to prove "not just that truth was on [their] side, but also certainty".[52] Given the widespread esteem for geometry, it is hardly surprising that these philosophers would draw their epistemological models from mathematics, since this would give their arguments a veneer of certainty. This was despite the fact that they knew well that the axioms they developed were not quite self-evident but were simplified assumptions about the "physical aspects" of their sciences.[53]

As mentioned in the previous chapter, this correlation between

---

50   Lloyd and Sivin, *The Way and the Word*, 173.
51   Lloyd, *Adversaries and Authorities*, 130.
52   Lloyd and Sivin, *The Way and the Word*, 173.
53   Good examples of such postulates would be Archimedes' assumption that all fluids are perfectly homogeneous, or Galen's presumption that the "opposites are cured by opposites". Ibid. 167.

mathematics and epistemic certainty continued to dominate empirical investigations during the modern Scientific Revolution, with Kepler going so far as to assert that "geometry existed before the Creation, [and] is co-eternal with the mind of God". The 19th century, however, saw the gradual overshadowing of the geometric approach by statistical analysis. The value of statistics first came to the fore in 1854 when John Snow employed it to demonstrate contaminated water as the major cause for cholera.[54] Its scientific importance was confirmed in the 1940–50s when it was used successfully by Sir Bradford Hill to prove the efficacy of *Streptomycin* and PAS in tuberculosis treatment, and that smoking was a major cause of lung cancer.[55] Since then, Randomised Controlled Trials (RCTs) have been taken for granted as the norm for assessing the efficacy of all new medical therapies. The rise of evidence-based medicine in the 1980s further established the legitimacy of statistics by applying it to conduct systematic reviews and meta-analyses of RCTs. RCTs and evidence-based medicine, of course, have become yet additional benchmarks for biomedical physicians to assess the efficacy of Chinese medical therapies. The methodological issues pertaining to this, however, are long drawn and often contested by Chinese physicians. Due to the complexity involved, they will be discussed in Chapter 10 instead.

To conclude our survey of the use of mathematics in Greek and biomedicine, I would like to reflect briefly on the general application of statistics in medical research. First of all, it should be clear by now that the Western preoccupation with "creating medical science after the image of mathematics" was motivated primarily by the ancient Greeks' desire for demonstrating certainty in their knowledge. Once this assumption gained momentum, it was pretty much taken for granted even as Galenic medicine evolved into its modern counterpart. Secondly, whether it was geometry or statistics, the same problem which troubled the Greeks has remained: that

54   Bynum, *History of Medicine*, 194–96.
55   James Le Fanu, *The Rise & Fall of Modern Medicine* (London: Abacus, 2014), 47–73.

is, mathematical exactness and certainty can never be transposed to the physical sciences (including medicine) without a necessary simplification of particular aspects of the physical reality itself.[56] For example, several groups of system biologists have, in recent years, employed computer simulation to develop very impressive models of the heart. Despite the complexity and life-likeness of such virtual hearts, it is a sobering thought that these models are still far from depicting how the heart actually works. This is because the current models are based only on 2% of the estimated 5,000 genes involved in the electrical and mechanical behaviour of the heart.[57]

This brings us to our third point. Intrinsic to statistical analysis is the logic of induction. As a scientific model, statistical induction operates on the premise that *just* as a phenomenon occurs in a sample group, *so also* would it occur in a population that is characteristically similar to the sample. Besides the fact that statistical models are not deductive and therefore, strictly speaking, cannot be used to demonstrate causality, the robustness of a model is also highly dependent on the assumptions made about the model constructed, all of which are determined by the scientists' experience, training, epistemic biases, financial and time constraints, and other factors.[58] For example, most trials are usually conducted using "ideal patients" who are "often less sick than real-world patients and on fewer other drugs" and thus respond better to treatments. Many of these trials are held in Third World countries, where the patients, demographically speaking, may not be similar to the actual patients who will use the drugs eventually. In both cases, it is an open question whether the drugs approved based on these parameters could be equally effective for real-world patients in the developed countries. Often the

---

56   Lloyd and Sivin, *The Way and the Word*, 167.
57   Noble, *Music of Life*, 85–86.
58   See Rosenberg for further discussions on the application of statistical induction. Alex Rosenberg, *Philosophy of Science: A Contemporary Introduction* (London: Routledge, 2003), 38–40.

pressures of time and the characteristics of certain diseases mean that many trials cannot adequately assess the real-world outcomes (such as heart attacks or survival rates) of a drug before it is submitted for approval. Consequently, what most trials settle for are improvements in surrogate outcomes, such as reductions in blood pressure or improvements in blood tests. Again, it remains to be seen whether the success with surrogate outcomes actually translate to actual improvements in real-world outcomes, which, clearly, matter more to both physician and patient.[59] As we shall see in Chapters 9 and 10, biomedical and Chinese medical assumptions about the human body, diagnosis and therapy vary quite significantly. If biomedical premises are introduced (as it so often happens) in a Chinese medical RCT, the results derived may not well reflect the efficacy of Chinese medical diagnosis and therapy, even if these turn out to be positive.[60]

More seriously, medical science in recent years has often privileged statistical knowledge over and above clinical experience and judgement. Indeed, the latter has sometimes been regarded as "less reliable and inferior". This, lamented Le Fanu, is regrettable since "clinical trials [often] cannot answer the sort of complex questions that frequently crop up in medical practice". More importantly, he observed that "statistically derived knowledge ... has consistently been shown to be unreliable, promoting the patently absurd as proven fact". For instance, when clinical trial findings are scrutinised critically, they have "been shown to result in the adoption of an ineffective treatment in 32 per cent of cases and the rejection of a useful treatment in 33 per cent of cases."[61]

---

59   Bradford Hill himself cautions that whenever incorrect or inadequate assumptions are made about the nature of the problem, the statistical study will be in "danger of drawing false inferences and conclusions". He also provides a list of criteria which should be expected of any RCT, which are helpfully summarised in Le Fanu, *Rise & Fall of Modern Medicine*, 71–72. For the problem of surrogate outcomes, see Goldacre, *Bad Pharma*, Kindle Location 2060–109.

60   Hai Hong, *The Theory of Chinese Medicine: A Modern Explanation* (London: Imperial College, 2014), x.

61   Le Fanu, *Rise & Fall of Modern Medicine*, 431.

All these limitations are notwithstanding the fact that clinical findings have increasingly shown an uncanny bias for the pharmaceutical companies sponsoring their research.[62] This growing alliance between what should have been independent parties is, of course, a cause for much concern among medical professionals. This development and the concerns it raises have been well described by Marcia Angell, the Chief Editor of the *New England Journal of Medicine*.

> Until the 1980s, researchers were largely independent of the companies that sponsored their work. Drug companies would give a grant to an academic medical centre, then step back and wait for faculty researchers to produce the results. They hoped their product would look good, but they had no way of knowing for sure. They certainly did not attempt to tell the researchers how to run their clinical trials. Now, however, companies are involved in every detail of the research—from design of the study through analysis of the data to the decision whether to publish the results. That involvement has made bias not only possible but extremely likely. Researchers don't control clinical trials anymore. Sponsors do.[63]

Much has been said regarding the significance of mathematics in the evolution of the Western medical tradition. It is timely to now ask the comparative question: "Was mathematics similarly esteemed and co-opted in Chinese sciences, including medicine?" Just as in the

---

62   There are three variants of the drug, olanzapine, which is used to treat schizophrenia. These are manufactured by Eli Lilly, Janssen and Pfizer. Independent researchers have reviewed the studies in which the three products are compared. As it turns out, the trials paid for by Eli Lilly presents its product as superior to Janssen, while those funded by Hanssen concludes that it was better instead. A similar bias was observed in the trial sponsored by Pfizer! Ibid., 472.

63   Marcia Angell, *The Truth about the Drug Companies: How They Deceive Us and What to Do about It* (New York: Random House, 2004), 100.

case of anatomy and ontology, this interest in mathematical certainty has not been a concern for ancient Chinese sciences. Take Chinese astronomy, for example.

> Although classical astronomers continually sought greater accuracy in establishing eclipse cycles and other calendrical constants … they did not attempt to prove a view of the physical dispositions of the heavenly bodies, let alone show that things must be so and could not be otherwise.[64]

This is not to say that the Chinese lacked an interest or ability in mathematics.[65] By the Han period (206 BC–AD 220), several mathematics treatises had been composed, such as the *Arithmetic Classic of the Zhou Gnomon* (*Zhoubi Suanjing*, 周髀算经), the *Nine Chapters on Mathematical Procedures* (*Jiuzhang Suanshu*, 九章算术) and the *Book of Mathematical Procedures* (*Suanshushu*, 算术书). To these we may add the many writings that employed mathematics in their fields, such as those that addressed astronomy, calendars and tables, as well as divination.[66] Judging by how the Chinese employed mathematics, it is evident that the distinction between "the study of nature" and mathematics was not their concern. "Rather, each discipline dealt with the quantitative aspects of the phenomena it covered as and when the need arose." More importantly, what preoccupied the Chinese was "to explore the unity of mathematics [across the various disciplines] and to extend its range [by means of analogy]".[67]

Unlike the Greeks, the vast expanse of China was united under the Qins (221–206 BC) as early as the third century BC. While the

---

64   Lloyd and Sivin, *The Way and the Word*, 173.

65   For a historical survey of Chinese Mathematics, see Jean-Claude Martzloff, *A History of Chinese Mathematics* (New York: Springer, 2006).

66   Lloyd, *Disciplines in the Making*, 45–46.

67   Ibid., 54–56.

Qin dynasty was short-lived, it proved influential for Chinese culture and science in the long run.

First of all, its model of centralising the government in the imperial capital (rather than to leave the Dukes to rule their respective counties, as in the Zhou dynasty) would be adopted by subsequent dynasties from the Hans right to the Qings. This centralisation, as Unschuld noted, sensitised the Qins and their successors to the importance of effectively managing the supply of food and resources to the capital. Without this, the well-being of the capital and the country would be threatened.[68]

Secondly, the Qins' legalistic and harsh approach towards government was immensely unpopular and quickly repudiated when the dynasty was overthrown. In its stead, Confucianism was adopted as the new ideology of government—a model which more or less persisted until the Qing dynasty. According to the Han Confucians, cosmic harmony was to be attained when the emperor abided by the Heavenly Mandate through a consultative relationship with his Confucian officials. Moreover, this mutuality and reciprocity was to be extended to and to govern all hierarchical relationships from the emperor and his officials, right down to the husband and his wife, and the parent and his child.[69] When operating in tandem with one another, both models must have impressed upon the Chinese the importance of managing the relationships between different entities in life, whether this was in logistics, government or familial relations. Once this mental image caught on, it should not surprise us that the Chinese would regard mathematics not so much as a subject to be studied *in abstracto*, but more in terms of its relations and applications to other disciplines. As we shall see in Chapters 6 to 8, Chinese medicine would operate by a similar premise. Not only did it see no need to mathematise its methodology, but it also felt quite free to

---

68   Paul U. Unschuld, *What Is Medicine: Western and Eastern Approaches to Healing* (Berkeley, CA: University of California Press, 2009), 51.

69   Lloyd, *Adversaries and Authorities*, 124–25.

employ concrete but rather subjective metaphors in both its theories and diagnostics—a practice that would have been unimaginable for the Greeks.

Conclusion

In view of the above, it should be clear that, contrary to popular expectations, modern biomedicine is neither value-neutral nor ideologically unbiased. Rather, its intellectual roots run deep, and may be traced to the philosophical concerns of the Pre-Socratics, the classical philosophers, most notably Plato and Aristotle, and also the Hellenistic and Late Antique physicians, such as Praxagoras and Galen. Three major concerns have been raised in this chapter. The first is the Greeks' teleological understanding of anatomy. As they saw it, anatomy is not merely a mess of entrails and tissue. Instead, if one were to scrutinise it properly, one would be able to discern in it the intricate design of the Creator. This teleological conviction gained currency among the Greek physicians eventually and played an important role in forging the close relationship between anatomy and medicine. The ties between the two would persist, even in modern-day biomedicine.

The second legacy that the Greeks bequeathed to biomedicine was their ontological perspectives of medicine. Underlying Galen's doctrine of humours was the Greek understanding that the humours, or for that matter, all things, were constituted by the four elements. While the rise of biomedicine saw the eventual demise of humoral theory, this ontological view of the human body and disease continued unabated. In fact, it compelled biomedical physicians to continue seeking the most "basic unit of medical understanding of disease", first in anatomy and later, in the cell, the DNA and germs. Third and finally, the Greeks' desire for epistemic certainty was a key reason why they adopted the methods of geometry for their study of medicine. Once the idea gained traction, mathematics was taken for granted as a crucial or, in fact, the preferred means of establishing medical knowledge.

Philosophical language and categories have always been empowering, enabling us to articulate and frame our concerns, and also helping us to develop creative answers for our questions. The same, however, can also be restrictive, since they compel us to look at problems, issues, and even reality from a limited perspective, to the exclusion of others. In this process, many answers to unasked questions have been inadvertently excluded, and blind spots introduced into our epistemic paradigms. This phenomenon is not unique to Greek philosophy, of course, but is intrinsic to all kinds of philosophical discourse, whether Eastern or Western. In the case of Greek philosophy, it has done well and much to help biomedicine construct valuable perspectives of human physiology and disease, and to develop many more life-saving therapies. On the other hand, it has also taught its adherents to interpret human well-being and sickness in particular ways that may not only limit its future progress, but render other medical traditions incongruent to biomedical eyes. This, I suggest, is the reason why biomedicine has often found Chinese medical philosophy, theory and practice bewildering or even implausible. By and large, biomedicine has failed to recognise that, when it judges Chinese medicine to be "unscientific", what it is actually demanding Chinese medicine to do is to conform to the epistemic biases and expectations of Greek philosophy. In the light of our studies above, biomedicine's privileging of its Greek epistemic legacy can only be understood as an implicit form of cultural imperialism, which remains, unfortunately, mostly unrecognised by its followers.

How then should we proceed? If biomedicine is to engage Chinese medicine constructively, it must first seek to understand the philosophies underlying Chinese medical theories and practice, before identifying ways in which the two medical traditions can dialogue with one another. All these should be conducted in a spirit of mutual learning, with respect for each other's epistemic assumptions, without requiring one to conform or submit to the philosophical expectations of the other. This premise is that which has been adopted by the author and will be developed in the rest of this book.

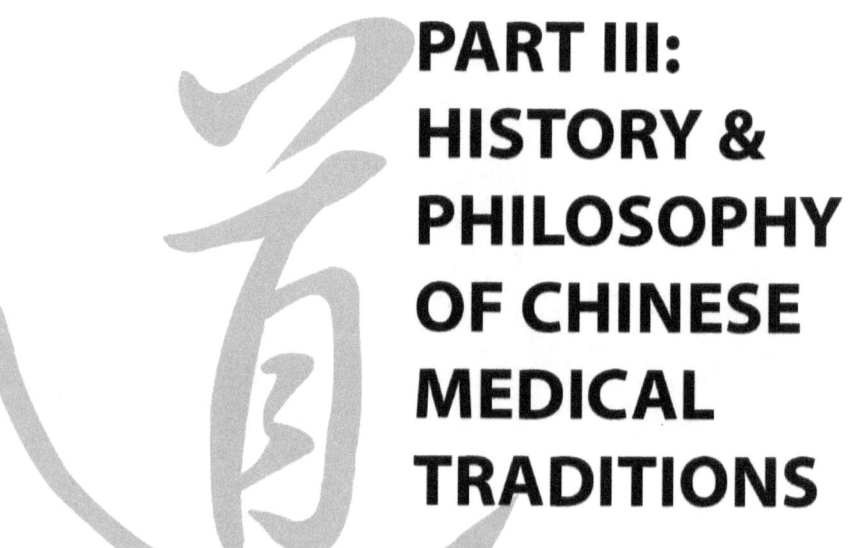

PART III: HISTORY & PHILOSOPHY OF CHINESE MEDICAL TRADITIONS

Over the last three chapters, we have surveyed the historical developments of both Greek and modern medicine, before evaluating the philosophies assumed by them. Our goal is not only to learn how we arrived at where we are (in terms of modern medicine), but also to recognise the philosophical and epistemic biases which these traditions have bequeathed to us (who are mostly trained in modern science). This self-knowledge, as we have emphasised time and again, is crucial for any fruitful dialogue with Chinese medicine. This is because it cautions us against any pre-judgement of the Chinese medical tradition, while, hopefully, reminding us to be more patient and open-minded in our engagement with the Chinese tradition.

This brings us to Part 3 of this book. What we shall do here is similar: map out the historical, philosophical, theoretical, and empirical background of Chinese medicine, so that we can bring the two medical traditions into dialogue in Part 4, or Chapters 10 and 11. Briefly, Chapters 6 and 7 will survey the historical developments of Chinese medicine from the Pre-Han period to the 20th century. Chapter 8 will consider the medical discourses of both Western and Chinese medical traditions through the analytical lenses of cognitive linguistics or, more specifically, the contemporary theory of metaphors. It would then be seen that philosophy plays a significant role in how each tradition conceptualises health, disease and well-being, and this is mostly why their understanding of aetiology and therapy differs so dramatically. However, as was mentioned in the Introduction, some readers may find this Chapter rather technical and can skip it to go on to the next Chapter without losing the flow of the metanarrative. Finally, Chapter 9 provides a basic introduction to Chinese medical theory and practice. As and when possible, medical case studies will be presented to help readers have a better grasp of how Chinese medicine operates in practice.

6

THE HISTORICAL DEVELOPMENT OF CHINESE MEDICINE I:

FROM PRE-HAN TO TANG ERAS

Misunderstanding Chinese Medicine

An oncologist once advised his patient not to take Chinese medication while undergoing chemotherapy, lest the former affected the efficacy of the latter. When asked whether she could drink wolfberry and red date tea instead, the doctor readily agreed since, in his mind, these were food, not medication. This distinction would have come across as odd for Chinese medical doctors since wolfberry and red dates are ingredients commonly used in Chinese medical therapies.[1] Not a few years ago, *The Straits Times'* Senior Writer, Andy Ho, criticised the

---

1   This is not to say that Chinese medical herbs do not interfere with biomedicine therapy. That a medical herb is regarded as either "Chinese" or "Western" is but imposing a cultural category on the herb itself. This does not negate the fact that different herbs will interact differently with one another, some beneficially, while others lethally. See, for example, the unfortunate case when a patient unknowing consumed Cordyceps before her surgery and suffered fatal post-op bleeding. Amir Hussain, "Cordyceps 'likely led to post-op bleeding'", Text, *The Straits Times*, 27 May 2016, http://www.straitstimes.com/singapore/courts-crime/cordyceps-likely-led-to-post-op-bleeding.

Singapore Medical Council for allowing doctors to refer patients to TCM practitioners, especially acupuncturists. As he saw it, this was a regrettable development, since acupuncture was a therapy offered by "shamans and blood letters", not by "the Chinese physician in days of yore". That is, acupuncture was never mainstream Chinese medicine. Ho goes on to explain that acupuncture is problematic on two counts. First, there is no positive clinical trial evidence for its efficacy.[2] Second and, perhaps, more importantly, its theories of *qi* and the meridians are based on a flawed Chinese astrology.[3] Again, Ho's distinction between the "Chinese physician" and the acupuncturist would have been strange for TCM physicians. This is because the two share essentially the same beliefs in *qi* and meridians in their diagnostic and therapeutic practices.

In his *A Biblical Approach to Chinese Traditions and Beliefs*, Daniel Tong advises Christians to avoid TCM therapies altogether. Apart from his belief that TCM theories have no biomedical basis, he fears that these theories (particularly, the ideas of *qi* and *yinyang*) are tainted by Daoist ideas and may, therefore, expose its users to demonic influence.[4] While Sinologists will agree that these ideas are important for the Daoists, most will also find Tong's conclusions inaccurate.[5] The reason being that the same ideas, as we shall see, were taken for granted even by the Confucians, and were incorporated into Chinese medical theory before the advent of religious Daoism. In fact, as we shall see, the development of classical Chinese medicine was actually more indebted to Confucianism than Daoism.

In view of the above, it is clear that many criticisms of Chinese medicine are often based on a partial or an erroneous understanding of the medical tradition. The reasons for this are many. Up until recently,

---

2   This is an often-debated topic and will be addressed later in Chapter 10.

3   Andy Ho, "Pinning down Acupuncture: It's a Placebo", *The Straits Times*, 2011.

4   Daniel Tong, *A Biblical Approach to Chinese Traditions and Beliefs* (Singapore: Genesis, 2003), 108–24.

5   Sinology refers to the academic study of Chinese thought and culture, such as Chinese history, poetry, literature, philosophy, music and medicine.

English scholarship on Chinese medical theories and histories has been few and far between.[6] Even those well-known among Sinologists are often unknown to, let alone consulted by, popular discussions about Chinese medicine.[7] Furthermore, a fair and accurate assessment of Chinese medicine requires not only Sinology but also a familiarity with the development of Western scientific philosophy, its influence on Greek and modern medicine, and how these scientific paradigms impinge on our analysis and understanding of Chinese medicine. In other words, what is often thought of as a mere biomedical study of TCM's efficacy—subject its therapeutic claims to clinical trials and let's see whether it is effective—is actually an inter-disciplinary project that requires a multi-prong approach to the study of the two medical traditions. This, by and large, has been the aim of this book.

Thus far, we have examined the historical and philosophical roots of the Western medical traditions in Chapters 3 to 5. We shall now do the same for Chinese medicine, beginning, first of all, with its historical developments. The history of Chinese medicine can be divided into three significant epochs: the Han, Song and the late-Qing to modern periods. Our survey will, more or less, be structured around these milestones. The present chapter will focus on the first, by tracing the evolution of Chinese medicine from its origins in the Shang dynasty to its first zenith in the Han dynasty when classical medical theory was first formalised. It then concludes by considering the subsequent medical developments until the late Tang period. Chapter 7 will cover the second and third epochs. It will begin with the Song medical renaissance, when we witness the integration of Chinese pharmacology with classical medical theories, and how this gave rise

6   If one is to judge from the bibliographies of such critics, it appears that they have relied primarily on English sources, and not Chinese scholarship on the subject.

7   Daniel Tong's *A Biblical Approach to Chinese Traditions and Beliefs* is a good example. While it was published in 2003, it made no reference to several important works on Chinese medicine, such as Joseph Needham's *Celestial Lancets: A History and Rationale of Acupuncture and Moxa* (1980), Paul Unschuld's *Medicine in China: A History of Ideas* (1985) or Shigeshisa Kuriyama's *The Expressiveness of the Body and the Divergence of Greek and Chinese Medicine* (2002).

to a flowering of Chinese medicine lineages during the Song-Jin-Yuan eras. The third epoch, which is the late-Qing and modern eras, is no less important. It is here that we shall see how Chinese medicine was transformed by its encounter with its Western counterpart.

Spiritual Healing from Shang Dynasty Onwards

Contrary to popular expectations, the Chinese medical world was diverse and pluralistic from the outset. Like its Greek counterpart, secular and religious forms of healing often co-existed, inter-mingled, and sometimes competed with one another.[8] The earliest evidence for Chinese therapeutic activities may be found on the oracle bone inscriptions from the Shang Dynasty (1766–1122 BC). Here, we encounter a world of spiritual healing, where one's illnesses were due either to one's dead ancestors, the deified ancestor known as *di* (帝), or evil wind-spirits (*xiefeng*, 邪风).[9] The Zhou dynasty (1100–221 BC) saw further modifications to this spiritual aetiology, with the spirits of the dead, demonic spirits, worm spirits (*gu*, 蛊), or even homeopathic magic becoming the new pathological agents. "When a person falls ill", as Han Feizi (280–233 BC) put it plainly, "it means he has been injured by a demon".[10]

A wide range of therapeutic options were available against these malevolent spirits. Besides the ritual offerings of animals, the ancients also had recourse to summoning aid from deities, exorcisms, spells, incantations, talismans, amulets, prayers, or even the use of drugs. The idea of magic correspondence was also common, where specific days or times of the day were seen as most suitable for the performance of various exorcist rituals. Such spiritual therapies would remain popular throughout much of the imperial period, even with

8   Vivienne Lo and Michael Stanley-Baker, "Chinese Medicine", in *The Oxford Handbook of the History of Medicine*, ed. Mark Jackson (Oxford: Oxford University Press, 2013), 150.

9   Paul U. Unschuld, *Medicine in China: A History of Ideas* (Berkeley, CA; London: University of California Press, 1985), 17, 25.

10   Ibid., 37.

the advent of secular Chinese medicine from the Han dynasty (206 BC–AD 220) onwards. Often, these remedies were included even in the physician's therapeutic toolkit. For example, 27 or 10 percent of the prescriptions found in the Han medical treatise, *Prescriptions Against Fifty-Two Ailments* (*Wushier Bingfang*, 五十二病方, 168 BC) are spells against spiritual attacks. The medical compendium, *Qian Jin Yi Fang* (千金翼方), written by the famous Tang physician, Sun Simiao (孙思邈, AD 581–682), identified a further list of 32 drugs as effective against diseases caused by demonic spirits.[11] By and large, religious healing remained popular right until the late Qing dynasty. It continues to be practised in some quarters of Chinese society even till this day.[12]

The Emergence of *Yinyang*, *Wuxing* and *Qi* Theories

The late Zhou era saw the disintegration of the nation into several independent states that were often at war with one another (thus, the Warring States period). In response to this national crisis, several schools of thoughts emerged—Confucian, Daoist, Legalism and others—each vying to develop a political philosophy that will resolve the socio-political chaos at hand. This period of decline was also taken generally as the time when the Chinese moved towards "more humanistic and rationalistic understandings of the world and the place of human beings in it".[13] As readers will realise, this transition coincided, quite remarkably, with the Greeks' move towards non-mythological or naturalistic explanations of nature. In the case of the Greeks, what transpired was an ontological approach towards the

---

11   Ibid., 35–46, 52–53. For further discussion on therapeutic magic in the early Han period, see Donald John Harper, *Early Chinese Medical Literature: The Mawangdui Medical Manuscripts* (London: Kegan Paul International, 1998), 148–83.

12   Bridie Andrews, *The Making of Modern Chinese Medicine, 1850–1960* (Vancouver: UBC Press, 2014), 29–32.

13   Robin Wang, *Yinyang: The Way of Heaven and Earth in Chinese Thought and Culture* (Cambridge: Cambridge University Press, 2012), 163.

study of nature, science and medicine. For the Chinese, however, their re-conception of the world did not take an ontological turn. Instead, a different epistemic paradigm emerged and took root by the Han dynasty. Thereafter, it would transform Chinese thought and culture for the centuries to come, including its perspectives of science and medicine. This epistemic paradigm is none other than the theory of *yinyang*.

Evidence for the incorporation of *yinyang* theory in Han medicine is ample. The earliest are medical texts unearthed from the Mawangdui tombs (马王堆古墓, 168 BC) in Changsha, Hunan. Among these is a treatise called *Ten Questions* (*Shiwen*, 十问), where we have the legendary kings, Yao (尧) and Shun (舜), discussing health and well-being.[14]

> Yao asked Shun: In all that is under heaven, what is the most valuable? Shun replied: Life is most valuable. Yao said: How can life be cultivated? Shun said: Investigate *yinyang*.
>
> 尧问于舜曰：「天下孰最贵？」舜曰：「生最贵。」尧曰：「治生奈何？」舜曰：「审夫阴阳」。

As to what the investigation of *yinyang* entails, one has to turn to a later Han text, the *Yellow Emperor's Inner Canon* (*Huangdi Neijing*, 黄帝内经). Here, we have yet another emperor, Huangdi, declaring that the True or Ideal human being (*zhenren*, 真人) is one who lives according to the principles of heaven and earth (提挈天地) and abides by the rhythms of *yinyang* (把握阴阳). In so doing, he enjoys longevity and is able to live as long as the heaven and earth.[15]

---

14 Vivienne Lo notes that ancient cultural heroes, such as the legendary kings, Yao, Shun, Huangdi and the Divine Farmer (*shennong*, 神农), were often employed by the Han writers as the spokesmen for their writings, particularly in the field of medicine. Lo and Stanley-Baker, "Chinese Medicine", 151.

15 余闻上古有真人者，提挈天地，把握阴阳，呼吸精气，独立守神，肌肉若

But what is *yinyang* theory? How did it originate and come to dominate Chinese thought and culture? The first usage of the two words can be found in the Zhou texts, the *Book of History* (*Shangshu*, 尚书, c. 500 BC) and the *Book of Odes* (*Shijing*, 诗经, c. 600 BC). In the former, *yin* was employed to refer to the northern side of a mountain or a body of water, while *yang* to the southern side.[16] In the latter, the same words described the shady and sunny sides of a hill respectively.[17] It would seem, therefore, that *yin* and *yang* were never ontological or distinct entities to begin with, but functional categories that enabled one to delineate an entity's relationship with its geographic and chronological context.[18] Furthermore, judging by Zhuangzi's (370–287 BC) remarks, the same words also convey the ideas of rhythm and movement in life:

> Those who know the joys of Heaven, during their life conform to the ways of Heaven, and at death transform with things. In their stillness they possess the same virtue as *yin*, and in their movement they flow the same as *yang*.[19]

> 知天乐者，其生也天行，其死也物化。静而与阴同德，动而与阳同波。

Given their ability to describe the rhythms of and the relationships

---

一，故能寿敝天地，无有终时，此其道生。《素问。上古天真论》

16   The legacy of this idea continues till this day. The city of *Huayin* (华阴) in Shanxi is thus named because it is located on the northern side of *Hua* mountain. It is noteworthy, however, that a city located on the western or northern side of a body of water will be named *yang* instead. Thus we have the city of *Luoyang* (洛阳) which is located north of the *Luo* river. Wang, *Yinyang*, 25.

17   "Viewing the scenery at hill, looking for *yinyang*" (既景迺冈, 相其陰陽).

18   For example, the side of a hill facing eastwards (the geographic context) is *yang* only from the morning to early afternoon (chronological context). This is due to the fact that the sun only shines on this side of the hill during these few hours (both geographic and chronological context).

19   Zhuangzi, *Way of Heaven* (*Tiandao*, 天道).

between humanity and the cosmos, it did not take long before *yinyang* thought was incorporated into Chinese astrology. The Chinese calendar, for example, was developed to advise the ancients on the times most desirable for planting, harvesting and even religious rituals. The *Zuo's Commentary* or *Zuozhuan* (左传, late fourth century BC) observed that, by the Spring and Autumn period, the officer in charge of astrology was already using *yinyang* as a means of explaining weather conditions and seasonal changes. Not surprisingly, diviners also began to incorporate *yinyang* thinking into their practices. Not all approved of such applications, of course. When asked whether unusual phenomena, such as stars falling or trees groaning, were portents of future ominous events, Xunzi (荀子, 298–238) replied otherwise, explaining that while such unusual events were due to "a modification of the relation of Heaven and Earth or a transmutation of the *yin* and *yang*…. We may [only] marvel at them, but we should not fear them".[20]

Despite Xunzi's concerns, it appears that a *yinyang* school, led by Zou Yan (鄒衍, 305–240 BC), emerged during the Warring States period and began to adopt *yinyang* theory as a paradigm for fortune telling and divination—a practice that continues among contemporary Chinese geomancers.[21] During the late Qing period, this gave much cause for modern Chinese intellectuals, such as Liang Qichao (梁启超, 1873–1929), to denounce *yinyang* theory as the root of superstitious thinking in Imperial China.[22] This is also the reason why many Christians remain apprehensive about *yinyang* theory till this

---

20   Quoted from Wang, *Yinyang*, 30.

21   Unfortunately, we have no extant writings for this *yinyang* school. What is to be known about the school and its founder, Zou Yan, are to be found in the brief biography composed by the Han Historian, Sima Qian's (135–86 BC), in his *Records of the Grand Historian* (*Shiji*, 史记). Ole Bruun and Stephan Feuchtwang, *Fengshui in China: Geomantic Divination between State Orthodoxy and Popular Religion* (Copenhagen: NIAS Press, 2011), 248, 263.

22   Bruun and Feuchtwang, 248, 263.; Qichao Liang, "The Origin of Yinyang and Wuxing", in *The Debate on Ancient History* (古史辩), ed. Jiegang Gu, vol. 5 (Shanghai: Shanghai Guji Press, 1982), 343.

day. It is to be noted, however, that the same school also applied *yinyang* thinking in scientific and technological studies, thereby rendering it a philosophical means for demythologising or naturalising the Chinese understanding of the world.[23] It is this strand of *yinyang* philosophy that the Han physicians would employ when they developed a secular or natural approach towards medicine.

Before we discuss the evolution of Han medicine, we need to understand two other important pre-Han ideas. They are the concepts of *wuxing* (五行) and *qi* (气). This is because the *yinyang* theory that the Han physicians adopted was not the same as that conceived by Zou Yan, but a Han epistemic paradigm that integrated all three ideas of *yinyang*, *wuxing* and *qi*.

The concept of *wuxing* originated from the Zhou period, quite independent of *yinyang* thinking. The earliest reference appeared in the *Book of History*, where we are told that the damming up of the inundating waters apparently "threw into disorder the arrangement of the *wuxing*". Later, in the *Zuozhuan*, *wuxing* was interpreted as the elements or agents which can be used by humankind:

Imitate the brightness of heaven; go along with the nature of the earth. [The Heaven and earth] will produce their six *qi* and [you] may use their *wuxing*.[24]

则天之明，因地之性，生其六气，用其五行。

From the onset, *wuxing* referred to the five elements of metal (*jin*, 金), wood (*mu*, 木), water (*shui*, 水), fire (*huo*, 火) and earth

---

23   Unlike Confucius, Zou Yan was apparently very popular and honoured among the Wei, Zhao and Yan kings of the late Zhou/ Warring states period. Donald Harper speculates that this could be due to Zou Yan's stature as a teacher of occult and scientific knowledge, and, therefore, a "master of the ultimate secrets of the cosmos". These skills would also have come in handy for warfare, as compared to Confucius' political and moral ideals. Harper, *Early Chinese Medical Literature: The Mawangdui Medical Manuscripts*, 50; Wang, *Yinyang*, 35–36.

24   *Zuozhuan, Zhao Lord Year 25* 《左传，昭公二十五年》.

(*tu*, 土). Despite their similarity with the Greeks' four elements, the *wuxing* is better translated as the *Five Phases* or *Five Agents*. This is because what is important about *wuxing* is not the elements themselves but the relationships they denote. This relational logic is already evident in Zou Yan's *Theory of the Beginning and Ending of Five Forces* (*Wude Zhongshishuo*, 五德終始说) where he appropriates the idea of *wuxing* to explain the rise and fall of the earliest Chinese dynasties.[25] According to him, the Xia dynasty was characterised by wood and was thus overcome by the Shang dynasty (symbolised by metal). The Zhou dynasty, in turn, was denoted by fire and this was why it defeated the Shang but was later extinguished by the waters of Qin.

While Zou Yan was most likely the first to marry *yinyang* and *wuxing* thinking, his application illustrated but one aspect of *wuxing* theory. A more comprehensive expression of this idea, as generally understood in Chinese science and medicine, was that articulated by the Sui scholar, Xiaoji (蕭吉, d. 501). According to Xiao, there were two sets of relationships intrinsic to the *wuxing*: *xiangsheng* (相生, mutually generating) and *xiangke* (相克, mutually conquering).

The generating sequence is: water generates wood; wood generates fire; fire generates earth; earth generates metal; and metal generates water. The conquering sequence is: water conquers fire; fire conquers metal; metal conquers wood; wood conquers earth; and earth conquers water.[26]

In other words, the idea of *wuxing* enabled the Chinese to describe the systematic relationships between multiple entities by drawing attention to how two paired entities complemented or opposed one another.

We turn now to the theory of *qi* (气). The relationship between *qi* and *yinyang* was forged much earlier around the fifth century BC.

---

25   Despite the lack of extant writings by Zou Yan, scholars have often attributed this theory to him.

26   Wang, *Yinyang*, 38.

The *Sayings of Zhou*, for example, speaks of a *qi* of heaven and earth that "does not lose its order". Indeed,

> if it goes beyond the order, the people are in confusion. *Yang* bends over and cannot go out; *yin* rushes and cannot distil away, so there is an earthquake.[27]

Clearly, an order or disorder in the cosmic *qi* was taken here as no less than an ordering or disordering in the cosmic *yin* and *yang*. The association of the two concepts was likewise assumed in the *Zuozhuan*. Here, Heaven is spoken of as having six *qi*,

> which go down and produce the five flavours, develop into the five colours, are verified in the five notes but when overflowing produce the six diseases. The six *qi* are *yin*, *yang*, wind, rain, darkness and brightness. They separate into the four seasons and fall into sequence as the five nodes. If overstepped then they cause disasters.[28]

天有六气，降生五味，发为五色，征为五声，
淫生六疾。六气曰阴、阳、风、雨、晦、明也。
分为四时，序为五节，过则为灾。

Qi was also used regularly to denote and relate different biological, ethical and cosmological ideas. Mengzi, for example, spoke of the will "as the general of the *qi* and the *qi* as the fullness of the body" (夫志、气之帅也；气、体之充也).[29] Later, he even ascribed moral connotations to *qi* by regarding his *surging qi* (*haoran zhiqi*, 浩然之气) as accompanied by justice and the *Dao* (其为气也，配义与

27   *Sayings of the States* 1, *Sayings of Zhou* 1. Quoted from Dainian Zhang and Edmund Ryden, *Key Concepts in Chinese Philosophy* (Beijing: Foreign Languages Press, 2002), 46.
28   *Zuozhuan* 10, *Zhao* 1. Quoted from Zhang and Ryden, 47.
29   *Mencius* 2, *Gongsun Chou A*.

道) and engendered by the accumulation of justice (是集义所生者).[30] Zhuangzi likewise perceived *qi* as that which subsists in the body but is to be distinguished from one's heart or mind. Elsewhere, he added that this internal *qi* may be differentiated from the "one *qi* of heaven and earth". Nonetheless, the two are intimately related since the change in *qi* creates a form and the change of form, in turn, gives life.[31] As he explained,

> [T]he coming to life of human beings is but the gathering of *qi*. It gathers and so they come to life; it scatters and so they die. … Thus the myriad things are One. Thus it is said, "There is but one *qi* running through heaven and earth.[32]

人之生，气之聚也。聚则为生，散则为死。… 故万物一也。通天下一气耳。

Han Confucian Philosophy and Medicine

After centuries of chaos, China was finally unified by the Qins in 221 BC. The dynasty was short-lived, however, and was soon succeeded by the Hans in 202 BC. In spite of this, the Qins would leave behind two legacies that would prove influential for the subsequent development of Han medicine.

From Qin Legalism to Han Confucianism

When the Qins united the country, it adopted Legalism as its political philosophy. In accordance with its principles, Shi Huangdi governed the country with an iron hand and meted out severe laws and punishments to the populace. Understandably, Legalism became immensely unpopular and was repudiated soon after the Hans took

---

30   Ibid.
31   *Zhuangzi* 4.26–28, 6.68, 18.17–18.
32   Ibid., 22.10–13.

over. In its place, Confucianism was favoured and adopted as the new imperial ideology. Han Confucianism, however, differed from its Zhou predecessors in that the Han scholars were not contented merely with implementing Confucius' political and moral vision in the new dynasty. Rather, they were also interested in forging a philosophy or, indeed, a cosmology that would explain the inter-relations between all reality, that is, the Chinese triad of Heaven, Earth and Humankind (*tiandiren*, 天地人). This concern is well expressed by Lu Jia (陆贾, d. 170 BC):

> Heaven gives birth to a myriad of things; the Earth nurtures them; the sages complete them. When our deeds and virtues accord with the Heaven and Earth, the practice of the Way (*Dao*) emerges.[33]

> 天生万物，以地养之，圣人成之。功德参合，而道术生焉。

To express this new cosmology, the Han Confucians integrated the Daoist, Confucian and other pre-Qin conceptions of *yinyang*, *wuxing* and *qi*. In so doing, they developed a dynamic epistemic paradigm that enabled them to describe how the myriad of things were generated from the interaction of *yinyang* and how this, in turn, correlated all entities in the cosmos—heaven, earth and humanity—and rendered them interdependent with one another.[34] As Dong Zhongshu (179–104 BC) explained in his *Luxuriant Gems of the Spring and Autumn Annals* (*Chunqiu Fanlu*, 春秋繁露),

> the *qi* of heaven and earth unites and becomes one, separates into *yinyang*, divides into the four seasons, spreads out into

---

33   Lu Jia, *New Discourses* (*Xinyu*, 新语), 1.
34   William Theodore De Bary, Irene Bloom, and Wing-tsit Chan, *Sources of Chinese Tradition*, vol. 1 (NY: Columbia University Press, 1999), 283–84; Mark Csikszentmihalyi, *Readings in Han Chinese thought* (Indianapolis, IN: Hackett, 2006), xvi–xviii.

the *wuxing*.[35]

天地之气，合而为一，分为阴阳，判为四时，
列为五行。

Like their Greek counterparts, the Han Confucians' doctrine of the correlated triad allowed them to demythologise and re-envisage the Chinese cosmos as "a constant flux of transformation, always regenerating itself as its constituents spontaneously change".[36] The two cultures, however, differed in a fundamental way. Unlike Greek philosophy, Han Confucianism developed in a context where the Han rulers offered their scholars court protection in return for their support and allegiance. Out of this mutuality emerged a new social order, where "hierarchical relationships that apply all the way from emperors and their ministers, to fathers and sons" were understood as reciprocal, interdependent and analogous to one another.[37] The significance of this bilateral correlation logic cannot be understated. After finding its way into every aspect of Chinese sciences and cosmology, it became, until recently, the primary worldview by which the Chinese understood their world. Namely, as a grand synthesis where all things subsist in *yinyang* relationships of "mutual interdependence and reciprocity" and that none can exist "in isolation from the other".[38]

The Qin-Han Political Model
When Shi Huangdi (260–210 BC) unified China, he consolidated his

---

35   *Luxuriant Gems of the Spring and Autumn Annals* 58, *The Mutual Generation of the Five Agents*. (春秋繁露 58: 五行相生). Quoted from Zhang and Ryden, *Key Concepts in Chinese Philosophy*, 100.

36   G. E. R. Lloyd and Nathan Sivin, *The Way and the Word: Science and Medicine in Early China and Greece* (New Haven, CN; London: Yale University Press, 2002), 198.

37   G. E. R. Lloyd, *Adversaries and Authorities: Investigations into Ancient Greek and Chinese Science* (Cambridge: Cambridge University Press, 1996), 125.

38   Ibid., 121.

power by centralising the government in the capital. This led to the relocation of some 120,000 aristocratic families to Xianyang. Prior to this, Zhou settlements and cities were largely small, dispersed, and self-sufficient. When the Qins moved all the nobility to the capital, they inadvertently created a densely populated city that required a reliable and efficient supply of food and supplies from all over the country. By necessity, this demanded the creation of a whole network of depots, palaces, road, canals, granaries, and agricultural production centres to support the capital's burgeoning needs. When the Hans took over, the same political-economic model was maintained and soon taken for granted by subsequent dynasties. As Unschuld points out, this "newly structured social and economic environment" was an experience that the Chinese never had previously.[39]

> It was an experience of being an organism consisting of several units, where each unit contributed to the well-being of the whole. All units were connected by a network of roads. Only if the traffic on these roads ran smoothly, if a person could travel without hindrance and transport goods from one place to another, was this state organism in order.[40]

The corollary is that any failure or "blockage" in the system would reduce the supplies to, or even become catastrophic for, the cities supported by the logistics network. Similarly, repairs or improvements to any node in the network would benefit not only its vicinity, but also all the cities in the system.

As we shall see, the above logistics system would provide, for the Han physicians, a powerful mental model by which to imagine human physiology. Briefly, the human body would be conceived as no less than a system of production centres, storage facilities and

---

39   Unschuld, *Medicine in China*, 79–80.
40   Paul U. Unschuld, *What Is Medicine: Western and Eastern Approaches to Healing* (Berkeley, CA: University of California Press, 2009), 51.

transport networks operating in unison to provide for the body's needs. Any failure or imbalance in any of the nodes or connecting pathways would likewise result in a deterioration of, or sicknesses in, the body. As for the new *yinyang* paradigm, it would become, for the Hans, the philosophical language by which they can articulate the systemic relationships between these depots, palaces and other nodes in the human physiology. Just as an imbalance in the *yinyang* of socio-political relationships can wreak havoc in the kingdom, so also can an imbalance in the physiological relationships body bring illnesses to the human being.

Han Medical Theories and the Doctrine of Systematic Correspondence

Having addressed the philosophical and epistemic foundations of Han medicine, we turn now to the classical medical theories that evolved during the Han period. For the most part, our discussions will focus on the *Huangdi Neijing Suwen* or the *Yellow Emperor's Inner Canon* (hereafter, *Suwen*).[41] The *Suwen* is commonly regarded as the most important classic in the Chinese medical canon, whose medical theories still dominate Chinese medical thinking today. Whenever relevant, references will also be made to other Han medical texts, such as the *Mawangdui* writings, and the *Classic of Difficult Issues* (*Nanjing*, 难经, first century AD). We shall also briefly examine a late Han medical text that would become influential from the Song Dynasty

---

41   The *Huangdi Neijing* consists of two texts: the *Suwen* (素问) and *Lingshu* (灵枢). Since most of the key medical theories are found in the *Suwen*, it would be the focus of our discussion. The *Suwen* is most likely a compilation of health and medical care ideas from the Zhou to Han period. While it is evidently a Han composition, its history of transmission is unclear. The earliest known edition is based on the *Neijing* commentaries written by Quan Yuanqi (全元起, sixth century AD) and Wang Bing (王冰, ninth century AD). The *textus receptus* on which all current texts are based is the *Huangdi Neijing Suwen* published by the Song imperial authorities in the 11th century. Paul U. Hermann Tessenow and Zheng Jinsheng Unschuld, *Huang Di Nei Jing Su Wen: An Annotated Translation of Huang Di's Inner Classic—Basic Questions*, 2 (Berkeley: University of California Press, 2011), 11.

onwards: Zhang Zhongjing's (张仲景) *Treatise on Cold Damage and Miscellaneous Disorders* (*Shanghan zabinglun*, 伤寒杂病论).

Philosophy of Psychosomatic Well-Being

The Han understanding of psychosomatic well-being was best expressed in *Suwen's* opening dialogue between the Yellow Emperor, Huangdi (黄帝), and Qibo (岐伯). Here, we have the emperor asking his advisor why the ancients enjoyed longevity and lived beyond a century old, while the people nowadays weaken and wane before they even reach the age of 50. This then set the stage for Qibo to articulate *Neijing's* philosophy of health and well-being:

> The people of high antiquity, those who knew the Way (*Dao*), they modelled [their behaviour] on *yin* and *yang* and they complied with the arts and the calculations. [Their] eating and drinking was moderate. [Their] rising and resting had regularity. They did not tax [themselves] with meaningless work. Hence, they were able to keep physical appearance and spirit together, and to exhaust the years [allotted by] heaven. Their life span exceeded one hundred years before they departed.

> The fact that people of today are different is because they take wine as an [ordinary] beverage, and they adopt absurd [behaviour] as regular [behaviour]. They are drunk when they enter the [women's] chambers. Through their lust they exhaust their essence, through their wastefulness they dissipate their true [*qi*]. They do not know how to maintain fullness and they engage their spirit when it is not the right time. They make every effort to please their hearts, [but] they oppose the [true] happiness of life. Rising and resting miss their terms. Hence, it is [only] one half of a hundred

[years] and they weaken.[42]

上古之人，其知道者，法于阴阳，和于术数，食
饮有节，起居有常，不妄作劳，故能形与神俱，
而尽终其天年，度百岁乃去。今时之人不然也，
以酒为浆，以妄为常，醉以入房，以欲竭其精，
以耗散其真，不知持满，不时御神，务快其心，
逆于生乐，起居无节，故半百而衰也。

For Qibo, there were two rubrics for medical wisdom. The first involved the knowledge of the *Dao* or, in this case, human physiology, and how it operated by the principles of *yinyang*. This included an understanding how human well-being is related intricately to the *Dao* and *yinyang* of the world. The second pertained to the ethical lifestyle that one must abide by in order to enjoy psychosomatic well-being. This entailed a life of moderation, where one shows restraint in one's desires and consumption, and lived in tandem with one's biological cycle and natural environment, such as changes to the seasons or weather patterns. If one should do otherwise, one would find oneself exhausting one's *qi* or life prematurely, and not attaining the longevity one could have enjoyed.

While this idea of living in harmony with the Dao was clearly influenced by philosophical Daoism, Confucian ideals also loomed large behind Han medical thinking.[43] This could be seen, first of all, in how the *Neijing* appropriated Xunzi's theory of government.[44] Just as "the true ruler begins to put [his state] in order while [a condition of] order [still prevails]" and "does not wait [until] insurrections [have already erupted]", so also

---

42   *Neijing* 1 (Translated from Unschuld, 30–33).

43   By philosophical Daoism, we mean the teachings of *Laozhuang*, that is, Laozi's *Daodejing* and *Zhuangzi*. While the *Laozhuang* philosophy would be adopted by religious Daoism during the late Han period, it remains distinguishable from their religious successors. More would be said about these differences later.

44   Unschuld, *Medicine in China*, 63.

the sages do not treat those who have already fallen ill, but rather those who are not yet ill. They do not put [their state] in order only when revolt [is underway], but before an insurrection occurs.[45]

是故圣人不治已病，治未病，不治已乱，治未乱，此之谓也。夫病已成而后药之，乱已成而后治之，譬犹渴而穿井，斗而铸锥，不亦晚乎。

This idea of treating an illness before it develops has come down to contemporary Chinese medical discourse as the three-fold categorisation of physicians: the Upper, Middle and Lower Physicians (*shangyi, zhongyi* and *xiayi*, 上医、中医、下医).[46] Of the three, the most inferior physicians are the *xiayi* since they treat diseases (下医治病). Superior to them are the *zhongyi* who are capable of treating the human being (中医治人). That is to say, they are able to tune or adjust (*tiao*, 调) a patient's physical health so as to strengthen it and to prevent diseases from becoming full blown.[47] The best physicians, however, remain the *shangyi* who have the ability even to govern the state for the well-being of the people.

Han Political System as Model for Chinese Physiology
The second dominant Confucian ideal has already been mentioned, that is, the imposition of the Han political-economic hierarchy upon the human body. According to the *Suwen*, there are 11 organs (or organ systems) in the human body, which are divided into the two

---

45 *Suwen* has bequeathed to Chinese medicine an emphasis on disease prevention. That is, to treat and improve a person's health so that he would not be afflicted by graver diseases. Currently, it is not uncommon to see Preventive Medical clinics (治未病诊所) in China that offers such treatment. *Suwen* 2 《黄帝内经问。四气调神大论》

46 The Chinese characters, *zhongyi*, are the same as those which are now used to denote "Chinese medicine".

47 For a description of the clinical process of *tiao*, see Yanhua Zhang, *Transforming Emotions with Chinese Medicine: An Ethnographic Account from Contemporary China* (Albany: State University of New York Press, 2007), 105–57.

categories of five *zang* (五藏) and six *fu* (六腑).[48] The former are the heart, lungs, liver, spleen, and kidneys while the latter are the small intestine, large intestine, gall bladder, stomach, bladder and triple burner (*sanjiao*, 三焦).[49] More will be said about how these organ systems operate in chapter 9. What is important to note, at this point, is that the terms *zang* and *fu* referred originally to the "storage facilities" or "storage houses" in the Han distribution systems. Presumably, the two types of organs mimicked the Han politico-economic model by "fulfill[ing] functions in the human body that were considered to parallel those functions associated with the *zang* and *fu* in the national economy".[50] Furthermore, just as the Han storage facilities were linked and supplied by transportation channels, so also were the *zangfu* of the body connected to one another by 12 meridians or *jingluo* (经络).[51] To the Chinese mind, the health of the nation's distribution system was closely bound to an efficient or ceaseless flow of goods and supplies through the system. This idea was, more or less, transposed to medical thinking, where the ceaseless and efficient flow of *qi* and blood (*qixue*, 气血) through the body's *zangfu* and *jingluo* was also regarded as imperative for one's psychosomatic well-being.[52] The corollary, of course, was that whenever there was

---

48   The earlier Mawangdui texts, *Zubi Shiyimai Jiujing* (足臂十一脉灸经) and *Yinyang Shiyimai Jiujing* (阴阳十一脉灸经) speaks of 11 vessels, some categorised as *yang* while others as *yin*. These ideas still differ significantly from the later ideas of *zangfu* in the *Neijing*. Unschuld, *Medicine in China*, 74.

49   *Suwen* 23.

50   Elsewhere, *Suwen* 8 applies the government hierarchy to the *zangfu* organs and assigns political roles to each organ. For example, the heart is the ruler while the lung the chancellor. In so doing, this lends greater credence to the application of the socio-economic model upon the *zangfu*. Paul U. Unschuld, *Huang Di Nei Jing Su Wen: Nature, Knowledge, Imagery in an Ancient Chinese Medical Text* (Berkeley, CA; London: University of California Press, 2003), 129–30.

51   Unschuld, *Medicine in China*, 81.

52   The dominance of this mental model can be seen in the *Lüshi Chunqiu* (吕氏春秋, third century BC), which asserts: "Flowing water and the pivot of a door do not rot because of their constant movement. The relationship between the form and *qi* is the same. If the form does not move, the essence (*jing*, 精) does not flow; if the essence does not flow, the *qi* will stagnate." Ibid., 82.

an impediment to the flow of *qixue*, illnesses would occur. This idea, that a change to a *zangfu* or a channel will either benefit or impair other *zangfu* or channels in the Chinese physiological system, is now known generally as the doctrine of systematic correspondence.[53]

Han Aetiologies

We turn now to the aetiological ideas common in Han secular medicine. According to the *Suwen*, diseases were mostly caused by attacks from without by the wind (a wind aetiology), and sometimes by an imbalance within, that is, in one's *qi*.[54]

> The wind is the origin of one hundred diseases (故风者，百病之始也).[55]

> I know that the hundred diseases are generated by the *qi* (百病生于气也).[56]

As the *Suwen* saw it, wind can enter the body through its skin pores and affect the flow of *qixue* in the meridians. Once the wind settled in the body, it affected its proper *qi* and, in so doing, harmed the *qi* in one or more of the *zangfu*. The condition of the *zangfu* thus deteriorated and illnesses occurred.[57] Besides this, *Suwen* 66–74 also recognised other natural environmental agents, particularly, "rain, water, frost, hail, snow, cold, coolness, summer heat, wind, dryness, dampness and dew… with the presence of specific *qi* and with well-defined states of illness".[58] As mentioned earlier, an immoral lifestyle,

---

53   The name was coined by Paul Unschuld in his *Medicine in China*.

54   As explained shortly, it is often wind attacks that lead to an imbalance in the internal *qi*. The former can therefore be taken as a cause for the latter. We note further that this concept is a marked difference from earlier Han medical etiologies, whereby bugs, either natural or demonic, are seen as the dominant causes of diseases. Unschuld, *Huang Di Nei Jing Su Wen*, 181.

55   *Suwen* 3.18.4.

56   *Suwen* 39.221.7.

57   Unschuld, *Huang Di Nei Jing Su Wen*, 187–88.

58   Ibid., 194.

such as immoderate or improper drinking, eating and sexual practices can also exhaust one's *qi*. As to how an impediment to one's *qi* can cause illnesses, it is well-illustrated in *Suwen* 47. Here, we encounter the case of a pregnant woman who suddenly became dumb. The reason given was that the uterus was tied to a network meridian joined to the kidneys. The kidneys, in turn, had another meridian (*shaoyinzhimai*, 少阴之脉) that led to the base of the tongue. Presumably, the growing body of the foetus had pressed against the uterus' meridian and, in so doing, blocked the exchange between the kidney and the mouth. In this case, no treatment was possible or necessary. The woman recovered once she delivered her baby.[59]

Diagnostics

We turn now to Han diagnostic approaches. Three were commonly discussed in the *Suwen*: inspection (*wang*, 望), inquiry (*wen*, 问) and pulse or meridian diagnosis (*qiemai*, 切脉).[60] During an inspection, a physician would observe a patient closely by paying attention to the changes in his facial colours. This was because, according to the *wuxing* logic, different colours denoted different illnesses. A yellow and red complexion, for example, signalled the presence of heat, while a green-blue colour and black represented pain.[61] Furthermore, these changes in colour also indicated a corresponding deterioration in the *zangfu*. Accordingly, the left cheek becoming red first suggested "heat disease in the liver", while the forehead becoming red first suggested "heat disease in the heart".[62] Besides facial colours, the physician would also be on the lookout for other pathological signs such as "sweating, coughing, shortage of breath, emotional outbursts, depressed speech, sadness, loss of appetite, severe exhaustion, a

---

59   For a further discussion of the case, see Unschuld, 239.

60   The word, *mai* (脉) have been translated in different ways. Paul Unschuld prefers the word, "vessel". Others have named it "tract" or "meridian". I have opted for the "meridian" since it is commonly used by TCM physicians.

61   *Suwen* 39.221.2.

62   Ibid., 39.129.1.

bloated face or abdomen, inability to stand upright, [and] panting".[63]

With regards to inquiry, a physician might enquire about non-observable physiological signs, such as eating patterns, colour of urine and so on. The inquiry can also be directed to the patient's social history since his social status and aspirations might have an adverse effect on his health. Among the three approaches, the *Suwen* devoted the most attention to pulse or meridian diagnosis. The aim here was to discern the palpitations of different meridians and, in this way, assess the conditions of the associated *zangfu*.[64]

Therapeutics

These three diagnostic approaches, when taken together, allowed the physician to arrive at a prognosis of the disease, whether it was mild, severe or terminal. For treatable diseases, chisel stones, needles and moxa (or moxibustion) were commonly prescribed. Blood-letting and cauterisation are also employed occasionally.[65] With regards to drug therapies, the *Suwen* mentioned the use of hot liquids and medicinal wines. Very few drugs, however, were actually identified by name.[66] That this was the case was surprising since the Mawangdui manuscripts demonstrated quite clearly that the Hans, by then, had accumulated a vast body of drug knowledge.[67] Equally intriguing was the fact that the later Han text and the first Chinese *materia medica*, the *Divine Husbandman* or *Shennong Bencaojing* (神农本草经, first century AD), contained a total of 365 drug prescriptions but made no mention of *yinyang* or *wuxing* theories or the meridians taught in the *Suwen*. Returning to the *Suwen*, its "seven comprehensive discourses" in Chapters 66 through 74 did show some attempts to apply

---

63   Unschuld, *Huang Di Nei Jing Su Wen*, 251.

64   The intricacies of pulse diagnosis will be explained further in Chapter 9.

65   *Suwen* 14.87.2, 24.156.1.

66   Ibid., 14.86.10.

67   In fact, a total of 283 prescriptions were documented in this period. Of the 224 drugs mentioned, "106 can be identified as of herbal, 65 as of animal, 9 as of human, and 15 as of mineral origin". Unschuld, *Huang Di Nei Jing Su Wen*, 286.

pharmacotherapy in the doctrines of systematic correspondence. Nonetheless, these teachings did not seem to have much influence until the Song dynasty. Taken together, the above evidence suggests that, between the Han to pre-Song era, a "pharmacology of systematic correspondence of individual substances" had yet to be fully conceptualised. This would happen eventually, but not before the Song rulers took a personal interest in and developed Chinese medicine from the 11th century onwards.[68]

Like the Mawangdui medical texts, the *Suwen* also commended dietetics as a form of medical therapy. The former, along with the Zhangjiashan (张家山, 196–186 BC) manuscripts, also provided extensive teachings on the philosophy and techniques of nurturing life (*yangsheng*, 养生). Practised by the aristocratic elite during the Western Han period, these techniques included a grain-abstinence diet (*bigu*, 辟谷), breathing techniques, sexual cultivation practices and therapeutic calisthenic exercises (*Daoyin*, 导引).[69] The latter, in particular, were the earliest forms of the *Qigong* exercises that are now popular worldwide.[70]

Before we conclude our discussion of the *Suwen* and the doctrine of systematic correspondence, we should note that the treatise was not the last word on the Hans' understanding of this doctrine and other related medical theories. Rather, the mature formulation of the two was to be found in a later treatise called the *Nanjing* (first century AD). Here, the teaching was not only assumed but developed quite extensively. Meridian diagnosis, for example, was clarified as an examination of the wrist. The *zangfu* were further divided into the *yin* and *yang* organs. In a similar vein, different parts of the body were also categorised into *yin* and *yang*—the left side and lower body being

---

68   Ibid., 287–88.

69   Vivienne Lo, "The Influence of Nurturing Life Culture on the Development of Western Han Acumoxa Therapy", in *Innovation in Chinese medicine*, ed. Elizabeth Hsu (Cambridge; NY: Cambridge University Press, 2001), 21–22.

70   Livia Kohn, *Chinese Healing Exercises: The Tradition of Daoyin* (Honolulu, TH: University of Hawaii Press, 2008), 36.

yin, while the right side and upper body were *yang*. In the area of diagnostics, the *wuxing* paradigm was employed to determine how a wind attack could deeply infiltrate a body and affect its different *zangfu* organs. As Unschuld pointed out, the *Nanjing* would overshadow the *Nejing* as the dominant medial treatise in the first millennium. It was only from the Song era onwards that medical commentators began to think otherwise and regarded the earlier *Neijing Suwen* as the more important text for Chinese medicine. It is this latter view that has held sway till this day. [71]

Cold Damage Disorders

The late Han period (late second to early third century AD) saw the empire descending into political chaos, with peasants revolting in the Yellow Turban Rebellion (*Huangjin Qiyi*, 黄巾起义, 184–205 AD) and senior officials conspiring against the emperor and one another. Not surprisingly, the populace suffered the most during this period. Besides the hardships of war, the Hans also found themselves plagued by a series of earthquakes, floods and epidemics. It was during this turbulent period that the famous Han physician, Zhang Zhongjing (张仲景, 150–220 AD) or Zhang Ji (张机), was born. Zhang began his career as the Chamberlain for Palace Revenues in Changsha (长沙), the southern end of the empire, before becoming a physician. Like most of the southern areas, Changsha was often afflicted by plagues which were often unknown to and neglected by the northern-oriented mainstream medicine. As a result, Zhang saw several members of his family fall victim to infectious diseases. Finding no remedies to these plagues, he began to study the ancient medical texts for himself and collected contemporary medicinal formulas that proved effective against these plagues, or Cold Damage Disorders. [72]

---

71   Unschuld, *Medicine in China*, 85–89.

72   Asaf Moshe Goldschmidt, *The Evolution of Chinese Medicine: Song Dynasty, 960–1200* (London; New York: Routledge, 2009), 293–95.

From these efforts emerged the fruit of his labours: his *Treatise on Cold Damage and Miscellaneous Disorders* (*Shanghan Zabinglun*, 伤寒杂病论) (hereafter, *Cold Damage Treatise* or *Shanghan Lun*).[73] The extant Treatise is divided into two sections:

> [A] Cold Damage part that concentrated on the treatment of acute febrile disorders by means of formulas, and a Miscellaneous Disorders part that discussed disorders of the viscera and the circulation tracts.[74]

The text, however, neither listed the "symptoms needed to deduce treatment, as was common in empirical symptom-specific practices", nor determined the manifestation types, which was the diagnostic approach of the *Neijing Suwen*. Rather, it mapped out the developmental stages of Cold Damage Disorders (*Shanghan*, 伤寒) into the Three-*Yin* and Three-*Yang* categories, known otherwise as the "Six Warps" (*liujing bianzheng*, 六经辨证). By organising the "signs and symptoms of diseases" into "syndrome-like groups according to the six-fold categorisation", the treatise thus enabled the physician to discern the stage of the disease, for example, whether it was "mature *Yang*" or "mature *Yin*", and to administer the appropriate treatments.[75]

Unfortunately, Zhang's treatise was lost soon after his death. Judging from the paucity of references to the text, it would appear that it was mostly unknown, let alone referred to or influencing the development of Chinese medicine from the post-Han to the pre-Song periods. Zhang's teachings did become prominent during the Song dynasty, when three versions of his *Shanghan Lun* were published by the imperial authorities, based on fragments or incomplete copies

---

73   Cold Damage, as Goldschmidt explains, "is defined by a vague group of symptoms that may correspond to anything from the common cold to typhoid". Ibid., 54.

74   It is commonly assumed that the original treatise consisted of six parts: "pulse diagnosis, Cold Damage Disorders, miscellaneous disorders, women's disorders, children's disorders, and dietary prohibitions". Ibid., 295.

75   Ibid., 295–96.

that survived under private ownership.[76] It is these efforts that would redefine Zhang as the preeminent physician of the Chinese medical tradition. As to the reasons for the Song authorities' interest, this will be taken up in Chapter 7, when we discuss the Song medical reforms.

Medical Developments from Post-Han to Tang Dynasty

When the late Han dynasty disintegrated into political anarchy, several peasant revolts broke out. These rebels were often religious groups that not only claimed direct contact with the divine (such as the deified Laozi or Huangdi), but also promised a new age of Great Peace (*Taiping*, 太平) for the people. It is from these religious movements that the first religious Daoist sects emerged: the Way of the Celestial Masters (天师道, 180s) and the Way of the Great Peace (太平道, c. 184), the latter of which was responsible for the Yellow Turban rebellion. In the centuries that followed, new religious Daoist groups would be formed, such as the Highest Clarity (*Shangqing*, 上清, c. 360s), Lingbao (灵宝, 390s) and Louguan (楼观, late fifth century AD) sects.[77]

Generally, these Daoist sects regarded Laozi and Zhuangzi (hereafter, Laozhuang) as their founding fathers. Indeed, the two were even esteemed as deities who could offer supernatural aid to these Daoists. These new sects, however, differed from Laozhuang in one important way. Judging from the *Daodejing* and *Zhuangzi*, it is clear that the two pioneers of philosophical Daoism regarded death as a natural part of life which one should accept and not seek to overcome. In his *Great and Venerable Teacher* (大宗师), Zhuangzi speaks of a Master Yu (*Ziyu*, 子輿), who was overcome by illness so much that his back became crooked and hunched. When asked

---

76   The three versions are the basis for all contemporary publications of the *Shanghan Lun*. Contemporary TCM scholars generally regard the *Baiyunge Zangben* (白云阁藏本) as the most reliable of the three. Goldschmidt, *The Evolution of Chinese Medicine*, 298–306; 张仲景 et al., 白云阁藏本伤寒杂病论 (河南: 中原农民出版社, 2013).

77   Livia Kohn, *Introducing Daoism* (London; New York: Routledge, 2009), 86–92.

whether he resented these changes, he replied:

> Why no, what would I resent?... I received life because the time had come; I will lose it because the order of things passes on. Be content with this time and dwell in this order and then neither sorrow nor joy can touch you. In ancient times, this was called the 'freeing of the bound'. There are those who cannot free themselves, because they are bound by things. But nothing can ever win against Heaven—that's the way it's always been. What would I have to resent?[78]

> 亡，予何恶！…且夫得者时也，失者顺也，安时而处顺，哀乐不能入也。此古之所谓县解也，而不能自解者，物有结之。且夫物不胜天久矣，吾又何恶焉？

Ironically, Zhuangzi's religious successors thought otherwise by regarding the pursuit of longevity and immortality (*chengxian*, 成仙) as their primary goals instead. Given their new health concerns, it was hardly surprising that the religious Daoists quickly developed a strong interest in secular medicine and became prominent in its subsequent development. The Daoist, Tao Hongjing (陶弘景, AD 456–536), for example, was well known not only for compiling the Scriptures of the Highest Clarity sect, but also the first Chinese *materia medica*, the *Divine Husbandman* (*Shennong Bencaojing*, 神农本草经), which was apparently lost after the Han period.[79] The longevity or *yangsheng* techniques long practised by the Han elite, such as eating *qi*, grain-abstinence, sexual cultivation, breathing exercises and therapeutic gymnastics, were also taken on board by the religious Daoists.[80] To

---

78   Zhuangzi, *The Complete Works of Zhuangzi*, trans. Burton Watson (New York: Columbia University Press, 2013), 48–49.

79   Unschuld, *Medicine in China*, 114

80   Ute Engelhardt, "Longevity Techniques and Chinese Medicine", in *Daoism Handbook*, ed. Livia Kohn (Leiden: Brill, 2000), 74–103.

these traditions, they added other forms of healing therapies such as visualisation meditation techniques, drinking talisman water, the summoning of divine help, and the compounding of elixirs (*waidan*, 外丹). It should be noted that not all medieval Daoists were enthusiastic about the adoption of secular medicine. At least in the case of the Celestial Masters, the use of drug and acupuncture therapies was expressly prohibited.[81] In light of these developments, it should be clear then that while religious Daoism employed secular Chinese medicine extensively, it is but one of its users. It is, therefore, incorrect to regard secular Chinese medical theory as Daoist, or to deem that it was influenced by religious Daoism.

Buddhism first entered China during the Han dynasty (c. 60s) and became popular over the next few centuries, gaining much support from both the gentry and even the imperial household.[82] Inadvertently, Indian traditions of healing were introduced to China with the Buddhist faith. Indian cataract surgery, for example, was first mentioned around the seventh to ninth century. Apparently, the great Tang physician, Sun Simiao, also incorporated some aspects of Buddhist healing into his writings.[83] Notwithstanding this, Indian medicine, on the whole, neither took root nor played an influential role in secular Chinese medicine.

Conclusion

Like most ancient cultures, the Chinese medical tradition, at its inception, was a mixture of both religious and secular healing

---

81   Engelhardt, 76; Kohn, *Introducing Daoism*, 140.

82   Such imperial patronage was not always consistent. When the monks of Shaolin assisted Emperor Li Shimin (600–649) in the military campaigns that led to the founding of the Tang empire, they were favoured in the courts. Sentiments soon turned against Buddhism in the later Tang period when the religion was perceived as superstitious and foreign to the nation. Meir Shahar, *The Shaolin Monastery: History, Religion and the Chinese Martial Arts* (Honolulu: University of Hawaii Press, 2008), 22.

83   Unschuld, *Medicine in China*, 150–51.

practices. With the emergence and integration of *yinyang*, *qi* and *wuxing* theories during the late Zhou to Han periods, Chinese physicians began to employ these theories to naturalise or demythologise Chinese medicine, and to develop a doctrine of systematic correspondence. While the doctrine managed to integrate Chinese physiology and medical diagnosis with acupuncture and moxibustion therapies, its relation to Chinese pharmacology remained unresolved at this stage. The Han period also saw the conceptualisation of Cold Damage Disorders by Zhang Zhongjing. Although Zhang's writings did not become influential in the centuries that followed, they would be regarded highly from the Song Medical Renaissance onwards, as we shall see. The same Renaissance would also play the important role of integrating the doctrine of systematic correspondence with pharmacology.

The post-Han period saw the rise of religious Daoism, whose reception of secular Chinese medicine was mixed. Although some Daoists became important physicians and innovators of the medical tradition, others repudiated it. With regards to Indian medicine, this entered China through the auspices of Buddhism. While some Indian healing practices were incorporated into Chinese medical practice, they played no important role in the development of secular Chinese medicine.

7

THE HISTORICAL DEVELOPMENT OF CHINESE MEDICINE II:

FROM THE SONG MEDICAL RENAISSANCE TO THE MODERN PERIOD

Introduction

At its zenith, the Tang dynasty (618–907) was the most cosmopolitan nation of its time. Unfortunately, the empire went into decline from the mid-8th century onwards and, finally, crumbled in the early 10th century. Not surprisingly, its education system fell into disrepute, along with the practice of medicine. The next 50 years, also known as the Five Dynasties and Ten Kingdoms period (五代十国), was a period of political upheaval, where dynasties succeeded one another rapidly, and a dozen other states were established in the south. It would not be until AD 960 when Emperor Taizu (960–976) would manage to reunite the country to establish the new Song dynasty (960–1279). In so doing, Taizu also set the stage for a Renaissance of Chinese medicine from the late 10th century onwards.

The Song Medical Renaissance

Among the first things Taizu did was to reconstitute the imperial educational system. Unlike most emperors before him, Taizu and his three successors had a personal interest and were, in fact, proficient in medicine. Taizu himself was conversant with moxibustion while Taizong (976–97) and Zhenzong (997–1022) were both well-versed in drug therapy. As for Renzong (1022–63), he proved not only astute in Chinese pharmacology, but also in acu-moxa therapy.[1] Given their strong interest in medicine, it was no wonder that, when the imperial libraries began to gather literary works to rejuvenate their collections, private medical manuscripts were collected as well. This marked the start of a new Song Medical Renaissance.

To begin, the new cache of manuscripts enabled the imperial libraries to revise ancient medical texts, such as the *Neijing* and *Nanjing*, for publication. In addition, they were able to reconstruct medical texts that were thought to be previously lost, such as the *Shanghan Lun*. Apart from these, new medical texts, particularly drug formularies, were also compiled, like the *Divine Doctor's Formulary for Universal Relief* (*Shenyi Pujiu Fang*, 神医普救方, 986), and the *Imperial Grace Formulary of the Great Peace and Prosperity Reign Period* (*Taiping Shenghuifang*, 太平圣惠方, 982).[2] The significance of these publishing efforts cannot be understated. By making available a wide range of medical texts for public reading, it allowed physicians to have access to, dialogue with, and eventually develop the medical theories and therapies taught in these texts.

In the area of acupuncture, a ground-breaking manual on the subject called the *Illustrated Canon Explaining Acu-moxa Therapy Using the Bronze Figure and its Acu-points* (*Tongren Yuxue Zhenjiu Tujing*, 铜人腧穴针灸图经) was published in 1026, along with

---

1   Asaf Moshe Goldschmidt, *The Evolution of Chinese Medicine: Song Dynasty, 960–1200* (London; New York: Routledge, 2009), 83–86.

2   Ibid., 93–95, 129–31.

a cast-bronze human model illustrating the acupuncture points. Prior to the Song dynasty, it appears that acupuncture was shunned by physicians, due to their concerns about the hazards of incorrect needling. By clarifying the acupuncture points and providing a model for training, the Illustrated Canon did much to re-establish acupuncture as a legitimate form of therapy and to improve the skills of the Song physicians.[3]

During the reign of Renzong (1022–63), the southern part of the empire was struck by a series of epidemics. In the earlier chapter, we learned that Zhang Zhongjing composed his *Shanghan Lun*, or *Cold Damage Disorder*, to address similar plagues which occurred during the late Han dynasty. The current epidemics, quite understandably, revived interest in the *Shanghan Lun*, and led eventually to the publication of three new revisions or reconstructions of the treatise. In due course, several commentaries on the *Shanghan Lun* and cold damage disorders were also written.[4] Together, these efforts did much to establish Zhang as one of the most influential teachers in subsequent Chinese medical history, and the study of cold damage disorders as an important sub-discipline in Chinese medicine.

With the publication of medical texts that were previously lost or limited in circulation, Song physicians now had easier access to and became more familiar with a wide range of classical medical doctrines and drug therapies. In due course, it was also apparent that the medical approaches, terminologies and even conceptions of diseases taught in the different ancient texts, such as the *Suwen* and *Shanghan Lun*, often differed from one another. This catalysed a gradual process whereby succeeding generations of Song physicians began to reconceptualise the relationships between the classical medical theories and drug formulas until Chinese pharmacology was finally integrated with the classical doctrines of systematic correspondence.

---

3   This was certainly the case during the Tang Dynasty. Goldschmidt, 113–20.
4   Ibid., 223–39, 284, 293–95.

These integration efforts began as early as the reign of Taizu when the *Newly Detailed and Definitive Materia Medica of the Kaibao Reign* (*Kaibao Xin Xiangding Bencao*, 开宝新详定本草) was published in 974. At this stage, the revision efforts were modest, focusing mainly on the correction of errors and verification of statements made in the Tang *materia medica*. A change of focus was observed in 1062, when the *Illustrated Materia Medica* (*Bencao Tujing*, 本草图经) of 1062 began to assess the knowledge of the ancients in the light of contemporary experience. For example, its authors concluded that the ancients were unaware that a drug's potency could vary significantly, depending on the climate and topography where it was grown.[5] It was Kou Zongshi's (寇宗奭) publication of his *Dilatations on Materia Medica* (*Bencaoyanyi*, 本草衍义) in 1119, however, that introduced a paradigm shift in Song medicine. For the first time, we saw detailed discussions on how drug therapies and formulas were related to the classical medical theories taught in the ancient canons. For example, "a direct connection between the five sapors of drugs and the climatic environment and its *qi*" was introduced, thereby linking a drug's therapeutic effect with the doctrine of Five Circulatory Phases and the Six Seasonal Influences (*wuyunliuqi*, 五运六气), first mentioned in the *Neijing Suwen* 67. Elsewhere, Kou also employed the classical categorisation of the Eight Rubrics (*bagang bianzhen*, 八纲辨证) and the Four Methods of Examinations (*sizhen*, 四诊) as the means for prescribing drug formulas. Kou's greatest contribution, however, remained his theory of channel tropism (*guijing*, 归经), where he described how different drugs can affect different meridians and *zangfu*. Channel tropism would be popularised in the centuries to come and is now taken for granted by most TCM physicians.[6]

With Kou's treatise, a new trajectory was introduced in Song medicine. Thereafter, writings on Chinese medical theory or drug formularies would always integrate the two fields. For example,

---

5   Ibid., 329–335, 341, 352–54.
6   Ibid., 536–39.

the largest drug formulary of the Northern Song dynasty: *A Sagely Benefaction of the Zhenghe Reign Period* (*Zhenghe shengji zonglu*, 政和圣济总录), frequently interwove discussions on classical medical theories with comments on drug formulas. Xu Shuwei's (许叔微, 1079–1154) *Original Formulary of Classified Manifestation Types for Popular Relief* (*Leizheng Puji Benshifang*, 类证普济本事方, 1144), likewise discussed the 25 major manifestation types (of illnesses) along with the relevant drug formulas that could heal these ailments. In addition to these, he even included several case histories to illustrate his new teachings. By the time we reach the Southern Song (1127–1279) and Jin periods (1115–1234), Zhang Yuansu (张元素, c. 1120–1200) could take for granted that a proper understanding of the *zangfu*'s systematic functions and its relation to the doctrine of systematic correspondence must precede any drug prescription.[7]

Besides the above developments in Chinese medical theory, the Song medical reforms also did much to change the gentry's perception of medical practice. Prior to the Song dynasty, the physician was generally regarded as an artisan, whose skills were passed down from a master to his disciple. Socially, he was also deemed to be of a lower class, equal only to the spirit-mediums and musicians. Not surprisingly, medicine was a vocation disdained and avoided by the gentry and aristocrats. When the Song reforms were introduced, an Imperial Medical Service was set up to build a network of medical schools in the capital, provinces and districts.[8] In so doing, medical training was institutionalised and took a form similar to Confucian learning. Henceforth, physicians, like their Confucian counterparts, could also boast of their own medical canon, such as the *Neijing* and *Shanghan Lun*. Like their Confucian counterparts, they also had to take qualifying examinations and could expect to be promoted

---

7   Ibid., 545, 567–69, 571–72, 586–88.

8   Emperor Huizong was particularly dismayed by the level of incompetency among many physicians in the country and regarded the schools as an important means of resolving this problem. Goldschmidt, 139, 153–60, 164–65, 171.

during the course of their careers. Most importantly, the imperial authorities also actively encouraged scholars who failed to make it for civil service to pursue a medical career instead. This was because they saw the medical vocation as equally vital for the nation's well-being. Thereafter, medicine was taken up more enthusiastically by the elite and the Confucian scholars. A new title called the "Literati Physician" or *ruyi* (儒医) was even created to differentiate these scholar physicians from their less-educated counterparts. In due course, the title became commonly used and continued to distinguish the scholarly class of physicians, right till the late Qing era.[9]

Besides the above, the Song reforms also did much to improve the medical infrastructure of the country. Imperial pharmacies were established to provide simple drugs and prescriptions for the populace. During epidemic seasons, these pharmacies also played an important role in relieving the sick. Besides this, relief hospitals were also set up to care for the sick, while poorhouses were built to accommodate the widowed and the orphaned.[10]

Song-Jin-Yuan to Early Qing Medicine: Diverse Branches from Common Roots

In the year 1127, the Jurchens defeated the Song rulers. The latter soon regrouped in the new southern capital of Lin'an (临安, present-day Hangzhou) and managed to endure for another century and a half as the Southern Song dynasty (南宋, 1127–1279). Despite its early success at overcoming the Jurchens and the Chinese, the Mongolian or Yuan Empire (1271–1368) proved to be short-lived and soon gave way to the Ming dynasty (1368–1644). The latter would be the last Chinese dynasty to reign in ancient China before they were defeated by another foreign tribe, the Manchurians, who ushered in the Qing Dynasty (1644–1912).

---

9   The Tang scholar, Han Yu (韩愈, 768–824), for example, regards medicine as an art that was despised by both the common folk and gentlemen. Ibid., 74, 153–56, 183–85.

10   Ibid., 204–206, 374–400.

During these turbulent centuries, secular medicine, by and large, operated within the medical framework that evolved during the Song reforms.[11] Commentaries on the *Neijing*, *Shanghan Lun* and other ancient texts continued to be written, even as new drug formularies and *materia medica* were published. With regards to the latter, the largest and most well-known remains Li Shizhen's (李时珍, 1518–1593) *Compendium of Materia Medica* (*Bencao Gangmu*, 本草纲目). The tome details the therapeutic attributes of 1,800 drugs, 11,000 prescriptions, and the application of 1,094 herbs in various drug therapies. The 16th century also saw an exponential growth in the number of medical case records or histories (*yian*, 医案). While the earliest case histories were compiled by Chunyu Yi (淳于意, 216–150 BC) during the Han dynasty, the genre remained uncommon and was limited in circulation even until the Yuan dynasty. During the Ming era, the number of case histories published grew significantly, such as the *Shishan Yian* (石山医案, 1519), *Xueji Yian* (薛己医案, 1529), *Wangkentang Yian* (王肯堂医案, 1562), *Sun Wenheng Yian* (孙文恒医案, 1573), and Nie Jiuwu's (聂久吾) *Qixiao Yishu* (奇效医述, 1616). Among these, the most famous was Jiang Guan's (江瓘, 1503–1565) *Case Histories of Famous Physicians* (*Mingyi Leian*, 名医类案, 1549), which not only documented over a hundred Pre-Ming medical case histories, but also included several of the author's.[12]

Despite the dominance of the doctrine of systematic correspondence and its associated therapies, the Jin-Yuan period did see several innovations that would give new emphases to the traditional theories or even take them towards new directions. Such was the case for the four master physicians during the Jin-Yuan era. Known popularly as the Jin-Yuan Four Masters (*Jinyuan Sidajia*, 金元四大家), their

---

11   As Unschuld observes, "until the beginning of the twentieth century, the concepts of systematic correspondence dominated Chinese medical literature and undoubtedly the approaches of educated practitioners and self-healing citizens". Paul U. Unschuld, *Medicine in China: A History of Ideas* (Berkeley, CA; London: University of California Press, 1985), 223; 李经纬 (Li Jingwei), 中医史 (*History of Chinese Medicine*) (Hainan: Hainan, 2007), 289–92.

12   李经纬 (Li Jingwei), *History of Chinese Medicine*, 287–88.

theoretical and therapeutic developments would inspire different currents or schools of thought (*pai*, 派) by the Qing era.[13] The first master was the Jin physician, Liu Yuansu (刘元素, 1120–1200), a contemporary of the earlier mentioned Zhang Yuansu.[14] Liu developed a theory of Warm Pathogen (*huore shuo*, 火热说) that advocated the reduction of the heart's fire and the improvement of the kidney's water (降心火，益肾水) as the means of treating warm pathogen disorders. His teachings eventually provided the foundational framework for the Warm Pathogen Current or School of Thought (*wenbing xuepai*, 温病学派) that would flourish during the Qing era. In contrast, Zhang Congzheng (张从正, 1156–1228) asserted that one should attack the evil or pathogenic *qi* (攻邪气) instead as the primary healing approach. In contemporary TCM, he is better known for his three methods of attacking the pathogenic *qi*. Namely, the three methods of inducing sweating, vomiting or defecation (*fahan yongtu xiexia sanfa*, 发汗、涌吐、泻下三法).

The third master, Li Dongyuan (李东垣, 1180–1251), emphasised the importance of nurturing the stomach-spleen viscera, or more accurately, the digestive system (*piweilun*, 脾胃论). As he saw it, earth (*tu*, 土) was the most important aspect of the body's Five Phases. This was because the stomach-spleen functional system, represented by earth, was responsible for transforming all food into the nutrients needed by the body (土为万物之母, 脾胃乃化生之源, 人以胃气为本). Consequently, if the stomach-spleen system was hurt or damaged, a variety of diseases would occur (内伤脾胃，百病由生).[15] As for Zhu Danxi (朱丹溪, 1281–1358), his

---

13   As Scheid explains, the word, *pai* (派), need not denote a school or faction because "its members do not always share a common theory directing research and practice". We shall be taking Scheid's cue by translating *pai* as "current" for the rest of this chapter. Volker Scheid, *Currents of Tradition in Chinese Medicine, 1626–2006* (Seattle: Eastland Press, 2007), 12.

14   In fact, Zhang came to fame by successfully treating the more senior Liu, when the latter was unable to diagnose and treat his Cold Damage Disorder successfully. 李经纬 (Li Jingwei), *History of Chinese Medicine*, 225.

15   Since 2000, modern medicine has begun to recognise the intimate relationship between

therapeutic philosophy posited that one often has an excess of *yang* and a deficiency in *yin* (阳常有余，阴常不足). For this reason, therapy should focus on nurturing the *yin* while reducing the fire or *yang* (*ziyin jianghuo zhifa*, 滋阴降火之法). This approach marked the beginning of yet another school of thought called the Nurturing Yin Current (*Ziyinpai*, 滋阴派).[16]

Compared to Western medical history, it is evident that Chinese medical historiography tends to give more emphasis to the contributions of famous Chinese physicians and their lineages. While figures such as Galen, Robert Koch and Louis Pasteur may be familiar to biomedical physicians, most will have trouble recalling that Alexander Fleming was the scientist who discovered penicillin or that hip replacements were invented by John Charnley. What is for sure is that they would neither attribute medical schools of thought to these figures (with the exception of Galen) nor esteem them as sages. This, however, is not the case for the Chinese's conception of their medical sages, such as Bianque (扁鹊, d. 310 BC), Huatuo (华佗, c. 140–208), Zhang Zhongjing, or the master physicians mentioned above. For example, it is not uncommon for biomedical physicians working in Chinese societies to receive calligraphies as gifts of gratitude with the words, the *Reincarnation of Huatuo* (*Huatuo Zaishi*, 华佗再世), that esteem the physician as no less than the famous Han physician. This Chinese sentiment could well be due to the Confucian emphasis on revering one's ancestors and teachers, and upholding what they have passed down.[17] It is for this reason that a recent survey of

---

one's digestive system and one's psychosomatic health. It has been established that diseases as diverse as eczema, poor immunity, dementia, cancer and other psychological illnesses can be due to digestive problems to start with. See Giulia Enders, *Gut: The Inside Story of Our Body's Most Under-Rated Organ* (Rearsby, Leicester: WF Howes, 2017).

16   李经纬 (Li Jingwei), *History of Chinese Medicine*, 225–33.

17   A case in point is the Zhang Zhongjing Drug Formulary International Conference (仲景经方国际论坛) held recently in Dengzhou, Henan. The event saw three senior TCM physicians accepted as official disciples of Tang Zuxuan, a specialist in Zhang Zhongjing's medicine. "河南举行仲景传人师承大典", accessed 21 December 2017, https://kknews.cc/culture/jvx6b5l.html.

medical traditions and lineages in the Jiangsu province identified not only several famous physicians in the Wuzhong district (吴中区) but also medical families, the lineage of whom could be traced all the way back to the 13th-century Southern Song Dynasty. These included the earliest Ge family (*geshi shiyi*, 葛氏世医), the Zheng family of gynaecologists (*zhengshi fuke*, 郑氏妇科), the Jin family of paediatricians (*jinshi erke*, 金氏儿科), the Min family (闵氏) famous for bone injuries and re-setting (*gushang*, 骨伤) and the You family (尤氏) renowned for its acu-moxa therapy. Most intriguingly, one can still find a number of descendants from these families (such as the Zheng, Min and You lineages) still practising the family tradition today.[18] Apart from these, Jiangsu was also home to a number of scholar physicians (*ruyi*), the most famous being the *Menghe* current or lineage (孟河学派), whose adherents would prove influential in the modernisation of contemporary Chinese medicine.[19]

Three further developments in Ming-Qing medicine are noteworthy. The first was the popular use of variolation (*rendou jiezhongshu*, 人痘接种术) as a means of inoculating the Chinese from the threat of smallpox (*tianhua*, 天花) from the 16th century onwards.[20] The second was the anatomical discoveries of the Qing physician, Wang Qingren (王清任, 1768–1831). After observing dismembered corpses left to rot during the plagues, and personally examining the bodies of executed criminals, Wang came to the conclusion that the anatomy taught in the ancient and contemporary medical texts was far from accurate. While he did not make much headway in redefining Chinese anatomy, his discoveries anticipated the future evolution of Chinese medicine in the 20th century, which would see Western anatomy incorporated into Chinese medical

---

18 陈仁寿 (Chen Renshou), 江苏中医：历史与流传派传承 (*Jiangsu Chinese Medicine*) (Shanghai: Shanghai Science and Technology Publishing, 2014), 82–83.

19 For a more detailed discussion of the *Menghe* Current, see Scheid, *Currents*.

20 李经纬 (Li Jingwei), *History of Chinese Medicine*, 257.

knowledge.[21] Finally, acupuncture practice would encounter a major setback in 1822 (the second year of *Daoguang*, 道光二年), when the Qing authorities banned the use of acupuncture in the imperial hospitals as a practice unworthy of gentlemen and the aristocratic elite.[22] The reason for this is unclear. It could well have been due to the authorities' concerns that assassins might use acupuncture needles as weapons against the foreign rulers. Notwithstanding this, the evidence for a decline in acupuncture practice in the 18th to 19th centuries is mixed. On the one hand, we have Xu Dachun (徐大椿) lamenting, in his historical survey of Chinese medicine, that acupuncture was a rare art, with few competent in it and young physicians unable to find instructors to train them.[23] On the other, we have several Jiangsu physicians administering it, such as the famous Menghe physicians and the You family of acupuncturists (尤氏针灸).[24] You acupuncture, for example, began in 1880 and continues to be practised in the family till this day.[25]

Encounters with Western Medicine: Further Evolution and Transformation

The advent of the 19th century saw the Qing Empire slide into an irreversible political decline. Internally, it suffered from weaker governance, lower tax income and continued uprisings from different religious and local sects, such as the White Lotus sect (*bailianjiao*, 白莲教), Heaven-Earth society (*tiandihui*, 天地会) and the Taiping sect (*Taiping Tianguo*, 太平天国). Externally, China was also frequently bullied by foreign aggressors. The Chinese defeat at the First Opium

---

21   Unschuld, *Medicine in China*, 212–15.

22   "针灸一法，由来已久，然以针刺火灸，究非奉君之所宜，太医院针灸一科，着永远停止。"李经纬 (Li Jingwei), *History of Chinese Medicine*, 353.

23   Bridie Andrews, *The Making of Modern Chinese Medicine, 1850–1960* (Vancouver: UBC Press, 2014), 197–98.

24   Scheid, *Currents*, 157.

25   In fact, as of 2009, You acupuncture has been recognised as a non-material culture legacy of the Jiangsu province. 陈仁寿 (Chen Renshou), *Jiangsu Chinese Medicine*, 86–88.

War (1836–1839) saw the country ceding the island of Hong Kong to the British. Decades later, a similar story was replayed with Taiwan being handed over to Japan after the Chinese lost the Sino-Japanese War (1894–1895). The sorest defeat, however, was the invasion by the Eight Nation Alliance (*baguo lianjun*, 八国联军), that led to the sacking of the Forbidden City (1900).[26] In response to these national catastrophes, many Chinese began to seriously doubt the legitimacy of the Qing government and their own culture, and started to seek, in different ways, to employ Western science and culture to rejuvenate the country.

The earliest attempt at this was the self-strengthening movement (*ziqiang yundong*, 自强运动). Initiated after the Second Opium War (1860), its supporters sought only economic and military reforms as the means of strengthening the empire. China's defeat at the Sino-Japanese war, however, proved this to be inadequate and encouraged Liang Qichao, Kang Youwei (康有为, 1858–1927) and others to pursue a more radical renewal programme—the Reform Movement (*weixin yundong*, 维新运动). This second movement did not make much headway, unfortunately. Instead, anti-Manchu sentiments soon welled up, giving rise to the revolution of 1911 and the overthrow of Qing rule. Peace did not prevail, however, as China lapsed rapidly into a chaotic Warlord period (1916–1927) that convinced many that the old Chinese culture and society must be abandoned entirely if they were to rebuild a new China. The May 4th (*wusi yundong*, 五四运动, 1919) and New Culture Movements (*xinwenhua yundong*, 新文化运动, 1916–1928) were thus born. Among their proponents, many advocated a "wholesale Westernisation" (*quanpan xihua*, 全盘西化) of China and the replacement of Confucius with Mr Science (*Sai xiansheng*, 赛先生), or as some put it, the "Scientisation of China" (*zhongguo kexuehua*, 中国科学化). Not all were supportive of such radical reforms, however. While recognising

---

26   Harold Miles Tanner, *China: A History Volume 2* (Indianapolis: Hackett, 2010), 60–69, 76–79, 90–92.

the need for reforms, the National Essence Current (*guocuipai*, 国粹派), nevertheless, called for the preservation of the national essence (保存国粹).[27] As we shall see, these different political and cultural pressures will play a pivotal role in determining how Chinese medicine will be transformed in the 20th century.

In Chapter 1, we mentioned that Chinese healing practices in the 19th century were very diverse. According to Qiu Jisheng's (裘吉生) "Medical Customs of Shaoxing" (1915), Chinese healers included spirit-mediums, temple priests, itinerant doctors (*jianghuyi*, 江湖医), toothworm removers (*xiaoyachong*, 消牙蟲), and drug peddlers (*caoyaodan*, 草药担). Besides these, there were also the physicians associated with the government, such as the official doctors (*guanyi*, 官医), military doctors (*junyi*, 军医) and welfare agency doctors (*shantangyi*, 善堂医). Finally, to be distinguished from these were the classical Chinese physicians (*zhongyi*, 中医) who specialised in a variety of ailments, such as pox, eye diseases, throat diseases, paediatrics, surgery or internal medicine.[28] Even among the practitioners of classical medicine, standards varied significantly, with some doctors more well-versed with the classical traditions, while others quite inept in or even misinterpreting them. Unlike the Song era, medical training was rarely conducted in schools or institutions, but more commonly through apprenticeships. This, of course, posed a serious constraint on the proliferation of Chinese medical knowledge since most physicians would prefer to transmit their learning to a few selected disciples rather than to benefit the Chinese medical community at large.[29]

The first Chinese exposure to Western healing came in the form of an apothecary shop opened in 1820 by John Livingstone, a physician of the East India Company, and Robert Morrison (1782–1834), the first Protestant missionary in China, and translator of the first Chinese

27   Scheid, *Currents*, 175–77; Unschuld, *Medicine in China*, 243.
28   Andrews, *Making of Modern Chinese Medicine*, 28–44.
29   Scheid, *Currents*, 191–93.

Bible.[30] At this stage, European medicine was still in transition. Many of the discoveries that would define modern biomedicine, such as germ theory, cell theory, antisepsis, public hygiene, and antibiotics therapy, had yet to be discovered. This was probably why Morrison and Livingstone were still quite happy to purchase drugs from local physicians and even learn native forms of healing. Western medicine proper entered China via the medical missionaries, the first being Peter Parker (1804–1888), who opened a clinic in Canton in 1835. Despite initial doubts whether missionaries should be engaged in medical work, more financial resources were soon poured into this work, so much so that 362 missionary hospitals were in operation by the end of the century.[31]

During the intervening decades, medicine in Europe saw significant progress. Not surprisingly, Western physicians' regard for Chinese medicine also declined correspondingly. Take, for example, the remarks by Benjamin Hobson (1816–1873), an English medical missionary who worked in Macau, Canton and Shanghai:

On Chinese and Western Medicine:

The sciences of today, as for instance the writings on astronomy, mathematics, and geography, are more sophisticated than in former times; why should medicine be an exception? ... In the West, medical scholars must pass a series of examinations. Those who take a degree will have a title and may then go out to practice. ... Medical scholars in China are men who train themselves. They do not add any tokens of distinction [to their names]. This is the first

---

30   The 17th-century Jesuit missionaries did attempt to disseminate their knowledge of European anatomy and physiology, but were unsuccessful in convincing the Chinese. Louis Fu, "The Protestant Medical Missions to China: The Introduction of Western Medicine with Vaccination", *Journal of Medical Biography*, 21 (2013): 112–17.

31   Unschuld, *Medicine in China*, 235–39.

reason of their being unsophisticated. ... [A]ll Western physicians comprehend the mysteries of the organs and of the blood vessels. Chinese who study medicine do not even have one single such [experience]. Old physicians who have [practiced for] decades still do not know the shape of the organs. If they are confronted with a strange and incurable symptom, they will never know where the origin of the illness was. This is the second reason of their being unsophisticated.[32]

Ironically, by the early 20th century, it was the standards of missionary hospitals that were called into question. A 1920 study by the China Medical Missionary Association revealed that 80 percent of the missionary hospitals in rural and urban areas had startling deficiencies, such as the lack of running water and sterilisation of bedding and mattresses. These inadequacies stood in sharp contrast with the newer hospitals built by the Chinese or foreign secular agencies, such as the Peking Union Medical College (*Beijing Xiehe Yiyuan*, 北京协和医院) funded by the Rockefeller Foundation. They also paled in comparison with the Japanese and European hospitals, which well-travelled Chinese were more familiar with by now.[33] Notwithstanding such change in fortunes, the challenge and dominance of Western medicine ushered in by the missionaries were here to stay, and would elicit different responses from Chinese physicians.

Among the earliest to familiarise himself with Western medicine was Zhang Xichun (张锡纯, 1860–1933). Unlike later TCM physicians, Zhang did not subordinate Chinese medical theory or epistemology to Western medicine. Rather, he sought to understand the latter through the lenses of the former. For example, when he discussed tuberculosis (*feijiehe*, 肺结核), he did not dismiss bacteria

32   Ibid., 236–37.
33   Ibid., 241–42.

as a cause of the disease but argued that germs alone were insufficient cause for the illness. When he used Western drugs (creosote and menthol) to create his own concoction, he formulated his drugs on the principles of Chinese pharmacology. That is, he categorised and administered these drugs according to their nature (*xing*, 性) and taste (*wei*, 味).[34]

A more intriguing "cross-fertilisation" of the Chinese and Western medical traditions is Cheng Dan'an's (承淡安, 1899–1957) development of scientific acupuncture. Cheng was trained in both Chinese and Western medicine, but was soon convinced of the merits of acupuncture after his father used it to cure him of a severe back problem in 1923. In the decade that followed, Cheng not only set up his own acupuncture practice and published extensively on the subject, but also visited the Tokyo College of Acupuncture (1934) for more insights. Here, he saw how Western anatomy and physiology were used "to create a new understanding of how acupuncture worked", whereby the meridians were conceived as a "function system that encompassed the nerves, blood vessels and lymph glands of Western medicine". Thereupon, he began to draft an acupuncture manual that integrated the teachings of the Song treatise, *Illustrated Canon Explaining Acu-moxa Therapy Using the Bronze Figure and its Acu-points*, with Western anatomy. In doing so, modern Chinese acupuncture was "invented".[35] In the decades that followed, Cheng would continue to modernise different aspects of acupuncture and moxibustion practice. He is still most well-known, however, for his *Chinese Acupuncture and Moxibustion Therapeutics* (*Zhongguo Zhenjiu Zhiliaoxue*, 中国针灸治疗学, 1932), which is regarded as the most important work on the subject in the last century.

Despite the above examples of promising medical dialogue, the different reform movements soon made their presence felt on Chinese medicine negatively. In 1915, Chen Duxiu (陈独秀, 1879–

34   Andrews, *Making of Modern Chinese Medicine*, 133–35.
35   Ibid., 200–2.

1942) denounced Chinese medicine as unscientific in the journal, *New Youth* (*xinqingnian*, 新青年 1915):

> Our [own] physicians do not know science. They do not understand human anatomy and what is more, they do not analyse the nature of medicine. As for bacteria and communicable diseases, they have not even heard of them. They only talk about the five phases, their production and conquest, heat and cold, *yin* and *yang*, and prescribe medicine according to the old formulas. All these nonsensical ideas and reasonless beliefs must basically be cured by the support of science.[36]

This opposition soon gained political clout when some Western physicians and their allies gained control of the Ministry of Health at Nanjing in 1928. Within a year, they had passed a proposal for "Abolishing Old-Style Medicine in Order to Clear Away the Obstacles to Medicine and Public Health". The Chinese medical physicians responded with unprecedented speed and unity by forming the National Union of Medical and Pharmaceutical Association (*Quanguo Yiyao Tuanti Zonglian Hehui*, 全国医药团体总联合会) to lobby against the proposal. They were not only successful in this venture but also managed to convince the Republican government to establish an Institute of National Medicine (*guoyiguan*, 国医馆), so as to oversee the scientisation of Chinese medicine.

In the next two decades, more modern-styled Chinese medical schools would be built, numbering more than 160 schools, colleges and teaching institutes by 1945. Several Chinese medical journals were also published during this period. Unfortunately, most of these developments were short-lived, due to a lack of funding. Nonetheless, the top three Chinese medical colleges in Shanghai still managed to do much better than their top three Western counterparts, by educat-

---

36   Scheid, *Currents*, 199.

ing more than twice the number of students.[37] The impact of these Republican developments on the subsequent transformation of Chinese medicine cannot be understated. This modernisation project, explains Scheid, required Chinese medical physicians

> to accept the visions and principles of modernity, science and nationhood.... The result was a reconfiguration not only of institutions, but also of epistemologies and memories, of the goals according to which Chinese medicine should be developed, and of what it meant to be a physician.[38]

Among the modernisers of Chinese medicine were Zhang Taiyan (章太炎, 1869–1936) and Lu Yuanlei (陆渊雷, 1894–1955). Both were adamant that the medical philosophies of *yinyang* and the five phases should be abandoned as "groundless speculation". Instead, Chinese medical research should now focus on using science "to prove the real efficacy [of Chinese medicine], to account for what is already known [by tradition], and to introduce it [science] into [Chinese medical practice] in order to discover what is not yet known".[39] In time to come, Lu's emphasis on the use of the *Shanghan Lun* as the primary guide for Chinese medical practice would

> pave the way for the organisation of contemporary Chinese medicine around the paradigm of pattern differentiation and treatment determination (*bianzhenlunzhi*, 辨证论 治) that continues to dominate Chinese medical practice today.[40]

---

37   Ibid., 193–94, 200–1.

38   Ibid., 202.

39   Ibid., 219.

40   This epistemic change, argues Rhonda Chang, can be limiting or even problematic for clinical practice. This is because physicians trained under this new scheme can no longer employ the logic of *yinyang* and *wuxing* to diagnose and treat more complex syndromes. Ibid., 220; Rhonda Chang, "Making Theoretical Principles for New Chinese Medicine", *Australian*

After the communist victory in 1949, the evolution of Chinese medicine went through several twists and turns, some positive, while others turbulent. Between the years 1949–1953, Mao Zedong and his Chinese Communist Party (CCP) leaders declared that they were still committed to "uniting Chinese and Western medicine". In practice, however, this meant that Chinese physicians could continue their practice only if they participated in the government's mass action programmes for disease prevention and demonstrated a basic proficiency in Western medicine. That the CCP was still biased against the Chinese physicians was also evident in the new licensing examinations introduced in 1952, which tested them largely on Western medical knowledge. Not surprisingly, most Chinese physicians failed and many would leave practice altogether. The years 1954–1966 saw the tide turn for Chinese medicine. During this period, Mao threw his weight behind the discipline and called for all to "take Chinese medicine seriously, to do research to rectify it, and to go further in developing Chinese medicine". In an attempt to create a new medicine (*xinyi*, 新医) that would unite Western and Chinese medicine, the government introduced a legislation in 1955 that required Western physicians to learn Chinese medicine (*xixuezhong*, 西学中).

In the same year, the Academy of Chinese Medicine (*Zhongyi Yanjiuyuan*, 中医研究院) was established, and in the year following, four new Chinese medical colleges were set up in Shanghai, Guangzhou, Chengdu and Beijing.[41] In addition, an administrative infrastructure was put in place to supervise research, education and the practice of Chinese medicine, even as Chinese medical departments were introduced in some Western hospitals. As for famous physicians and those from medical lineages, they were also strongly encouraged or, indeed, pressurised, to share their personal

---

and New Zealand Society of the History of Medicine, Health and History, 16, no. 1 (2014):66–86.
41   These remain the most important Chinese medical colleges in China.

knowledge and expertise so as to benefit more students and the larger Chinese medical community.[42]

Then came an unfortunate turn of events: the Cultural Revolution of 1964–1974. During this decade, many of the renowned physicians who had contributed to the modernisation of Chinese medicine were branded as "forces of evil", and subjected to all sorts of torture and abuse. Needless to say, they were also prevented from carrying out scholarly work or medical practice. Some of these doctors even committed suicide while others perished from the physical or emotional trauma. The most notable of these were Ma Zeren (马泽人, 1894–1969), Ma Shushen (马书绅), Qin Bowei (秦伯未, 1901–70) and Lu Shouyan (陆瘦燕, 1909–1969).

The death of Mao saw the end of the Revolution and the phenomenal rise of Premier Deng Xiaopeng (邓小平, 1904–1997). Deng soon initiated a programme that not only revitalised the Chinese medical sector but also encouraged the development of medical practices from non-Han minority groups. Thereafter, different developmental approaches were adopted for Chinese medical research and practice. Some began to re-emphasise their family traditions and practices, while others pursued the integration of Chinese and Western medical practice with renewed vigour.[43] To be sure, Chinese medicine, in many ways, still lives under the shadow of its Western counterpart, with the latter dictating much of the terms of engagement. Medical training, for example, is no longer based on the classical medical canon, such as the *Neijing* and *Shanghan Lun*, but upon systematically compiled textbooks, not unlike those used in training Western physicians. In practice, many Chinese physicians are often compelled to rely on their Western medical training and operate as second-rate Western medical physicians. This is because patient expectations often penalise the use of Chinese medicine. As some doctors explained,

42   Scheid, *Currents*, 300–4.
43   Ibid., 313–14.

[I]f someone died in your care… and you had relied on Chinese medicine alone, no authority would defend you against almost certain accusations of neglect by the family of the deceased. If you used only Western medicine, no one would dare to blame you.[44]

In spite of this, Chinese medicine has grown in confidence in recent years. Some physicians, for example, have left the public healthcare system to pursue what they see as a more traditional approach to Chinese medical practice and training.[45] Others have also made headway in developing a Chinese Emergency medicine, thereby attempting "a colonisation of what is widely regarded as the exclusive domain of Western medicine".[46] Recently, Jiangxi Chinese Medical University (*Jiangxi Zhongyiyao Daxue*, 江西中医药大学) also began to train a batch of medical students using more traditional modes of learning. That is, they use the traditional classics, such as the *Suwen* and *Shanghan Lun*, rather than the standard TCM textbooks as the means of instruction. Increasingly, biomedical hospitals in China are also becoming more open to offering TCM treatments. Besides employing TCM therapies in physiotherapy, some have even begun to set up TCM clinics in their premises. More recently, President Xi Jinping's government initiated a series of new policies to develop TCM pharmacology. These include the conservation and development of Chinese drug sources, promotion of pharmacological research, and

44   Volker Scheid, *Chinese Medicine in Contemporary China: Plurality and Synthesis* (Durham, NC ; Oxford: Duke University Press, 2002), 95.

45   A good example is Xu Wenbin (徐文兵 1966–), a well-known TV commentator of Chinese medical culture. A critic of the Westernisation of Chinese medical training, he left the public healthcare system to set up his own clinic and training school instead. See "厚朴中医", accessed 12 May 2016, http://www.hope.org.cn/; "徐文兵-树立正确的人生观与价值观(上)_医道修行_新浪博客", accessed 12 May 2016, http://blog.sina.com.cn/s/blog_62030a540101cfaz.html.

46   A case study of Emergency TCM will be given in Chapter 9. Scheid, *Chinese Medicine in Contemporary China*, 267.

the cultivation of TCM drug specialists.[47] As China matures as a global economic power and re-emphasises its historical and cultural roots, it is quite likely that this new confidence in Chinese medicine will develop and introduce further changes to the Chinese-Western medical dialogue.[48]

Conclusion

The establishment of the Song dynasty ushered in a new epoch and renaissance for Chinese medicine. Due to the support of imperial authorities, numerous ancient and new medical texts and *materia medica* were compiled and published. Medical practice was also reconceived as a vocation worthy of the aristocracy and gentry. More importantly, these developments and reforms led eventually to the integration of Chinese pharmacology with the doctrine of systematic correspondences, and a renewed interest and respect for Zhang Zhongjing's Cold Damage Disorders. They also set the stage for further medical innovation and diversification from the Jin to the Qing dynasties. The 19th century saw Chinese medicine encountering its Western counterpart for the first time. The series of national catastrophes that occurred in the same period soon compelled many Chinese to adopt Western science and culture as the means of strengthening the country. Inevitably, the value of Chinese medicine was questioned, with some calling for its rejection, while others, its modernisation. After a series of setbacks, Chinese medicine was endorsed by both the Chinese Republican and Communist authorities as an important cultural heritage that, nevertheless, required much modernisation.

---

47   "习近平签署主席令，《中医药法》正式颁布！（附全文）", accessed 21 December 2017, http://mp.weixin.qq.com/s/9H1OrpFPs9tEmLPCJd5mlA.

48   Despite such optimism, one major challenge to the growth of TCM is deteriorating quality (and thus medical efficacy) of many Chinese herbs. This is due to different reasons, including poor cultivation or processing of herbs, the excessive use of pesticides on cultivated herbs, or even the sale of counterfeit herbs. "中药疗效为何越来越低？真相往往很残忍！", accessed 21 December 2017, http://mp.weixin.qq.com/s/8fFAKYsG3XVuKCCnpMUX9A.

Since then, Chinese medicine has continued to evolve itself through dialogue with Western medicine, and remains a prominent aspect of the pluralistic healthcare system in present-day China.

8

METAPHORS AND THE CONCEPTION OF HEALTH AND ILLNESS IN WESTERN AND CHINESE MEDICINE

Language, Metaphors and the Conceptualisation of Ideas

The human brain is a computing machine.[1] The genome is a book of life. Human society is like the animal kingdom, where only the fittest survive. These are metaphors familiar to the general public, and often taken seriously by them. One reason why these metaphors—the computer, the book or animals—work is that they are concrete subjects, familiar to most people. When employed as metaphors of more abstract ideas, such as how the brain, the genome or human society works, they make it easier for people to appreciate the latter concepts. There are, however, pitfalls to such use of metaphors. Take, for example, the "book of life" metaphor. Popularised by Richard Dawkins and other Neo-Darwinians, it assumes that everything

---

1   For a critique of this metaphor, see Robert Epstein, "Your Brain Does Not Process Information and It Is Not a Computer—Robert Epstein | Aeon Essays", *Aeon*, accessed 21 March 2017, https://aeon.co/essays/your-brain-does-not-process-information-and-it-is-not-a-computer, and Giorgos Zarkadakes, *In Our Own Image: Savior or Destroyer?: The History and Future of Artificial Intelligence* (New York; London: Pegasus Books, 2016).

which can be known about a living organism can be found in and is dictated unilaterally by the DNA.[2] Once we know "all about the lowest level elements, genes and proteins", they claim, "everything about the organism [such as the pathways, cells and organs] would be clear to us".[3] Recent physiological research, however, suggests that an organism's physiology is not dictated substantially, let alone entirely, by its genome. Rather, the genome is but an organ of the body that interacts multilaterally with an organism's cells, organs, and even its environment.[4] For this reason, argues system biologist Denis Noble, the genome should be better understood as a "CD", or "database" of life, from which an organism draws the data necessary for sustaining its complex physiological processes.[5] All this goes to show how important metaphors are in helping us conceptualise and understand the world. At the same time, it also cautions us to be circumspect about how metaphors operate, and which we should use. When properly conceived, a metaphor allows us to peer deeper, as it were, into the mysteries of this world. When misconstrued, however, it limits our understanding, or even misleads us from the truth.

---

2   The metaphor became particularly prominent in the early 2000s, when the human genome project was first completed. Richard Dawkins, *The Selfish Gene* (Oxford; New York: Oxford University Press, 1989); "DNA Scientists Write 'Book of Life'", *Mail Online*, accessed 9 June 2016, http://www.dailymail.co.uk/news/article-176587/DNA-scientists-write-book-life.html.; "Reading the Book of Life", BBC, 30 May 2000, sec. Human genome, http://news.bbc.co.uk/2/hi/in_depth/sci_tech/2000/human_genome/760893.stm.
3   Denis Noble, *The Music of Life: Biology beyond Genes* (Oxford; New York: Oxford University Press, 2008), 5.
4   Recent research has demonstrated that different aspects of an organism and its environmental factors not only effect its genome but the same effect may be transmitted to its future generations. See James Alan Shapiro, *Evolution: A View from the 21st Century* (Upper Saddle River, NJ: FT Press Science, 2011), 91; Ian Sample, "Motherly Love May Alter Genes for the Better", *The Guardian*, 14 February 2007, http://www.theguardian.com/science/2007/feb/14/medicalresearch.genetics.; Oded Rechavi, Gregory Minevich, and Oliver Hobert, "Transgenerational Inheritance of an Acquired Small RNA-Based Antiviral Response in *C. elegans*", *Cell* 147, no. 6 (9 December 2011): 1248–56, https://doi.org/10.1016/j.cell.2011.10.042.
5   Noble, *Music of Life*, 10, 15.

In the previous chapters, we have seen how important social, political, and environmental factors were in the evolution of Western and Chinese worldviews. In the West, ontological concerns became primary, and truth claims came to focus on the knowledge of the "dot" (to use our earlier analogy), and how we can justify such knowledge using mathematical principles. In the case of the Chinese, making sense of the relationships between the "dots" became paramount. Understanding the complex system of relationships shared by the "dots" was soon presumed as necessary for every field of Chinese science, including medicine. In this chapter, we shall take this thesis further by arguing that the same metaphysical differences play a critical role in shaping medical discourse and conceptions in both Western and Chinese medicine. This has to do mostly with how the metaphysical preference of each tradition leads them to develop different metaphors for conceptualising health, illnesses, aetiologies and therapies. To demonstrate this, we shall first consider how metaphors operate as a linguistic tool for conceptualisation. Here, we shall employ the discipline of cognitive linguistics, particularly its contemporary theory of metaphors.[6] Thereafter, we shall apply this theory to both medical traditions, so as to elucidate how the medical concepts of biomedicine and Chinese medicine came to differ so radically.

The Contemporary Theory of Metaphors: An Overview

Prior to the 1980s, it was commonly held that "literal and figurative (or metaphorical in its broad sense) language" can be easily distinguished, the former being the language used largely by the

6   Cognitive linguistics is an interdisciplinary branch of linguistics studies. It examines "the relation of language structure to things outside language". Specifically, "cognitive principles and mechanisms not specific to language, including principles of human categorization; pragmatic and interactional principles; and functional principles in general, such as iconicity and economy". "About Cognitive Linguistics—Cognitive Linguistics", accessed 4 January 2018, http://www.cognitivelinguistics.org/en/about-cognitive-linguistics.

physical sciences.[7] Since then, the work of cognitive linguists has shown, quite conclusively, that metaphors play a significant role in the conceptualisation of any form of knowledge, including science.[8] Metaphors, as George Lakoff and Mark Johnson explain, are "pervasive in everyday life". In fact, "our ordinary conceptual system, in terms of which we both think and act, is fundamentally metaphorical in nature".[9] The reason for this is due to the nature of language itself.

> Language structure depends on (and itself influences) conceptualisation, the latter being conditioned by our experience of ourselves, the external world, and our relation to that world.[10]

In other words, our human embodiment and interaction with our environment is the concrete basis by which we conceptualise and understand abstract knowledge and ideas.

Conceptual Metaphors

Whenever we articulate an idea or a concept, some form of metaphor is assumed inevitably in our linguistic expression. These metaphors are known commonly as conceptual metaphors. Conceptual metaphors, explains Ning Yu, are "systematic mappings" of one domain of experience (the "source domain") to another domain of experience (the "target domain").[11] Take, for example, the conceptual metaphor, LOVE IS A JOURNEY. It operates by mapping the entities or characteristics within a more concrete source domain (journey) to correspondences in a more abstract target domain (love).[12]

---

7   Ning Yu, *The Contemporary Theory of Metaphor: A Perspective from Chinese* (Amsterdam/ Philadelphia: John Benjamins, 1998), 10.

8   Dawkins' "Book of life" metaphor is a good example.

9   George Lakoff and Mark Johnson, *Metaphors We Live by* (Chicago: University of Chicago Press, 1980), 3; Yu, *The Contemporary Theory of Metaphor*, 20.

10   Yu, *The Contemporary Theory of Metaphor*, 13.

11   Ibid., 14.

12   Mark Johnson, "Conceptual Metaphor and Embodied Structures of Meaning: A Reply

Source Domain		Target Domain
Journey		Love
Travellers	Mapped	Lovers
Common destination	to	Common goals
Impediments to travel		Difficulties in relationship

This mapping then becomes the basis for a whole host of metaphorical linguistic expressions (MLEs), or the varied and particular expressions of a conceptual metaphor. In the case of LOVE IS A JOURNEY, these include:

a. Look how far we've come.
b. It's been a long, bumpy road.
c. We're at a crossroads.
d. We may have to go our separate ways.

Once a conceptual metaphor takes hold, it is often taken for granted, so much so that its users may not even realise they are assuming the conceptual metaphor, let alone being cognizant of what it is. Hence, when someone tells his partner, "we may have to go our separate ways", he is unlikely to be aware that he is assuming LOVE IS A JOURNEY.

To appreciate just how prevalent conceptual metaphors are in our daily conversations, and how often we are unaware of their existence, consider the MLEs on the following page, and their corresponding conceptual metaphors. In all likelihood, we would be familiar with, or have even used the MLEs listed in the left-hand column. Yet, we may not realise that we are actually presuming the conceptual metaphors listed in the right-hand column.

---

to Kennedy and Vervaeke", *Philosophical Psychology* 6 (1993): 413–22.

Metaphorical Linguistic Expressions	Conceptual Metaphor
This gadget will *save* you hours. You're *wasting* my time. You're *running* out of time.	TIME IS MONEY
Your claims are indefensible. He attacked every weak point in my argument.	ARGUMENT IS WAR

Two Categories of Metaphors

Over the last four decades, linguistic research has unearthed a whole host of conceptual metaphors. Generally speaking, these can be categorised into two main groups: The Event Structure metaphor and the Great Chain of Being metaphor.[13] The former describes how events, actions or relations may be conceptualised metaphorically. Examples include LOVE IS A JOURNEY, LIFE IS A JOURNEY, ARGUMENT IS WAR, CHANGES ARE MOVEMENTS and MEANS ARE PATHS.[14] The latter enables us to envisage abstract ideas in terms of concrete or structured images. Common examples are IDEAS ARE OBJECTS, THE BRAIN IS A MACHINE and PEOPLE ARE ANIMALS. The table on the facing page outlines the linguistic characteristics peculiar to each group.[15]

Image Schemas

In the course of their research, Lakoff, Johnson and other cognitive linguists also observed that domain mappings within conceptual

---

13   Whether this categorisation is true beyond the English-speaking world is still debatable among scholars. With regards to Chinese linguistic studies, scholars have unearthed both significant similarities and differences between English and Chinese metaphors. Cf. Yu, *The Contemporary Theory of Metaphor* and Perry Link, *An Anatomy of Chinese: Rhythm, Metaphor, Politics* (Cambridge, MA: Harvard University Press, 2013), 183–214.

14   Zoltán Kövecses, *Metaphor: A Practical Introduction* (New York: Oxford University Press, 2010), 151.

15   Ibid., 151, 163.

Attributes	Great Chain of Being Metaphor	Event Structure Metaphor
Structures the world as	*Things* or entities "that have stability in space and over time".	*Relations* or conceptual links between two or more entities.
Linguistic code	Nouns	Verbs, adjectives, prepositions or conjunctions.
Assumes	A hierarchy of beings that can be analogous to one another.	Physical concepts such as location, force or motion may function as metaphors for events.
Operates by	Attributing a property of a more concrete thing to an abstract idea.	The above concepts are metaphors for "states that change, causes that produce changes, change itself, action, purpose of action, etc."
Examples	THE MIND IS A MACHINE, PEOPLE ARE ANIMALS.	LIFE IS A JOURNEY, CHANGES ARE MOVEMENTS, MEANS ARE PATHS.

metaphors are always mediated by what they call Image Schemas. Image schemas are imaginative, pre-conceptual and non-propositional (or non-ideological) organising structures or patterns. Based on the "recurring aspects of our human bodily experience", image schemas enable us to organise the relationships mapped from entities in the source domain to those in the target domain.[16] In general, there are two types of image schemas: those depicting structure, and those depicting spatial orientation or relations. Examples of each group are given below:[17]

---

16   Mark Johnson, *The Body in the Mind: The Bodily Basis of Meaning, Imagination, and Reason* (Chicago: University of Chicago Press, 2013), xxxvii.

17   Yu, *The Contemporary Theory of Metaphor*, 24–25.

Image Schema	Examples
Those depicting structure	CONTAINER, PATH, LINKS & OBJECTS
Those depicting spatial orientation or relation	UP-DOWN, FRONT-BACK, MOTION, SOURCE-PATHOGEN, SCALAR, FORCE

To illustrate how an image schema works, consider the following conceptual metaphors.

1. GOOD IS UP; BAD IS DOWN.

Here, the image schema for depicting what is good and bad is UP and DOWN respectively. Once GOOD is associated with UP, and BAD with DOWN, we can then construct the following MLEs:

- Things are looking up.
- We hit a peak last year, but it's been downhill ever since.
- He does high-quality work.
- This is low-grade petrol.

2. IDEAS ARE OBJECTS

Here, ideas are organised using the image schema, OBJECTS. That is, ideas are regarded as object-like entities which can be invested with spatial qualities, such as being moved around, or filling up another entity. Thereupon, we can construct the following MLEs:

- You gave me a good idea.
- You have a good idea.
- Don't fill his mind with silly ideas.

The Study of Chinese Metaphors

The contemporary theory of metaphors was largely developed in the English-speaking world. In recent years, many scholars have examined the extent to which the theory is applicable to the Chinese language. Thus far, Ning Yu, Perry White and others have concluded

Conceptual Metaphors	Image Schema	Metaphorical Linguistic Expression
GOOD IS UP, BAD IS DOWN	UP-DOWN	Things are looking *up*. We hit a *peak* last year, but it's been downhill ever since. He does *high*-quality work. This is a *low*-grade petrol.
IDEAS ARE OBJECTS	OBJECTS	You *gave* me a good idea. You *have* a good idea. Don't *fill* his mind with silly ideas.

that both languages share a remarkable number of similarities in their conceptual metaphors. Some interesting differences have also been noted, which may be traced to differences in their cultural and political environments, particularly the Western bias for ontology.[18] A few scholars have even applied the theory to their analysis of Chinese medical discourse. Ning Yu, for example, has studied the Chinese conception of the Gall Bladder. He points out that the image schema of container was used to depict the gall bladder as a container of courage, whereby courage is a kind of *qi* contained within the gall bladder.[19]

---

18   See, for example, Ning Yu, *The Chinese Heart in a Cognitive Perspective: Culture, Body, and Language* (Berlin, NY: Mouton de Gruyter, 2009) and Link, *An Anatomy of Chinese*, 231–32.

19   In view of the Chinese medical understanding of *qi*, it is questionable whether it should be conceived as a kind of gas enclosed within the gall bladder, as Ning argues, or denotes the functional well-being of the gall bladder, as it relates to the other Chinese organs. As we shall see, this chapter favours the second interpretation. Ning Yu, "Metaphor, Body, and Culture: The Chinese Understanding of Gallbladder and Courage", *Metaphor and Symbol* 18, no. 1 (2003): 13–31.

Sonya Pritzker, on the other hand, has used the theory to investigate how modern and Chinese medicine conceptualise depression, or *yu* (郁), so as to elucidate their differences.[20] What has yet to be considered extensively is the way Western and Chinese metaphysical assumptions influence the theories, aetiologies, and therapies of their respective medical traditions. This will be done in the remaining part of this chapter. As we shall see, the influence is considerable, and this is also why both traditions differ so dramatically in their conceptions of health, illnesses and therapy.

Western Medical Conceptual Metaphors

To facilitate our comparison of Western and Chinese medical metaphors, and the ways they shape medical discourse, we shall limit our discussion to the key conceptual metaphors employed in the two traditions. We begin with three main conceptual metaphors commonly used in biomedical discourse on human physiology, aetiology and therapy. They are:

1. GENES AND CELLS ARE BUILDING BLOCKS.
2. HUMAN BUILDING BLOCKS (CELLS, TISSUES, ORGANS) ARE MACHINES.
3. SICKNESSES ARE BATTLES.

*Conceptual Metaphor 1: **GENES AND CELLS ARE BUILDING BLOCKS***

In biomedicine, cells, tissues and organs are assumed to be the basic building blocks of the human body. While this theory differs from the humoral doctrine of Galenic medicine, the two traditions still share a similar bias, namely, their common belief that the human body

---

20   Sonya Pritzker, "The Role of Metaphor in Culture, Consciousness, and Medicine: A Preliminary Inquiry into the Metaphors of Depression in Chinese and Western Medical and Common Languages", *Clinical Acupuncture and Oriental Medicine* 4 (2003): 11–28.

should be made up of some kind of elements or building blocks. This ontological assumption is the basis for our first biomedical conceptual metaphor: GENES AND CELLS ARE BUILDING BLOCKS. In this case, entities in the source domain (bricks or other kinds of building blocks) are mediated by the image schema of OBJECTS and mapped to the target domain. The end result is given below:

The above is then the basis for the following MLEs that we often encounter in biomedicine.

- There are about 19,000–20,000 protein-coding genes in the human body.
- The human body is made up of more than 200 different types of cells.

Source Domain	Mapped to (Using OBJECT Image Schema)	Target Domain
Building blocks		Genes
Building blocks		Cells

Conceptual Metaphor 2: *HUMAN CELLS AND ORGANS ARE MACHINES*

In biomedical theory, cells, tissues and organs are not only the building blocks of the body. They are regarded also as "living units of structure and function".[21] To put it differently, these cells and organs are envisaged as some kind of machines, or containers with functional attributes. Using the CONTAINER image schema, what we know about machines (source domain) are mapped to cells and organs (target domain).

Accordingly, we can speak of cells and organs as having functions. So, when we describe the functions of blood, we use MLEs like:

---

21   Valerie C. Scanlon and Tina Sanders, *Essentials of Anatomy and Physiology* (Philadelphia, PA: F. A. Davis, 2015), 4.

- Red blood cells are known as *carriers* of oxygen.
- White blood cells *destroy* pathogens by *producing* antibodies.

Likewise, when we describe an organ, such as the kidney, we say:

- The kidney *performs* multiple functions, including waste *excretion*, *balancing* the level of water in one's body, and *regulating* the body's blood pressure, red blood cells and acids.

Source Domain		Target Domain
Tools and machines	Mapped to (Using CONTAINER Image Schema)	Organs and cells
Machine functions		Organ and cellular functions
Machine attributes		Organ and cellular attributes

If organs are some kind of machines, their health would depend on the extent of their functionality. Aetiologically speaking, illnesses then occur whenever the functions of a cell or an organ deteriorate. It is on this premise that we have aetiological MLEs such as:

- Defective genes.
- Kidney or organ failure.
- Cancers are abnormal cell growth.
- Lesions on an organ are evidence of organ sicknesses.

If illnesses are due to abnormalities in one's physiological building blocks, one way of treating these sicknesses would be by repairing these elements. This is exactly what gene therapy sets out to do. Thus, we have therapeutic MLEs such as:

- Gene therapy seeks to replace or inactivate a mutated gene.

- Gene therapy introduces a new gene to a body to help it fight a disease.[22]

To be sure, biomedicine does not just focus on the organs or cells. Indeed, there is much systematic thinking in biomedical physiology. During their training, every medical student is required to learn all the main physiological systems, such as the skeletal system, muscular system, integumentary (skin) system, nervous system, endocrine system, lymphatic system, respiratory system, vascular system, digestive system, urinary system and reproductive system. While the functions of these systems are often dominated by a single organ, there are some systems where multiple organs are involved. For example, the kidney is the main organ in the urinary system, while multiple organs, like the stomach, gall bladder, pancreas, liver and intestines, must operate in tandem for healthy digestion. Having said this, biomedical treatment and therapy remain rather organ centred, or focused on specific systems. This can be seen in the wide range of medical specialties we now have, such as dermatology, cardiology, neurology, urology, nephrology, immunology, and ophthalmology.[23] In each specialty, diagnosis and therapy are focused primarily on specific organs or physiological systems, rather than on how the different organs and systems may interact with each other. Such an emphasis is understandable, given the ontological prejudice of the above conceptual metaphors.

Conceptual Metaphor 3: SICKNESSES ARE BATTLES

Besides cellular or organ malfunction, illnesses can also be due to attacks by external agents such as bacteria and viruses. Over the

---

22   Genetics Home Reference, "What Is Gene Therapy?", *Genetics Home Reference*, accessed 3 June 2018, https://ghr.nlm.nih.gov/primer/therapy/genetherapy.

23   Another important reason for specialisation is that each specialty has become so complicated that a physician can only cope by focusing on a specialised field of knowledge. Atul Gawande, "The Problem of Extreme Complexity", in *The Checklist Manifesto: How to Get Things Right* (London: Profile Books, 2009).

last century, this language of warfare, or the warfare metaphor, has dominated biomedical thinking on aetiology and therapy, thus giving rise to our third Conceptual Metaphor: SICKNESSES ARE BATTLES.[24] Based on this paradigm, sicknesses can be cured only when these external enemies are eliminated. Most intriguingly, this warfare mentality has proved influential even in oncology. Here, cancer tumours are regarded as no longer part of the human patient but agents external to and hostile to her. Ironically, they must be destroyed even at the expense of other normal human cells.

Conceptual Metaphors 1 and 2 enable us to map building blocks and cities to the cells/ organs and the human body respectively. Using the OBJECTS image schema, Conceptual Metaphor 3 objectifies enemies and maps them to bacteria, viruses or cellular abnormalities. Just as enemy attacks damage cities, so do bacterial, viral or tumour attacks hurt the bodies. These then provide the grounds for MLEs such as:

- The antibiotics will kill or inhibit bacteria.
- We need more effective antibiotics against the superbugs.
- Immunotherapy targets and blocks the spread of cancer cells.

Yinyang, Qi and Wuxing Motifs in Chinese Medical Discourse

Having mapped the main conceptual metaphors assumed in modern biomedical discourse, we turn now to those utilised in Chinese medicine. Unlike its Western counterpart, Chinese medical discourse lacks a concern for ontology. Instead, the key philosophical concepts employed in Chinese medical theories are the ideas of *yinyang*, *qi*, and *wuxing*. Readers were briefly introduced to these ideas in the last two chapters, when we looked at how they were applied in Chinese

---

24   The warfare metaphor is characterised by "the systematic search for the microbial "cause" of each disease, followed by the development of antimicrobial therapies". Forum on Microbial Threats, *Ending the War Metaphor: The Changing Agenda for Unraveling the Host-Microbe Relationship—Workshop Summary* (Washington, D.C.: National Academies, 2006), 2.

Source Domain	Mapped to (Using OBJECT Image Schema)	Target Domain
Building blocks of a building or city		Human cells & organs
Building or city		Human body
Enemies		Bacteria or viruses
Warfare attacks		Bacteria or virus attack
Abnormalities in building (e.g. rust or corrosion)		Abnormalities in cells or organs (such as tumours or genetic defects)
Damaged building blocks		Damaged organs and bodies

medical theory. Before we examine how these concepts operate in Chinese medical conceptual metaphors, we should give more thought to the semantics and linguistic functions of these motifs.

We consider, first of all, the idea of *yinyang*. Although the motif is based initially on one's spatial experience—*yang* being the side of a hill or the part of one's body that is exposed to the sun, and *yin* representing the opposite—it is also clear that *yinyang* does not have an absolute ontological referent. Rather, it is a relational category used to describe the relationships and interdependence between multiple entities in space and time.[25] This is evident in how the motif is used in two texts mentioned earlier in Chapter 6. The first is Zhuangzi's *Way of Heaven*, which speaks of

> those who know the joys of Heaven, during their life conform to the ways of Heaven, and at death transform

25   Robin Wang, *Yinyang: The Way of Heaven and Earth in Chinese Thought and Culture* (Cambridge: Cambridge University Press, 2012), 7–17.

with things. In their stillness they possess the same virtue as *yin*, and in their movement they flow the same as *yang*.[26]

Here, the *yinyang* motif is used not only to differentiate between two states of being—stillness (*yin*) and movement (*yang*)—but also to correlate the two since an entity can only be described as slow when compared with another that is moving faster than it. Likewise, Dong Zhongshu's *Luxuriant Gems of the Spring and Autumn Annals* employ the *yinyang* motif to differentiate entities which have separated themselves into *yin* and *yang*, and also to underscore the fact that the two were once united and thus related to one another:

> [T]he *qi* of heaven and earth unites and becomes one, separates into *yinyang*, divides into the four seasons, spreads out into the *wuxing*.[27]

天地之气，合而为一，分为阴阳，判为四时，列为五行。

With regards to the concept of *qi*, its semantic field has become so broad over the last 2,000 years that the word can no longer be translated adequately by "a single European word".[28] The earliest application of *qi* is in discourse about nature and cosmology, where *qi* can denote the vapours of food (*guqi*, 谷气), the air that we breathe (*kongqi*, 空气), or even the stuff that makes up the universe (as it is used earlier in the *Luxuriant Gems*). The second is in the conception of ethical ideas and emotions. Thus, someone with *haoqi* (豪气) is

---

26   Zhuangzi, *Way of Heaven* (*Tiandao*, 天道).

27   *Luxuriant Gems of the Spring and Autumn Annals* 58, *The Mutual Generation of the Five Agents* (春秋繁露 58: 五行相生). Quoted from Dainian Zhang and Edmund Ryden, *Key Concepts in Chinese Philosophy* (Beijing: Foreign Languages Press, 2002), 100.

28   Paul U. Unschuld and Hermann Tessenow, with Zheng Jinsheng, *Huang Di Nei Jing Su Wen: An Annotated Translation of Huang Di's Inner Classic—Basic Questions*, 2 (Berkeley, CA: University of California Press, 2011), 19–20.

taken to be upright and just, whereas someone with *nuqi* (怒气) is understood to be angry. The third is in Chinese medicine, where *qi* is used regularly to describe one's physiology. *Yuanqi* (元气) or original *qi*, for example, refers to the essence that is transmitted by parents to their children at conception.[29] *Zangfuzhiqi* (脏腑之气) or the *qi* of organs, on the other hand, refers to the functional activity of specific organs. Hence, *feiqi* (肺气) refers to the functional activity of the lungs, while *shenqi* (肾气) to that of the kidney.

Qi is also associated closely with blood (*qixue*, 气血) and commonly employed to describe the activity or flow of blood in the body. Besides these, references to *qi* can also be non-organ specific. *Jingluozhiqi* (经络之气) or the *qi* in one's meridians, for example, refers to the activity in the meridians. Similarly, *weiqi* (卫气) or protective *qi*, is that which protects the body from external pernicious influences.[30] Finally, *qi* can also denote the state of one's health or disease. For example, a person with a lack of *qi* (*qixu*, 气虚) is understood to be physically ill or weak, while someone described as having too much dampness or damp *qi* (*shiqi*, 湿气) must expunge this excessive dampness before his body can recover.

Despite its diverse applications in Chinese medical discourse, it appears that *qi* is understood primarily as denoting process or functional flow between entities. That is to say, one's spatial experience of *vapours flowing in motion* is transposed to the human body to describe its various physiological activities. Or, as Wang Weigong puts it, *qi*, in the physiological context, should be understood as denoting the functional activity (*gongnengxing*, 功能性) of one's organs, meridians or blood.[31]

---

29   The word, "essence" is used loosely here and need not be understood ontologically as referring to specific substances. More likely, original *qi* refers to the functional abilities that parents pass on to their children, such as hereditary attributes and so on.

30   Ted J. Kaptchuk, *Chinese Medicine: The Web That Has No Weaver* (London: Rider, 2000), 49–54.

31   Wang Weigong (王唯工), *Qi as a Musical Movement* (气的乐章) (臺北市; 臺北縣 三重市: 大塊文化出版 大和书报总经销, 2002), 44–45.

In Chinese medicine, the same logic is extended to the relationship between one's body and the environment. Here, the cosmic *qi*, or environmental influence, is regarded as having a functional impact on the body, for better or for worse. Regardless of whether it is the *qi* in one's body or that in the environment, we should recognise that, to the Chinese mind, *qi* is never understood in discrete or ontological terms. That is to say, there is no homogenous *qi* substance or element we should be looking out for. Rather, as Wang explained, *qi* may be associated with different ontological substances, depending on its physiological context. For instance, the concept of protective *qi* (*weiqi*) is most likely a reference to the functional strength of one's immune system, while environmental evil *qi* (*xieqi*, 邪气) could well refer to pernicious bacteria, viruses or poisonous fumes that could have a negative impact on the body's physiological functions.[32]

We turn finally to the concept of *wuxing* or five phases, whose literal meaning refers to the five elements of metal, wood, water, fire and earth (*jinmushuihuotu*, 金木水火土). In Chinese medical theory, these five phases are used commonly to denote one's body type (*tizhi*, 体质), or *zang* (脏) organs.[33] Since the concept of the five phases is most often applied in the diagnosis of *zang* organs, we will focus primarily on its application here. At first glance, the five elements seem to be interpreted ontologically, as referring to one of the five *zang* organs: metal representing the lungs, wood the liver, water the bladder, fire the heart, and earth the spleen. These associations are by no means arbitrary. Often, they are based on the similar functional attributes shared by an element and the organ it represents. For example, just as water flows downwards and irrigates

32   In saying this, I differ from many Chinese medical scholars who still presume *qi* to be an ontological metaphor. Ted Kaptchuk is a good example. While he agrees that "*qi* is not some primordial, immutable material", he continues to perceive it in ontological or elemental terms by conceptualising *qi* as "a kind of matter on the verge of becoming energy, or energy at the point of materializing". Wang Weigong, 49; Kaptchuk, *Chinese Medicine*, 43.

33   Li Caifeng (李彩风), *The Simplest Introduction to Chinese Medicine in History* (史上最简单,白话中医入门) (Xinbi: Popular Book, 2011), 26–30.

the land, so also the bladder enables bodily fluids to flow downwards and regulates the fluids in one's body. It is for this reason that water is regarded as representative of the bladder. In the case of wood, it is understood as denoting growth and flourishing, and is, therefore, a good representation of the liver. This is because the liver stores blood and is responsible for maintaining "the smoothness and harmony of movement throughout the body".[34]

However, not all the elemental-organ associations are as straight-forward or convincing. The lungs, for example, are represented by metal, but the rationale for this is not entirely clear. The reason why the two are still correlated, we believe, can be found in the logic of *wuxing* itself. As it turns out, the primary concern of *wuxing* is not so much the elements themselves but the relationships represented by the different pairs of elements.[35] This is why, whenever the concept is applied, the physician's attention is always focused on how each element (or organ) mutually generates (*xiangsheng*, 相生) or opposes (*xiangke*, 相克) one another. These different relationships are categorised in the table on the next page for ease of understanding.

When applied to Chinese medical theory, the *wuxing* concept allows the physician to infer different relationships between the *zang* organs. For example, whenever there is a deficiency in the spleen (earth), it is likely that the liver (wood) will be adversely affected. For this reason, when a physician treats the spleen, he should also fortify or strengthen the liver. This strengthening of the liver, in turn, will also have a beneficial influence on the spleen.[36]

Given the significance of the *wuxing* in ancient Chinese thought, it is most likely that efforts were made to correlate the metaphor with empirical medical evidence so that the latter would

---

34   Kaptchuk, *Chinese Medicine*, 81.

35   This is why many TCM books, including this, prefer to translate the "elements" as "phases" instead.

36   For a detailed explanation of the five phases theory, its application in Chinese medicine and criticisms of this model, see Kaptchuk, *Chinese Medicine*, 441–49.

Elements/Phases	Generates	Opposes
Water	(Nourishes) Wood	(Puts out) Fire
Wood	(Feeds) Fire	(Blocks up) Earth
Fire	(Creates fertile) Earth	(Melts) Metal
Earth	(Yields) Metal	(Dams up) Water
Metal	(Condenses) Water	(Chops down) Wood

cohere with Chinese cosmological ideas. Truth be told, Chinese physicians sometimes disagree as to which of these mutually generating and conquering relationships are helpful for medical diagnosis and treatment. Some have attributed these differences to the difficulties of mastering the *wuxing* theory for clinical practice. The more pessimistic, however, have simply concluded that the ancients' attempts to correspond the two schemes were not entirely satisfactory. The debate continues to this day.

Chinese Medical Conceptual Metaphors

Having clarified the semantic fields of *yinyang*, *qi* and *wuxing*, we shall now look at how they give rise to the conceptual metaphors assumed in Chinese medical discourse. Four main Chinese conceptual metaphors will be discussed here:

1. THE PHYSIOLOGICAL SYSTEM/NATURE IS A BINARY SCALE.
2. MOVING *QI* (AIR) IS CHANGE.
3. HARMONIOUS FLOW IS GOOD, BLOCKAGE OR EXCESS IS BAD.

4. THE HUMAN BODY IS AN IMPERIAL DISTRIBUTION COMPLEX SYSTEM.

Conceptual Metaphor 1: THE PHYSIOLOGICAL SYSTEM/ NATURE IS A BINARY SCALE

The premise of *yinyang* is that all things exist in binary pairs, with the entities in each pair dependent on and held in balance with one another. Each pair thus exists on a scale, where one point of the scale is understood only in relation to the other. This gives rise to the first Conceptual Metaphor employed by Chinese medicine: THE PHYSIOLOGICAL SYSTEM/NATURE IS A BINARY SCALE. This conceptual metaphor operates by mapping the more concrete *yinyang* phenomena in our daily lives, such as movement-stillness, hot-cold, light-darkness, and male-female, to every aspect of natural phenomena. These binaries are adjectival pairs and are mostly mapped from the source to the target domain by means of the SCALE image schema.[37] In the case of the male-female pair, each gender is objectified using the CONTAINER image schema, so that "male" is regarded as containing all characteristics associated with masculinity, while "female" as representing all that is feminine. Once the male-female pair is mapped to the target domain, we can then categorise all kinds of natural phenomena as having either masculine or feminine attributes. Since each entity in the binary pair is either complementing or opposing the other, their relationship is denoted by the FORCE image schema.[38]

---

37   The SCALE image schema is bidirectional, unbound, and situates the binary pair on two poles of a scale or continuum. Arthur Mettinger, "Contrast and Schemas: Anonymous Adjectives", in *Issues in Cognitive Linguistics: 1993 Proceedings of the International Cognitive Linguistics Conference*, ed. Christoph Eyrich and Stadler (Berlin: De Gruyter Mouton, 2011), 103–7.

38   A Force schema is "an image schema that involves physical or metaphorical causal interaction. It includes the following elements: a source and target of the force, a direction and intensity of the force, a path of motion of the source and/or target, and sequence of causation". Under the Force schema, the sub-categories that best depict opposition and complementation would be the Counterforce and Enablement Image Schema. "Force Schema", accessed 3

Source Domain	Mapped to (Using the following Image Schema)	Target Domain
Yinyang entities: - Movement (*yang*)-stillness (*yin*) - Hot (*yang*)-cold (*yin*) - Light (*yang*)-darkness (*yin*) - Male (*yang*)-female (*yin*)	SCALE SCALE SCALE CONTAINER	All phenomena can be categorised in binary pairs.
Different relations between each binary pair (*yinyang* entities)	FORCE (Counterforce or enablement)	All phenomena can be categorised in binary relations, either complementary or opposed to one another.

The concept of *wuxing* can be represented similarly. In this case, varied entities or phases in the source domain are mapped to counterparts in the target domain by the CONTAINER image schema. The mutually complementary or opposing relationships within each binary pair are likewise mapped by the FORCE image schema.

Based on the above, we then have the MLEs commonly employed in Chinese metaphysics:

- There is a masculine and a feminine side to all things.
- There is stillness and movement in all things.
- There is a fullness (*shi*, 实) and emptiness (*xu*, 虚) in all things.

December 2015, https://glossary.sil.org/term/force-schema.

Source Domain	Mapped to (Using the following Image Schema)	Target Domain
Each phase in the *wuxing* (metal, wood, water, fire, earth).	CONTAINER	Entities in nature, human organs or human phenomena.
The mutual relations of opposition or complementation between the phases.	FORCE (Counterforce or enablement)	All phenomena are related to one another, either in opposing or complementing relations.

- A strong heart (fire) is helpful for the spleen (earth) and the digestive functions associated with it.

Conceptual Metaphor 2: MOVING QI (AIR) IS CHANGE

While the *yinyang* and *wuxing* motifs provide helpful mental models for depicting relationships between entities, they do not quite describe how one entity actually influences another. This is where the concept of *qi* comes in: to depict the actual dynamics, movement or change occurring between each binary pair. This brings us to our second conceptual metaphor: MOVING QI (AIR) IS CHANGE. The concrete or physical basis of *qi* is the image of steam swirling above a bowl of rice.[39] This image is mapped to the target domain using the image schema of CIRCULAR FLOW STATE. Thereafter, all natural phenomena are imagined as influencing and generating one another by means of a swirling *qi*.

Based on Conceptual Metaphor 2, we have the following MLEs in Chinese physiology:

- Original *qi* (*Yuanqi*, 元气) is the pre-natal basis of

---

39   This can be inferred from the original character for *qi* (氣), which includes the Chinese character for rice (*mi*, 米).

Source Domain	Mapped to (Using the following Image Schema)	Target Domain
Swirling steam (*qi*) from a bowl of rice.	CIRCULAR FLOW STATE	Swirling *qi* that changes the universe and all entities.
Breeze and winds that accompany seasonal patterns.	CIRCULAR FLOW STATE	Swirling *qi* are the changing rhythms that generate or change all things, including the human body.
Each *wuxing* phase opposes or complements the other to give rise to new changes.	FORCE (Counterforce or enablement)	Opposing or complementing forces (signified by *qi*) in Nature give rise to changes in all things, including the human body.

human life, inherited from our parents. It is a "motive force" that flows through internal organs and facilitates transformation of *qi* and blood. It also determines the general health of the organs.[40]

- *Qi* flows through meridians (*jingluozhiqi*, 经络之气).
- *Qi* within and circulating through the lungs (*feiqi*, 肺气).
- Protective *qi* (*weiqi*, 卫气).

Conceptual Metaphor 3: *HARMONIOUS FLOW IS GOOD, BLOCKAGE OR EXCESS IS BAD*

If moving *qi* is the basis of life, physiological health must depend,

40   Giovanni Maciocia, *The Foundations of Chinese Medicine: A Comprehensive Text for Acupuncturists and Herbalists* (Edinburgh: Elsevier Churchill Livingstone, 2005), 48–49.

Source Domain	Mapped to (Using the following Image Schema)	Target Domain
Flow of water or air.	CIRCULAR FLOW STATE	Flow of *qi* in the universe.
Blockage of water or air leads to unhealthy phenomena (e.g. stale air or murky water).	FORCE (BLOCKAGE)	Blockage of *qi* leads to illnesses.
Excess of water or air leads to unhealthy phenomena such as floods or whirlwinds.	FORCE (COMPULSION)	Excess of *qi* leads to illnesses.

therefore, on how well or poorly this *qi* is flowing. In Chinese medicine, it is generally assumed that one's *qi* must flow harmoniously in order for one to be healthy. Whenever moving *qi* is blocked or in excess, illnesses occur. This gives us to our third conceptual metaphor: HARMONIOUS FLOW IS GOOD, BLOCKAGE OR EXCESS IS BAD. Here the flow of air or water is mapped to the flow of *qi* in the Universe using the CIRCULAR FLOW STATE image schema, while the blockage or excess of this flow is mapped to the blockage of *qi* using the FORCE image schema and its sub-categories, BLOCKAGE or COMPULSION.[41]

---

41   The COMPULSION Image Schema is derived from the experience of being pushed by water, wind or a moving crowd. Such compulsions occur in a distribution system whenever an excess in one point of the system leads to an overflow in another. "Compulsion Schema", *SIL Glossary of Linguistic Terms*, accessed 3 December 2015, https://glossary.sil.org/term/compulsion-schema.

On the basis of Conceptual Metaphors 2 and 3, we employ aetiological MLEs such as:

- That patient lacks *qi* or suffers from *qi* deficiency (*qixu*, 气虚).
- The condition of *qi* stagnation (*qizhi*, 气滞).
- Excess *qi* illnesses.
- Spleen digestive-transformation problems (脾运化失调).
- Accumulation of dampness in one's interior body, leading to significant weight gain (水湿内停, 体重加重).

Therapeutically speaking, we must either tonify or regulate the flow to treat illnesses arising from the lack of or sub-optimal flow of *qi* in the body. Thus, we have therapeutic MLEs like:

- To overcome lack one needs to change; with change blockages are unbocked; what flows smoothly then endures (穷则变、变则通、通则久).
- We need to regenerate organ *yinqi* in order to surge *yangqi*.
- Tonify the upright *qi* (*zhengqi*, 正气).
- Using the needles to move the *qi* (以针行气、运气).

Conceptual Metaphor 4: *THE HUMAN BODY IS AN IMPERIAL DISTRIBUTION COMPLEX SYSTEM*

As explained earlier, traditional Chinese sciences took for granted the metaphor of *yinyang* in their conceptualisation of complex systems in human lives, such as seasonal cycles, political relations, and distribution systems. These complex systems, as Paul Unschuld argues, then become the basis for our fourth Conceptual Metaphor: THE

Source Domain	Mapped to (Using the following Image Schema)	Target Domain
Imperial distribution entities.	CONTAINER	*Zangfu* organs.
Relationships between the above entities.	FORCE (Counterforce or enablement)	Relationships between *zangfu* organs.
Roads linking the above entities.	LINKS	Meridians connecting the *zangfu* organs.
Products flowing from one entity to another.	MOTION	*Qi* and blood flow through the meridians and *zangfu* organs.
Excess flows lead to distribution problems.	FORCE (Compulsion)	Excess flows lead to illnesses.
Impeded flows lead to distribution problems.	FORCE (Compulsion)	Impeded flows lead to illnesses.

HUMAN BODY IS AN IMPERIAL DISTRIBUTION COMPLEX SYSTEM.[42] Specifically, the different entities within the Chinese imperial distribution system, and their relationships with one another, are mapped to the *zangfu* organs and meridians within a human body. This then allows Chinese politicians and physicians to hypothesise that both systems are healthy when their processes are flowing optimally

---

42   See Chapter 6 for further discussion on how the Han political-distribution system became a mental model for Han medical physiology. Paul U. Unschuld, *Medicine in China: A History of Ideas* (Berkeley, CA; London: University of California Press, 1985), 79–80; Paul U. Unschuld, *What Is Medicine: Western and Eastern Approaches to Healing* (Berkeley, CA: University of California Press, 2009), 51.

or harmoniously. The corollary is that problems or illnesses occur whenever the flows between the different entities are impeded.

Aetiologically speaking, we then have MLEs such as:

- The meridians are blocked.
- The *qi* and blood flow are blocked.

If excesses or impediments are causes of illnesses, and all organs are related to one another in some way or another, medical therapy can then be conceived as either the removal of excesses or blockages, or the stimulation and treatment of one organ for the sake of another. This logic then gives rise to therapeutic MLEs such as:

- Warm the kidney to strengthen the spleen (digestive system) (温补肾阳，补脾阳).
- Nurture the *yin* to strengthen the *yang* (滋阴补阳).

Biomedical and Chinese Medical Discourse: A Comparative Evaluation

By analysing biomedical discourse through the interpretive lenses of contemporary metaphor theory, it should be clear that biomedicine's conception of the human body, as constituted by elemental building blocks, or more specifically, cells, tissues and organs, was influenced significantly by its ontological concerns. By investing these building blocks with functional properties, the same bias also leads biomedicine to attribute illnesses to the deterioration of one's cells or organs, or attacks by external agents. In linguistic terms, biomedical discourse has a clear bias for Great Chain of Being metaphors. The net result is that biomedical therapies are skewed towards restoring the ontology of the affected cells or organs by treating the defective parts of the cells or organs, or by attacking the enemy from without, that is, the pernicious bacteria, viruses and even cancer tumours.

In contrast, Chinese medical discourse assumes that all entities in the human body are related to and dependent on one another. Consequently, it is more inclined towards the Event Structure metaphorical system. The dominant metaphorical model it ends up with is the imperial distribution system. On this basis, psychosomatic health is understood as the result of efficient flows or movements between physiological entities, signified by the motif of flowing *qi*. Illnesses thus occur whenever such flows are impeded, inadequate or in excess. This aetiology then obligates Chinese medicine to conceptualise therapy largely in terms of restoring that efficient flow or balance in the relationships between entities in the body.

Driven by their metaphysical biases, the ways Western and Chinese medicine envisage aetiology and therapy cannot be more different. This becomes obvious when we consider the ways both traditions approach oncological treatment. In the case of biomedicine, the warfare metaphor has largely held sway. The cancerous tumour or bacteria is regarded metaphorically as the external enemy that should be destroyed at all cost.[43] This has given rise to a whole host of therapeutic strategies aimed at either destroying or inhibiting the tumour or bacteria, often at the expense of the patient's body.[44] Chinese medicine, on the other hand, envisages the possibility of a patient co-existing with his cancer (*yuai gongcun*, 与癌共存). What is entailed here is not an aggressive attack of cancerous cells, but an inhibition of its growth through strengthening the other parts of the body. In so doing, the patient's immunity and life are not

---

43　Several types of cancers, such as stomach cancer, and cervical cancer, are caused by bacteria or viruses. "Bacteria That Can Lead to Cancer | American Cancer Society", accessed 13 January 2018, https://www.cancer.org/cancer/cancer-causes/infectious-agents/infections-that-can-lead-to-cancer/bacteria.html.

44　The limitations of this metaphor have been recognized in recent years, with more biomedical physicians warning against the unnecessary use of antibiotics or arguing that the metaphor should be abandoned in view of the losing war against superbugs. Giulia Enders, *Gut: The inside Story of Our Body's Most Underrated Organ* (Vancouver, BC: Greystone, 2015), Kindle Location 2793.

threatened, and the disease is managed as a form of chronic illness. To date, this therapeutic approach has helped many cancer patients enjoy several years of quality life, with some even experiencing a gradual diminution of their tumours.[45]

Conclusion

The immense success of biomedicine, whether it is in improving our knowledge of human anatomy and physiology, or in the development of medical therapies, demonstrates, quite clearly, the merits of an ontological approach to medicine. There is, indeed, much that Chinese medicine can learn from its Western counterpart. Having said this, the above linguistic insights also remind us that biomedicine's tendency towards conceptualising medical reality in ontological terms may well have kept it from, as Lakoff and Johnson would put it, "focusing on other aspects of [in this case, medicine] that are inconsistent with that [ontological] metaphor". Most notably, modern medicine often takes a discrete or fragmented approach towards therapy and pays far less attention to how the interactions between one's DNA, cells, organs, physiological systems, and environment may affect one's overall health. A good case in point is the dermatologist's treatment of eczema. Quite often, his diagnosis and therapy would focus on the skin's condition. It would not occur to him that the disease could well be due to problems related to one's digestive system or skeletal structure. This should not come as a surprise, since the ontological approach to problem solving invariably restricts the scope of the medical problem to the skin and its attributes, rather than other physiological entities which may well affect the skin.[46]

---

45   "與癌共存", *Apple Daily* 蘋果日報, accessed 23 March 2017, http://hk.apple. nextmedia.com/news/art/20110821/15542977.

46   Intrinsic to Chinese medicine is a belief that skin diseases are often symptoms of organ deficiencies. Consequently, treatments of a skin ailment, like eczema, would focus on the organ system, such as the stomach and spleen (that is, the digestive system), rather than on the skin itself. This example by no means legitimises Chinese medicine, of course. Rather, it simply

Fortunately, the last 50 years have seen Western medical discourse slowly changing course and adopting the metaphor of dynamic systems or networks as a mental model. In cardiology, for example, physiologists have, quite remarkably, worked out the functional mechanisms for more than 100 proteins related to the heart. This has enabled them to develop virtual models of the organ. Having said this, these life-like models are still a far cry from the reality since the total number of proteins associated with the heart is estimated to be no less than 5,000![47] In other words, there remains much to be learnt about the human heart, in particular, and how it might relate to the other organs in the human body. It is an open question when we will have the knowledge necessary to inspire a new generation of biomedical therapies.

Beyond this, our present study also alerts us to the fact that the differences between biomedicine and Chinese medicine are due not merely to disagreements about terminologies or methods. To put it differently, this is not just a case of which tradition has a better definition of the kidney's attributes. Rather, the differences go far deeper to the epistemic and linguistic levels, that is, how the two forms of medicine differ fundamentally in their framing, articulating, and understanding of medical reality. It is hardly surprising, therefore, that the two medical worlds do not "talk" well with or, in many cases, actually misunderstand one another.

Recognising this is crucial for any profitable dialogue between the two medical traditions. At the very least, it should caution us not to hastily dismiss Chinese medicine as unscientific or inferior, or to judge it purely on biomedical grounds. This is not to say that we must, therefore, accept Chinese medicine as an effective form of medicine. The question of legitimacy is a separate matter which involves a wide range of careful considerations. These will be taken up in Chapter 10,

---

illustrates the fact that the metaphor we use to understand realities can significantly skew the way we perceive the world.

47   Noble, *Music of Life*, 86.

when we examine the current state of Chinese medical research and its dialogue with biomedicine. 道

9

CHINESE MEDICAL THEORIES, DIAGNOSES AND THERAPIES

Introduction

In the previous chapters, we surveyed the historical background of Chinese medicine, and examined how its metaphysical biases influenced the way it conceptualised medical theory, aetiology and therapy. In this chapter, we shall look at the actual practice itself, namely, the theories, diagnostic approaches and therapies commonly employed in contemporary Chinese medicine. Due to the growing popularity of Chinese medicine worldwide, there is, thankfully, no lack of introductory literature on the subject, whether in Chinese or major European languages. Our present aim, therefore, is simply to familiarise our readers with Chinese medical theory and practice to the extent that you may know what to expect if you so choose to consult a Chinese physician.

In this survey, we shall begin by introducing readers to the theories of Chinese physiology, before explaining how Chinese medicine conceptualises disease causation, or aetiology. Thereafter, we will explore the different diagnostic methods regularly practised by Chinese physicians, and briefly examine the therapies that one may encounter in a typical consultation. As and when possible, case studies will be employed to illustrate the medical theory, diagnostic and therapy discussed.

Physiology According to Chinese Medicine

Exterior Body

The human body, as Chinese physicians see it, may be understood as a system of inter-related relationships, commonly expressed by the language of *yinyang*. Among these diverse relationships, the first two distinctions are those between the front and back of the body, and between the upper and lower part (below the waist) of the body. Accordingly, the front part of the body is *yin* and the back is *yang*, while the bottom half is *yin* and the top half being *yang*. The rationale for this is due to the body's spatial context. The top and back parts of the body are more exposed to the sun and its heat (thus *yang*), while the bottom and front parts have less exposure (thus *yin*). This being said, some parts of the body can be *yin* in one instance and *yang* in another, depending on their relative position to one another. For example, the chest area is *yin* in relation to the head, but becomes *yang* in relation to the abdomen.[1]

Interior Body 1: The Organs

As for the organs within the body, they are divided likewise into *yin* and *yang* categories. The five *zang* organs (五脏)—the heart, lungs, spleen, liver and kidneys are *yin*—while the six *fu* organs (六腑)—the gall bladder, stomach, small intestines, large intestine, bladder, and triple burner (*sanjiao*, 三焦), are *yang*. In addition to these, there are six other Curious Organs (*qihengzhifu*, 奇恒之腑), namely, the brain, marrow, bone, blood vessels, uterus and gall bladder.[2] "The

---

1   Giovanni Maciocia, *The Foundations of Chinese Medicine: A Comprehensive Text for Acupuncturists and Herbalists* (Edinburgh: Elsevier Churchill Livingstone, 2005), 9.

2   The gall bladder is counted as a *yang* organ because "it is involved in the breakdown of impure food; [and] curious because it alone among the *Yang* Organs contains a pure substance: bile". Ted J. Kaptchuk, *Chinese Medicine: The Web That Has No Weaver* (London: Rider, 2000), 78.

Yin organs," as Ted Kaptchuk explains, "are thought of as being deeper inside the body [and less exposed to the sun], and are therefore *Yin* in relation to the *Yang* organs". Essentially, their function is to "produce, transform, regulate, and restore the fundamental textures—*Qi*, blood, essence, spirit and fluids". As for the *yang* organs, their role is to "receive, break down, and

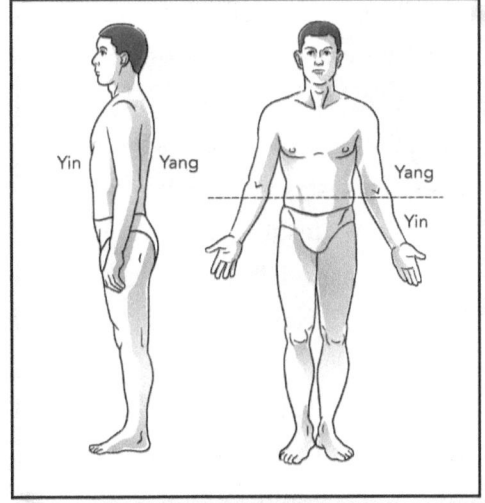

Figure 1: The Yin and Yang of the Body

absorb that part of the food that will be transformed into fundamental textures, and transport and excrete the unused portion".[3] Both in medical theory and practice, the *yin* organs are considered to be more important than their *yang* counterparts.

At this juncture, it is important to bear in mind that a Chinese physician does not conceive an organ in biomedical terms. In biomedicine, an organ is understood in terms of its anatomical functions and attributes, whereas in Chinese medicine, a reference to an organ is, essentially, a reference to a system of functions associated with the organ; an "organ system", if you will. Take the spleen, for example. According to biomedicine, it is a filter for blood as part of the immune system, where "old red blood cells are recycled", and "platelets and white blood cells are stored". It is also the organ that helps fight against certain forms of bacteria that causes meningitis and pneumonia.[4] In other words, it is an important aspect of one's immune system. Chinese medicine, however, conceptualises the spleen or *pi* (脾) differently. The spleen, as the Chinese physician

3   More will be said about these "fundamental textures" later.
4   "The Spleen (Human Anatomy): Picture, Location, Function, and Related Conditions", accessed 14 June 2016, http://www.webmd.com/digestive-disorders/picture-of-the-spleen.

sees it, is responsible primarily for digestion, whereby "the pure nutritive essences of ingested food and fluids [are extracted] and transform[ed]" into *qi* and blood. In other words, when the Chinese physician speaks of the spleen, what he has in mind actually is the digestive system of the body.[5] It is for this reason that the spleen is commonly discussed in conjunction with the stomach or *wei* (胃), which is responsible for "'receiving' and 'ripening' ingested food and fluid", that is, another aspect of digestion.[6]

Interior Body 2: The Fundamental Textures or Vital Substances

In addition to the organs, the Chinese body is also constituted by five "fundamental textures" or, as Giovanni Maciocia puts it, "vital substances".[7] These are *qi*, blood (*xue*, 血), essence (*jing*, 精), fluids (*jinye*, 津液) and spirit (*shen*, 神). According to Chinese medical theory, the latter four entities are but a continuum of *qi*. That is to say, each entity, in addition to the organs, is but *qi* in "different states of condensation and aggregation". *Qi*, in its most condensed state, forms the organs, while in its less condensed states, gives rise to the fluids, essence and blood. When *qi* is in its most rarefied form, it is no other than the spirit or *shen*.[8]

As mentioned in Chapter 8, we must be cautious about how we interpret the metaphor of *qi* in Chinese medical discourse. The primary inference here is not how the different vital substances share the same ontological basis or elements and, evolve from one state to another. In other words, this is not the case of ice melting into water or water evaporating into vapour, where all three states still share the same chemical constitution of H2O. Rather, the main inference of the *qi* metaphor is the process or functional activity of each *qi* stage,

---

5   Kaptchuk, *Chinese Medicine*, 79.

6   Ibid., 94.

7   Maciocia, *Foundations of Chinese Medicine*, 41.

8   Giovanni Maciocia, *The Psyche in Chinese Medicine: Treatment of Emotional and Mental Disharmonies with Acupuncture and Chinese Herbs* (Edinburgh: Churchill Livingstone, 2009), 4.

that is, how one stage generates or gives rise to the other. Thus, the optimal movement of *qi* is necessary for the creation of blood, while the transformation of the fluids is essential for the organs and so on. In other words, the *qi* metaphor underscores the systemic relationships and interdependence between each vital substance and, in this way, draws attention also to the unity intrinsic to these entities. Each entity is to be understood in relation to, and not in contrast with, let alone in opposition against, one another. In this way then, Chinese anthropology differs significantly from Greek anthropology, which generally postulates a sharp distinction between the soul and the body, where the latter is always subordinate to and dependent on the former.

• *Qi*

What then are these vital substances? What are their functions, medically speaking? As mentioned above and in the previous chapter, *qi* can represent a whole host of different substances and activities, depending on its physiological context. Besides denoting the relationships between the different vital substances, the *qi* metaphor is most often used to describe the different functional activities of the body. For example, when applied to the *zangfu* or meridians, it refers to the functional activity of the organ, whether it is optimal, in excess, or deficient. When conceived as *weiqi* or protective *qi*, it describes the extent to which one's immune system is operating well. As *yuanqi* (pre-natal or original *qi*), it refers to the nature (or the functional attributes of our physiology) which our parents bequeathed to us.

Due to the intimate relationship between the body and the spirit, one's psychological capacities, such as one's mental alertness and emotions, are assumed to be dependent on how well one's body is functioning. In *qi* terms, psychosomatic well-being is related to how optimal the flow of *qi* is in our body. For this reason, *qi* is generally regarded as *yang*, since it is associated with movement, strength, and positive emotions. In light of this, sicknesses occur whenever there is a disharmony in the *qi*. This can be due to a deterioration or stagnation in the functional activities of one's physiology, commonly known as deficient *qi* (*qixu*, 气虚) and stagnant *qi* (*qizhi*, 气滞) respectively, or a functional activity operating haphazardly or flowing in the reverse, rebellious *qi* (*qini*, 气逆).[9]

• *Blood (xue)*

The second "vital substance" of the body is blood (*xue*, 血). According to Chinese medical theory, blood is produced from nutritive *qi* (*yingqi*, 营气) and fluids, and is responsible for nourishing the organs and regulating the *qi*. Though distinct from *qi*, the two have "a mutually dependent and indissoluble relationship", where "*qi* is the commander of the blood, while blood is that which "gives birth to", or is the mother of *qi*" (气为血之帅, 血为气之母).[10] Pathologically speaking, sicknesses occur whenever there is a deficiency in the blood, there is blood stasis (the blood failing to move properly and stagnating), or the blood turns hot or heats up.[11]

• *Essence (jing)*

The third "vital substance" is *jing* (精), usually translated as "essence". The Chinese character, *jing*, is typically associated with the process of refinement or distillation. It is in this sense—*jing* as a refined substance—that the word is commonly understood in Chinese medicine. In Chinese medical theory, there are three types of *jing*. The first is the pre-natal essence (*xiantianzhijing*, 先天之精), which we inherit from our parents, while the second is the post-natal essence (*houtianzhijing*, 后天之精) which is derived from "ingested food and continuous physical, emotional and mental stimulation from a person's environment".[12] The third form is more specific and

---

9   Kaptchuk, *Chinese Medicine*, 46–52.
10   Ibid., 52–53; 李彩凤 (Li Caifeng), 史上最简单, 白话中医入门 (*The Simplest Introduction to Chinese Medicine in History*) (Xinbi: Popular Book, 2011), 103.
11   Maciocia, *Foundations of Chinese Medicine*, 64.
12   Kaptchuk, *Chinese Medicine*, 55–56.

refs to the kidney essence (*shenjing*, 肾精), which partakes of both pre- and post-natal essences and "determines growth, reproduction, development, sexual maturation, conception, pregnancy, menopause and ageing".[13]

• *Fluids (jinye)*

As for the fluids (*jinye*, 津液), they generally refer to the fluids found in living organisms. Specifically, *jin* denotes the "clear, light and thin-watery" fluids found in the space between and moisten the skin and muscles, while *ye* refers to the "more turbid, heavy and dense" fluids which are found in and moisten the brain, spine, bone marrow, joints and sense organs.[14]

• *Spirit (Shen)*

The fifth and final "vital substance" is the spirit (*shen*, 神). *Shen* "indicates the activity of thinking, consciousness, self-identity, insight and memory". It also denotes the five spiritual aspects of a human being, that is, the mind, the ethereal soul (*hun*, 魂), the corporeal soul (*po*, 魄), the intellect (*yi*, 意) and the willpower (*zhi*, 志). Since these spiritual aspects are taken as residing in the five different *zang* organs, it is commonly understood that a deficiency or illness in a *zang* organ will have a detrimental effect on one's psychological well-being. For example, Giovanni Maciocia has observed that among patients who suffer from depression, more than 99 percent of them suffer also from stagnation in their liver-*qi* and a deficiency in their spleen-*qi*.[15] The table below shows the different organ systems, and the spiritual aspects and psychological functions related to a specific organ system.

---

13   Maciocia, *Foundations of Chinese Medicine*, 46.

14   Ibid., 67.

15   According to Chinese medical anthropology, bodily illness may be due to psychological reasons (such as emotional distress) or physical reasons (such as poor diet, lack of exercise, or environmental factors). Regardless of the cause, the malfunction of a particular organic system is likely to precipitate a psychological illness. Maciocia, *Psyche in Chinese Medicine*, 393.

Organ System	Spiritual Aspect	Psychological Functions[16]
Heart	Mind (shen, 神)[17]	The activity of thinking, consciousness, self-identity, insight and memory.
Liver	Ethereal soul (hun, 魂)[18]	Intuition and creative inspiration.
Lungs	Corporeal soul (po, 魄)	Sensation, feeling, hearing and sight..
Spleen	Intellect (yi, 意)	Generating ideas and explicit memory.
Kidneys	Willpower (zhi, 志)	Memory capability and willpower.

Table 1: The Spiritual Aspects of the Zang Organs

The Meridians

The final aspect of the Chinese physiological landscape is the *jingluo* (经络), commonly translated as meridians. The meridians may be understood as invisible "channels or pathways that carry *qi* and blood", "an invisible lattice that links together all the fundamental textures and Organs", "regulat[ing] *Yin* and *Yang*, moisten[ing] the tendons and bones, benefit[ting] the joints". The meridians also "connect the interior of the body with the exterior", thus allowing the external

---

16   Ibid., 16, 29, 52, 67–69.

17   The word, *Shen*, has two meanings in Chinese psychology, the first representing the whole complex of the soul, and the second referring to the spiritual aspects of the heart.

18   K. E. Brashier, however, has challenged the medical distinction between *Hun* and *Po*, arguing that it is hardly employed by the Han populace when "envisioning post-mortem existence". K. E Brashier, *Ancestral Memory in Early China* (Cambridge, MA: Harvard University Press, 2011), 92.

treatments, such as acupuncture and moxibustion, to affect the interior body.[19]

In Chinese medical theory, the meridian system is made up of 12 meridians. Each meridian corresponds to the five *zang* and six *fu* organs, and the pericardium (*xinbao*, 心包), and traverses a significant part of the body. The lung meridian, (*shoutaiyin feijing*, 手太阴肺经), for example, runs from the tip of the right index finger to the lungs and

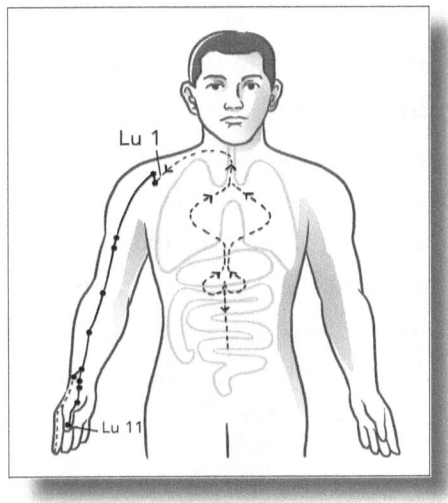

Figure 2: Lung Meridian

large intestine (see Figure 2). The stomach meridian (*zuyangming weijing*, 足阳明胃经), on the other hand, begins near the bridge of the nose and meanders downwards to the chest, past the stomach area before heading down to the big toe.[20]

In addition to the 12 meridians, there are eight Extra Meridians (*qijingbamai*, 奇经八脉), the most important being the Governing Vessel (*dumai*, 督脉) and Conception Vessel (*renmai*, 任脉). The first runs from the pelvic cavity upwards along the spine to the top of the head, while the second runs from the pelvic cavity towards the abdomen, chest, throat and finally the lip and eyes areas. Distributed throughout the 20 meridians are 365 acupuncture points. While contemporary Chinese medicine has increased this universe to at least 2,000 points, only 150 points are typically used in an acupuncture treatment.[21]

Both modern and Chinese medical communities have debated much over the objective existence of meridians and acupuncture

19   Kaptchuk, *Chinese Medicine*, 105–6.
20   For a more detailed discussion of each meridian, see Kaptchuk, 111–31.
21   Ibid., 108.

points. Traditionally, biomedicine has been sceptical about both theories, while some TCM physicians have even suggested that the meridian system should simply be understood as "an explanatory model that experience has found to be useful in the sense that in clinical situations the body behaves *as if* these pathways existed when the physician applies his needle".[22] More recently, the use of CT scans, MRI and other imaging technologies have provided strong evidence for the existence of both the meridians and acupuncture points. Through CT scan imaging, it has been observed that acupuncture points are characterised by

> a concentrated number of involuted microvascular structures. Non-acupuncture points, [however,] lacked the dense concentration of microvascular vessels and involuted structures found in acupoints.[23]

Another study using "an amperometric oxygen microsensor to detect partial oxygen pressure variations at different locations on the anterior aspect of the wrist" concluded that the "partial oxygen pressure is significantly higher at acupuncture points". As may be seen in Figure 3, which "maps the Lung, Pericardium and Heart channels and their associated local points", the "acupuncture points PC7 and PC6 clearly show high oxygen pressure levels as do the other acupuncture points in the region".[24]

More recently, clinical research using infra-red imaging technologies have demonstrated quite clearly the existence of the *du*

---

22   Hai Hong, *The Theory of Chinese Medicine: A Modern Explanation* (London: Imperial College, 2014), 118.

23   "CT Scans Capture Acupuncture Point Discovery", accessed 11 August 2016, http://www.healthcmi.com/Acupuncture-Continuing-Education-News/1418-ct-scan-acupuncture-point-discovery.

24   Ibid.

25   狄灵 et al., "红外热像仪观测" "督脉运行不畅", "颈腰椎病红外热像随机平行对照研究", 实用中医内科杂志, no. 12 (2014): 1–3.; 李婷婷, 魏明, and 李洪娟, "红外热像在中医学中的应用现状与展望", 北京中医药大学学报, 20, no. 4 (2013): 59–61.

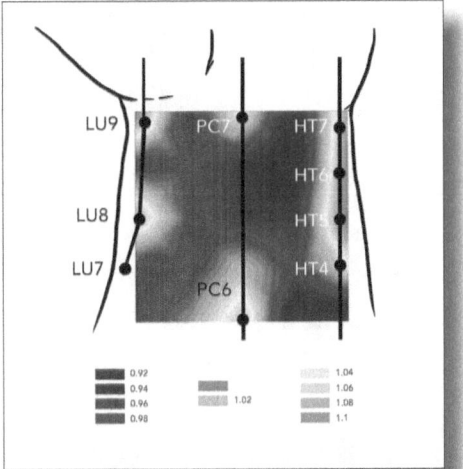

Figure 3: Oxygen variations at the wrist.

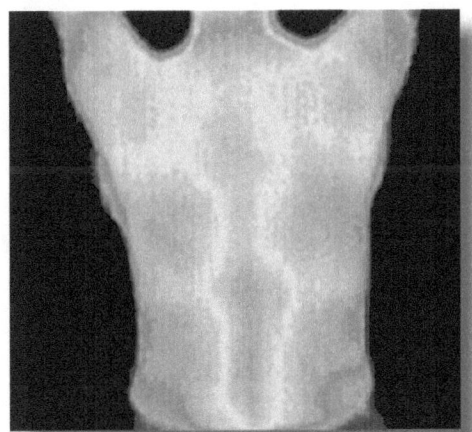

Figure 4: Infra-red imaging of *Du* meridian.

Figure 5: Infra-red imaging of left leg of a woman with liver cancer. Part of the liver meridian shows up as a white (hot) region.

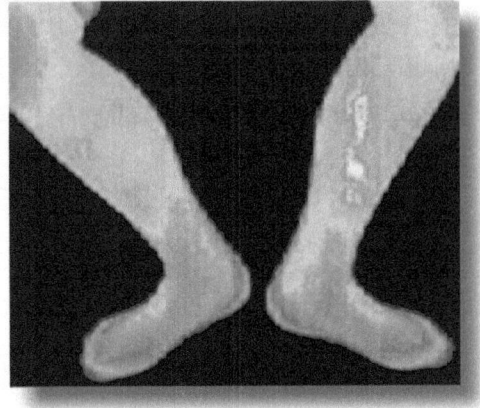

meridian (*dumai*, 督脉).[25] There is also growing evidence that other meridians, such as the liver and stomach meridians can be detected, at least partly.[26] The use of infra-red imaging in TCM research is still in its infancy, and shows great potential for applications in TCM clinical diagnostics.

Classical medical theory asserts that "disharmonies in an organ may manifest themselves in the corresponding meridians". Thus, pain along the heart meridian may indicate blood stasis or stagnant *qi* in the heart, while excess fire in the liver may cause redness in the eye, which is connected to the liver meridian.[27] The aim of Chinese medical therapy is to rebalance the *yinyang* within the meridians. This can be achieved, for example, by acupuncture or herbal drug therapy. More will be explained later about the diverse therapeutic approaches in this tradition. Before that, we need to consider the Chinese conception of disease and their causes, that is, Chinese aetiology.

Causes of Diseases

If health is the optimal functioning of or harmony within one's physiological systems, sicknesses must arise, therefore, from a disharmony within the same. However, a careful Chinese physician would not interpret the presenting disharmony as the cause of the disease. For instance, if one experiences tiredness, a lack of appetite and suffers from loose stools, the disharmony expressed may be a deficiency in spleen *qi*. This deficiency, however, should not be regarded as the cause of the disease. Rather, the cause of the disharmony should be found in the patient's dietary habits, environment, exercise regime and other aspects of his lifestyle.[28] For instance, the root cause for his spleen *qi* deficiency may well be due to the patient's habit of

---

26   "What Are Meridians? Can We See Them?", accessed 15 August 2016, http://www. acupuncturetoday.com/archives2004/mar/03lo.html.

27   Kaptchuk, *Chinese Medicine*, 107.

28   Maciocia, *Foundations of Chinese Medicine*, 237.

taking meals irregularly. For this reason, a good physician would not only treat the spleen *qi* deficiency, but also identify and rectify this underlying cause, so as to ensure a more permanent recovery.

According to Chinese medical theory, the causes of diseases may be categorised into four groups: the environment, the emotions, bodily constitution and one's way of life.[29]

Environment

We begin with the six pernicious influences (*liuyin*, 六淫), which take their names from six climatic phenomena: Wind, Cold, Fire/ Heat, Dampness, Dryness and Summer Heat (*feng han shu shi zao huo*, 风寒暑湿燥火). True to their names, these influences often denote external factors ("external pernicious influences") that adversely affect one's body. For example, the dampness of one's environment, be it the workplace or home, can infiltrate one's body. This, in turn, leads to an accumulation of damp *qi* (*shiqi*, 湿气) in the body, and a consequent deficiency in the spleen and digestive ability. In a similar vein, cold weather can attack the body, reduce body heat, and stiffen the muscles, thus giving rise to sudden chills, headaches and body aches.[30]

These six climatic phenomena can also function as analogies of one's pathological experience. For example, dampness (*shi*, 湿) is typically associated with wetness, heaviness and slowness. The following attributes often appear in one form or another in the symptoms of someone who suffers from a condition of Dampness: excretions that are copious and turbid; limbs that feel heavy and sore; a dislike for damp environments; or oozing skin eruptions. Likewise, Coldness (*han*, 寒) is generally associated with a lack of warmth, slowness or immobility. A person diagnosed as suffering

---

29   Diagnosing these four areas is commonly called *Distinguishing the Causes of the Disease* (*bingyinbianzheng*, 病因辨证). Hongzhou Wu, ed., *Learning Chinese Medical Diagnosis in 100 Days* (一百天中医诊断) (Shanghai: Shanghai Science and Technology Publishing, 2015), 3.

30   Kaptchuk, *Chinese Medicine*, 147–48, 152–53.

from Coldness will experience cold limbs, frequent urination, the need for extra blankets to keep warm and the lack of sexual desire. In both cases, these bodily symptoms may or may not be due to attacks from external dampness or coldness to begin with. Nevertheless, they would be taken by the physician as experiencing a damp or cold disharmony.

Seen from this perspective, it should be clear that the six pernicious influences may be understood either aetiologically, as an indication of the adverse effect that an environmental factor has on a body, or simply as a description of one's pathological condition (known otherwise as "internal pernicious influence").[31] Moreover, a patient may well suffer from multiple pernicious influences, whether external, internal or both.

Emotions (*qing*, 情)

As mentioned earlier, Chinese medical anthropology posits an intimate relationship between one's spirit and body. One's psychological

---

Summer Flood Disaster and Onset of Heat-Dampness Pernicious Influence

Background: A volunteer spent a month working in a flood disaster relief project. It was summer season and the weather was very hot at the disaster zone. When he returned from his project, he found himself feeling lethargic, his limbs heavy, and his tongue fat with teeth marks.

Diagnosis: He was suffering from the pernicious influences of heat and dampness (*shushi*, 暑湿). The heat was due to the hot weather at the disaster location. The dampness arose due to prolonged contact with the flood conditions.

---

31   For a more detailed discussion of the different forms of pernicious influences, see Kaptchuk, 146–60.

abilities, in other words, are bounded closely with how well one's organ systems are functioning. The reverse is also true. Overexertion of one's emotions can likewise harm one's organs and health. Chinese medical theory has identified seven types of emotional strain (*qiqing*, 七情) that can adversely affect our organs. They are listed below, together with the organs they affect, the disharmony they cause and the symptoms that arise.[32]

Table 2: The Seven Emotions, the Organ Systems and Disharmonies

Emotions	Organ Systems	Disharmony	Common Symptoms
Joy (*xi*, 喜)	Heart[33]	Slows down *qi*.	Palpitations, over-excitability, insomnia, restlessness. Sudden joy is akin to shock.
Anger (*nu*, 怒)	Liver	Stagnation of liver *qi*/blood, rising of liver *yang*, or blazing of liver-fire.	Headaches, dizziness, neck stiffness, red blotches on front of neck, red face.
Worry (*you*, 忧)	Lungs & Spleen	Obstructs and causes *qi* to stagnate ("knots" the *qi*)	(Lungs) Uncomfortable feeling of the chest, slight breathlessness, tensing of shoulder, dry cough, weak voice. (Spleen) Poor appetite, slight epigastric discomfort, abdominal distension, tiredness, pale complexion.

32   Maciocia, *Foundations of Chinese Medicine*, 241–54.
33   It is noteworthy that recent research on *takotsubo cardiomyopathy*, a change in the shape of the heart's left ventricle, suggests that one in 20 cases of cases are caused by joy-induced stress. James Gallagher, "Moments of Joy 'Can Damage Heart'", *BBC News*, 3 March 2016, sec. Health, http://www.bbc.com/news/health-35710232.

Emotions	Organ Systems	Disharmony	Common Symptoms
Brooding/ Pensiveness (*si*, 思)	Spleen	Stagnates *qi* of the heart. Affects the spleen and "knots" the *qi*.	Poor appetite, slight epigastric discomfort, abdominal distension, tiredness, pale complexion.
Sadness (*bei*, 悲)	Lungs & Heart	Cramps and agitates the heart, leading to poor circulation of Nutritive and Defensive *qi*. Heat accumulates and dissolves the *qi*.	Breathlessness, tiredness, feeling of discomfort in the chest, depression or crying.
Fear (*kong*, 恐)	Kidneys	Affects the kidneys and makes the *qi* descend.	Nocturnal enuresis, incontinence of urine and diarrhoea.
Shock (*jing*, 惊)	Heart	Affects the heart and scatters the *qi*.	Palpitations, breathlessness, insomnia.

Excessive Brooding, *Qi* Stagnation and Blood Stasis

Background: A middle-aged female patient complained of swollen and hurting breasts, and chest pain near the rib cage area. Her periods were often irregular and accompanied with blood clots. She also confided that she was experiencing some "domestic issues" at home.

Diagnosis: Her excessive brooding (*si*, 思) led to an inefficient flow of her *qi* (*qiyu*, 气郁). This gave rise to two pathological problems. (1) An inefficient flow of liver *qi*. Since the liver stores blood (*changexue*, 藏血) and oversees the lung area (*zhufei*, 主肺), this led to pain in her breasts and chest (below her rib cage), and blood stasis and clots. (2) When her spleen was hurt, her spleen *qi* also stagnated (*qizhi*, 气滞). Since, the spleen governs the blood and oversees *qi* (统血主气), spleen *qi* deficiency magnified her blood stasis and clots.

Body Types and Constitution

Unlike biomedicine, which adopts a rather homogeneous view of human bodies, classical Chinese medicine takes a more heterogeneous understanding by dividing human beings into five body types (*tizhi*, 体质). These are categorised according to the five phases (*wuxing*): wood, fire, wood, metal, and water. More recently, due to the research of Wang Qi (王琦) and others, the Chinese Pharmaceutical Association (中华中医药学会) has issued a new set of guidelines for determining one's body type. According to the Chinese Medicine Body Type Categorisation and Differentiation (中医体质分类与判定), human bodies can now be categorised into nine types.[34] Despite using different categories, both systems concur that specific physical and psychological characteristics can be attributed to each body type. This, in turn, renders one body type more susceptible to some diseases than others.[35]

---

34   The nine body types are balanced (平和质), *qi* deficiency (气虚质), *yang* deficiency (阳虚质), *yin* deficiency (阴虚质), phlegm-dampness (痰湿质), heat-dampness (湿热质), blood stasis (血瘀质), *qi*-depression (气郁质), and allergic (特禀质) body types. These different body types can be ascertained through a diagnostic questionnaire, the Chinese Medicine Body Type Categorisation and Differentiation Questionnaire (中医体质分类与判定表). " 中医体质分类与判定自测表 - 中医药学百科", accessed 15 January 2018, http://zhongyiyao.h.baike.com/article-1344880.html.

35   Li, *Simplest Introduction*, 26–30.

Physiological-Environmental Conditions and Body Constitution

Background: A pair of 10-year-old twins came to Dr Diarra for consultation. The elder weighed only 30 kg, while the younger weighed 50 kg.

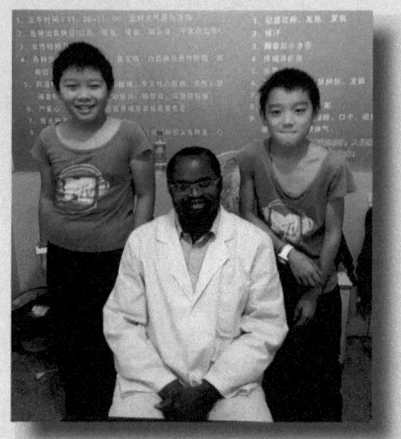

Diagnosis: Both suffer from spleen deficiency (*pixu*, 脾虚), which is due most likely to their pre-natal constitution (in view of the fact that they are twins). The two, however, experience different forms of spleen deficiency. The older brother suffers from spleen *qi* deficiency (气虚), leading to malnutrition, severe underweight and a lack of strength. The younger suffers from a deficient digestion and absorption ability (spleen transformation problems 脾主运化, 脾运化失调) and *yang* deficiency. Consequently, dampness accumulated in his interior body (水湿内停), leading to significant weight gain.

Therapy: The older brother was prescribed *Invigorating Spleen and Replenishing Qi* pills (*buzhong yiqi wan*, 补中益气丸) to strengthen his spleen *qi* (*bupiqi*, 补脾气). His younger brother was prescribed *Shenling Baigu San* (参苓白术散) to strengthen his *yang* (扶阳) and spleen (*jianpi*, 健脾), and to get rid of the dampness (*huatan*, 化痰).

In addition, every person is believed to be born with a specific body constitution. This depends largely on his "parent's health in general and their health at the time of conception specifically". This is also influenced by his mother's health during the course of her pregnancy. This physiological basis that one inherits from one's parents is known as "pre-natal" (*xiantian*, 先天) constitution.[36]

Way of Life

Finally, our lifestyles also play an important role in our health. [37]

a) Overwork, or "working excessively long hours for many years" often becomes a cause for disease as it involves irregular diets, emotional stress and a lack of rest. Such a hectic lifestyle often depletes one's *qi* severely.

b) Regular exercise is essential for a proper circulation of *qi*. The lack of it, therefore, will lead to *qi* stagnation and, oftentimes, Dampness in the body. It is to be noted that fitness need not correspond to health. A fit person may be able to run a marathon, but may still be unhealthy (that is, he could still suffer from a stroke).

c) In the case of men, excessive sexual activity can cause depletion in their kidney essence and is, therefore, regarded as a cause of disease. By "sexual activity" we mean "actual ejaculation for men". Sexual activities not culminating in these experiences would not be detrimental. Such activity should thus be moderated, according to the man's age, health and even the seasons. Interestingly, Chinese medicine also recognises that insufficient sex can also be a cause of disease and a moderate practice can benefit both genders.

d) Not surprisingly, insufficient eating, overeating, the conditions of

---

36   Maciocia, *Foundations of Chinese Medicine*, 267.
37   Ibid., 271–77.

eating (e.g., eating hurriedly) or eating the wrong types of food can be damaging to one's body.

e) Finally, one can also become sick due to poisons, physical trauma, wrong treatments and the use of recreational drugs.

Medical Diagnosis

Having considered the different ways in which one can fall ill, we turn now to the diagnostic methods commonly employed by Chinese physicians. In a typical Chinese medical consultation, a physician will apply the "Four Examinations" (*sizhen*, 四诊) of observation, smelling, interrogation (or questioning) and touching, commonly known as *wangwenwenqie* (望闻问切).

Four Examinations

The aim of the Four Examinations is to collate the diverse data related to the patient's sickness, so as to arrive at a pattern or an "image of the disharmony" experienced by him.

• *Observation (wangzhen, 望诊)*

When a patient first enters the clinic, her general appearance, that is, her physical shape and manner of behaviour, are observed. This is followed by the colour and quality of her face and skin. For example, the physician will note whether her face is red, pink, greenish, or pale; where is it wrinkled; and how the different hues are distributed on different parts of her face. As for her skin, the physician will note whether it is damp, dry or oily. Pathologically speaking, a white face that is lacklustre and withered signifies deficient blood, while a face that is entirely red is often a sign of excess heat.[38]

    Besides the skin, attention is also paid to the tongue. Specifically, both the "tongue material and the coating of the tongue" (*shetai*,

---

38   Kaptchuk, *Chinese Medicine*, 179.

舌苔) are examined.[39] Again, the colour of the tongue, such as the degree of redness, is noted, along with the thickness, colour, texture and general appearance of the tongue coating. For example, a very red tongue is a sign of a Heat condition in the body, while a very thick coating is almost always a sign of excess.[40] As in the case of the face, hues and textures on different parts of the tongue can be signs of deficiencies. The shape and contour of the tongue, along with any visible cracks can also be indicative of deficiencies in particular organs.

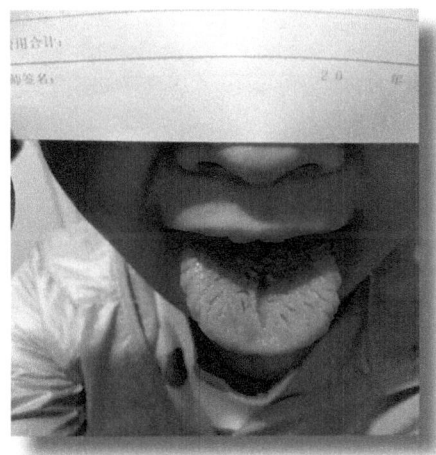

Figure 6: This patient's tongue has a deep groove or wrinkle (裂纹) in the middle, and multiple tongue wrinkles (舌纹) all over. The middle groove usually indicates problems with her stomach-spleen organ systems (that is, digestive problems). The multiple wrinkles suggest both *qi* and *yin* deficiency (气阴两虚).

Another area to be observed is the patient's secretions and excretions, that is, his phlegm, vomit, urine and blood. A clear and thin phlegm, for example, is usually a sign of a Cold pattern whereas a yellow sticky phlegm is usually a part of a Heat pattern.[41]

39　Tongue coating is also commonly translated as "moss" or "fur".
40　Kaptchuk, *Chinese Medicine*, 181–83.
41　Ibid., 185–86.

The Story of Bian Que's Observation Skills

Bian Que (扁鹊, 401–310 BC) is one of the most famous physicians in Chinese medical history, renowned for his ability to diagnose his patients simply by observation. It is said that he once met a prince, Lord Qihuan, and saw that he did not look well. When Bian Que advised Qihuan that 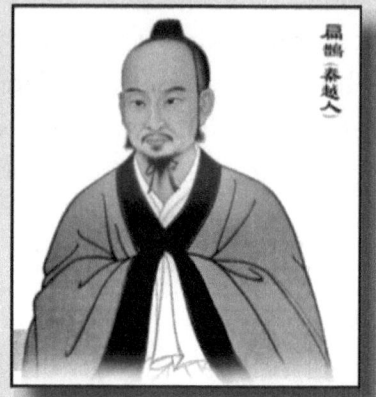 he should treat himself, lest his sickness worsened, the doctor was ignored.

Five days later, when Bian Que saw Lord Qihuan again, he noticed that the prince's illness had reached his blood and meridians (血脉) and advised treatment. Again, he was ignored. Yet another five days later, Bian Que saw the prince. This time, he exclaimed that the sickness had reached the prince's stomach and intestines. If he did not treat it then, it would be fatal. The prince was angered by his words and refused to listen. The fourth time Bian Que saw the prince, he feared the worst and immediately ran away. Curious at his behaviour, the prince asked his subjects to search out the doctor.

This was when Bian Que disclosed that the prince's illness was now fatal and could not be cured. True enough, five days later, the prince fell ill and Bian Que was nowhere to be found. Shortly after, the prince succumbed to his illness.

Dr Sun Guangrong Predicts a Woman's Death

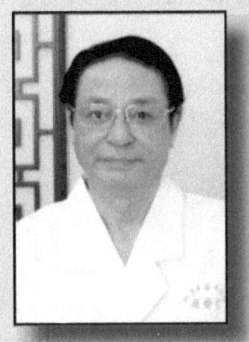

Background: Dr Sun Guangrong (孙光荣) is a National Master Physician (*Guoyi Dashi*, 国医大师) and the teacher of Dr Diarra. Sun once returned from a consultation looking rather glum. His colleague noticed and asked whether he was tired from the long walk back from his patient's house. Sun replied that the family was poor and could only afford to treat his young patient's sickness. Yet, it was the mother's sickness that was terminal. In fact, he predicted that she would die within the next 5–6 days. Astonished, the colleague enquired further about her condition.

Diagnosis: Sun explained that she suffers from bone flaccidity (*guwei*, 骨痿), judging from her syndromes—"house leaking" pulse (*wuloumai*, 屋漏脉), her flattened *renzhong* acu-point (人中平满), her completely flattened ankle and posterior tibia (脚踝、后胫骨都平了).[42] As the saying goes, "when the area between one's knees and foot flattens, the patient will die within five days" (足膝后平者，五日死). Sure enough, the poor lady passed away five days later.[43]

---

42   *Wuloumai* is one of the seven strange pulses. The pulse moves once in a long while and is uneven, slow and without strength. It feels like water leaking from a house's roof, dripping once in a long while. It is generally regarded as an indication that the patient's stomach *qi* and defensive *qi* have been exhausted and she is at her deathbed.

43   杨建宇, 明医薪传: 北京同仁堂中医大师孙光荣教授学术经验传承 (北京: 学苑出版社, 2010), 79.

• *Listening and Smelling (wenzhen,* 闻诊*)*

Here, attention is paid to the voice and respiration of a patient—whether his voice is coarse, or he has shortness of breath, or a weak, low voice. Wheezing may suggest mucus while a chronic loss of voice is usually a sign of deficiency.[44] With regards to smells, a foul, rotten, and nauseating odour often signifies heat, while the smell of fumes from bleach suggests cold and deficiency.

• *Interrogation or Asking (wenzhen,* 问诊*)*

Like the biomedical doctor, a Chinese physician would ask a series of diagnostic questions. For example, whether the patient feels hot or cold; how much he perspires; whether he has loose stools or constipation; whether he lacks appetite, feels dizzy, suffers from migraine; and what is the quality of his bodily pains, lifestyle and dietary habits.[45]

• *Touching and Pulse Diagnosis (qiezhen,* 切诊*)*

Finally, the physician would touch the different parts of the patient's body and his various acupuncture points. More commonly, he would diagnose the patient's sickness by feeling the palpitations at the patient's wrist. These palpitations, according to Chinese medical theory, arise from the 12 meridians linked to the left and right wrists, and provide a good indication of the health of the different organ systems. Three pairs of meridian palpitations can be detected on each wrist. On the superficial level, one can detect the palpitations of the small intestine, gall bladder and bladder on the left wrist. When we press deeper on the wrist, the palpitations of the heart, liver, and kidney organ systems can be detected. Likewise, at the superficial level of the right wrist, the palpitations of the large intestine/colon,

---

44   Kaptchuk, *Chinese Medicine*, 186.

45   A Ming physician, Zhang Jingyue (张景岳, 1563–1640), even composed a song, called the *Ten Questions* (十问歌) to summarise the different questions a physician should ask of his patient.

stomach and *sanjiao* can be detected. At the deeper level, those of the lungs, spleen and pericardium can be read.

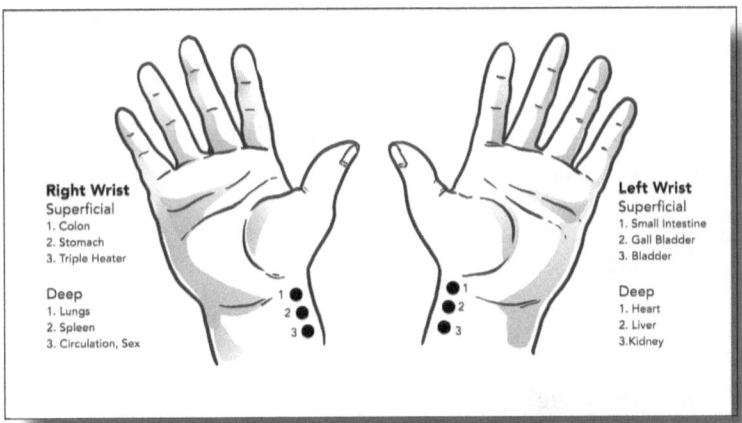

Figure 7: Meridian Pulse Diagnosis

Depending on the type of pulse detected at each organ system, the seriousness of the disease can be assessed. For example, a floating pulse (*fumai*, 浮脉) suggests a disharmony in the superficial parts of the body. A sinking or deep pulse (*chenmai*, 沉脉), on the other hand, indicates that the disharmony is internal and, therefore, more serious. In total, 18 different types of pulses can be detected at both wrists, thus making pulse diagnosis a complex discipline that requires much training and experience.[46]

Eight Principal Patterns (八纲辨证)

After detecting the different symptoms expressed by the patient, a physician must then interpret this complex of symptoms and signs to determine the patient's pattern of disharmony. For example, he could be suffering from a liver *qi* stagnation, a deficiency in spleen *qi*, or a Cold condition. Among the interpretative paradigms employed by Chinese physicians, the most popular is the *Distinguishing of the Eight*

---

46   For more details of the different pulses, see Kaptchuk, *Chinese Medicine*, 194–210.

Principal Patterns (*bangangbianzheng*, 八纲辨证), to be referred hereafter as the *Eight Principal Patterns*.

According to the *Eight Principal Patterns*, there are four pairs of disharmony patterns:

- Exterior (*biaozheng*, 表证) versus Interior (*lizheng*, 里证) Patterns.
- Deficiency (*xuzheng*, 虚证) versus Excess (*shizheng*, 实证) Patterns.
- Cold (*hanzheng*, 寒证) versus Hot (*rezheng*, 热证) Patterns.
- *Yin* (*yinzheng*, 阴证) versus *Yang* (*yangzheng*, 阳证) Patterns.

Predicting Blood Stasis through Pulse Diagnosis

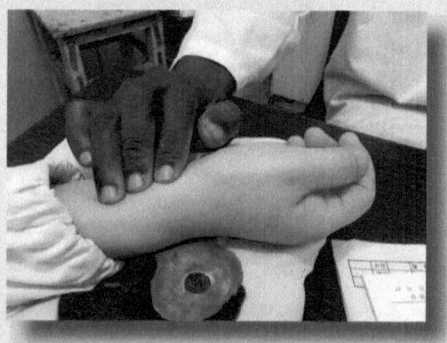

Diagnosis: A female patient was diagnosed with a *chi* pulse (*chimai*, 尺脉) that felt like an uneven or rough string (*xuanse*, 炫涩). This suggested that her lower torso (*xiajiao*, 下焦) had blood stasis or clots. She was advised to take an ultrasound scan which confirmed that there were blood clots in the same location.

• *Exterior/Interior Pattern* (表里)

The aim of distinguishing between the exterior or interior patterns is to assess the spatial location of the disharmony. Exterior patterns are usually due to external influences, while interior patterns are usually generated by internal disharmony. The former are often due to attacks by environmental factors (such as a sudden onset of cold weather), while the latter are often associated with a person's constitution, emotional life and chronic conditions.

• *Deficiency/Excess Patterns* (虚实)

An illness characterised by insufficient *qi*, blood and other vital substances, or by an inadequate activity in the *yin* or *yang* aspects of the organs is taken to be a Deficiency pattern. General signs include frailty, weak mobility, paleness and shallow breath. A pattern of Excess often occurs when a "Pernicious Influence attacks, when some bodily function becomes overactive, or when an obstruction causes an inappropriate accumulation of substances such as *qi* and blood". General signs of Excess patterns include a loud and full voice, heavy breathing, scanty urination, chest pains and thick tongue moss.[47]

• *Cold/Hot Patterns* (寒热)

When a patient's body lacks *yang* qi or suffers an attack by Cold Pernicious Influences, he will manifest a Cold disharmony pattern. Signs include slow, deliberate movements, a white face, fear of cold, cold limbs and watery stools. Heat disharmony, on the other hand, may be due to "a heat Pernicious Influence, hyperactivity of the body's *Yang* functions, or insufficient *Yin* or fluids, leading to a preponderance of *Yang*". Signs include delirium, talkative manner, high fever, red face and eyes, irritability, thirst and constipation.[48]

---

47   Kaptchuk, *Chinese Medicine*, 219.
48   Ibid., 219–20.

• *Yin/Yang Patterns* (阴阳)

Finally, the *Yin* or *Yang* pattern is a general categorisation of the illness at hand. *Yin* patterns are basically "combinations of signs associated with Interior, Deficiency, and Cold", while *Yang* patterns are associated with "Exterior, Excess and Heat" disharmonies. In reality, however, very few illnesses are entirely *Yin* or *Yang*. Most patients present a "complex mixture of Yin and Yang signs and symptoms". For this reason, explained Kaptchuk, the Eight Principal Patterns are "inadequate descriptions of clinical reality" and ought to be used only as a "preliminary guidance for further perceptual refinement".[49]

It should be noted that the *Eight Principal Patterns* is but one of the many diagnostic paradigms that a TCM physician can employ. Another common paradigm, which Dr Diarra uses frequently, is *Zangfu* Organ Pattern Diagnosis (*Zangfu Bianzheng*, 脏腑辨证). Here, the diagnosis will focus on whether a specific organ system suffers from a cold or hot pattern (*bianhanre*, 辩寒热), a deficiency or excess pattern (*bianxushi*, 辩虚实), an "according or contrary" to pattern (*bianshunni*, 辩顺逆) and life or death pattern (*bianshengsi*, 辩生死).[50]

Therapies

Once the Chinese physician determines the dominant patterns of disharmony, he then prescribes the therapies needed to treat the disharmony. While centuries of medical development have generated a wide range of possible therapeutic approaches, a typical physician would have access to a more limited range of options, depending on

---

49   Ibid., 221–22.

50   Under the "According to or Contrary to" Pattern, we observe whether the *yinyang* diagnosis gathered from other clinical observations coheres with or is contrary to one another or with the pulse diagnosis. Typically, a *yang* pattern should fit with a *yang* pulse. Should one look skinny but have a large pulse (*xingshou maida*, 形瘦脉大), for example, a contrary pattern is likely. 杨建宇, 明医薪传, 30–33.

his training and resources. What follows are brief descriptions of the main therapies that a patient can expect to encounter.

Drug therapy

The most common form of Chinese medical therapy is to prescribe drugs, which has "a direct, internal influence on the body's physiology".[51] Unlike the common biomedical drugs, which rely on a dominant active ingredient, most Chinese drug prescriptions are drug formulas, or, if you will, drug cocktails. The formulations of these prescriptions are governed by the logic of *junchenzuoshi* (君臣佐使). To illustrate how this logic operates, take Zhang Zhongjing's Cinnamon Twig Decoction (*guizhitang*, 桂枝汤), for example.

> Cinnamon twig as the ruler (*jun*, 君) expresses the therapeutic aim, which is to release wind-cold from the body's exterior layers of skin and flesh to the outside. The minister (*chen*, 臣), peony root, supports the ruler cinnamon by providing supplementary benefit to the *yin* (interior) of the body's *yin-yang* economy. Ginger root and jujube dates are the assistants (*zuo*, 佐), which modify the main drugs or moderate side effects. Licorice root is the envoy (*shi*, 使), directing the formula to the body's centre.[52]

Chinese drugs are processed in a wide variety of ways, some by roasting (with a liquid adjuvant; *jiu*, 灸), some by baking (*hongbei*, 烘焙), while others by steaming (*zheng*, 蒸) and stewing (*ao*, 熬).[53] As for the formulas, they are also made available in different forms, such as preparation (*jixing*, 剂型), cream (*rugao*, 乳膏), powder (*san*,

---

51   Maciocia, *Foundations of Chinese Medicine*, 1128.

52   Bridie Andrews, *The Making of Modern Chinese Medicine, 1850–1960* (Vancouver: UBC Press, 2014), 51.

53   Zhufan Xie, *On the Standard Nomenclature of Traditional Chinese Medicine* (Beijing: Foreign Languages Press, 2003), 242–43.

散), adhesive plaster (*gaoyao*, 膏药), tablets (*pian*, 片) and granules (*chongji*, 冲剂).[54] It should be clear by now that the *junchenzuoshi* model does not mean that a drug formula consists of only four drugs. Rather, there can be multiple herbs prescribed in each category. Dr Diarra, for example, often uses twelve herbs in his formulas, three herbs for each category.

Acupuncture

While acupuncture or needling (*zhen*, 针) is often regarded, at least in the West, as the dominant form of TCM therapy, it is most often used in conjunction with drug therapies. A typical treatment may see 20 to more than 100 needles inserted into the patient's acupuncture points. Not infrequently, it is administered along with moxibustion, where a lump of moxa is burnt at one end of the needle (warm needling or *wenzhen*, 温针). Some physicians even heat the needles before administering them, thus giving the name, "fire needles" (*huozhen*, 火针). As and when necessary, electric currents are passed through the needles to magnify the effects of needling ("electric needling", *dianzhen*, 电针).

Needling therapies operate by the logic that the treatment of the exterior body can have a positive influence on the internal organs and physiology. This could operate in different ways. The following are but a few examples.

To tonify the Upright *Qi*, acupuncture stimulates the *qi* of the Internal Organs to work better and therefore produce *qi* and blood; to expel pathogenic factors, acupuncture works mainly by moving *qi* of various organs. For example, in order to resolve Phlegm, acupuncture relies on the stimulation of the *qi* of the lungs, spleen, kidneys and triple burner so that fluids are transformed, transported and excreted.[5]

---

54   Ibid., 250.
55   Maciocia, *Foundations of Chinese Medicine*, 1128.

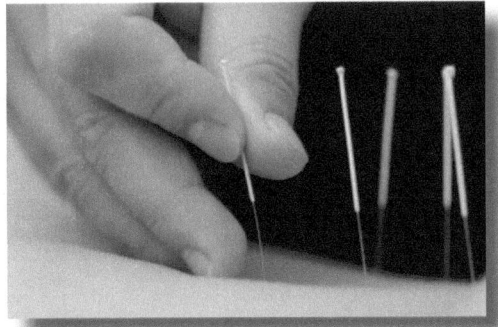

Figure 8: Acupuncture/ Needling

Figure 9: Needling with moxibustion

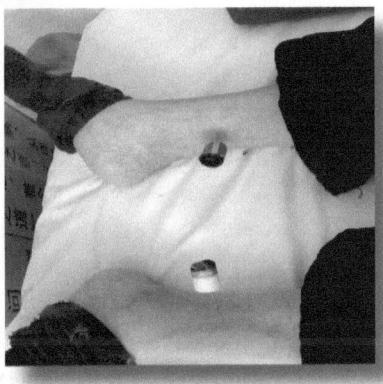

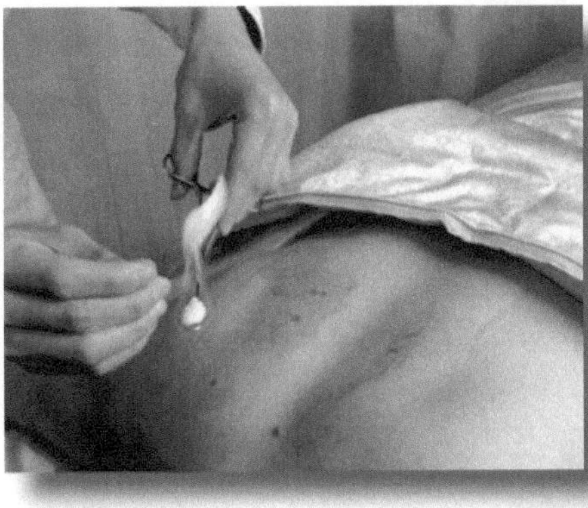

Figure 10: Fire Needling moxibustion

Figure 11: Electric Needling

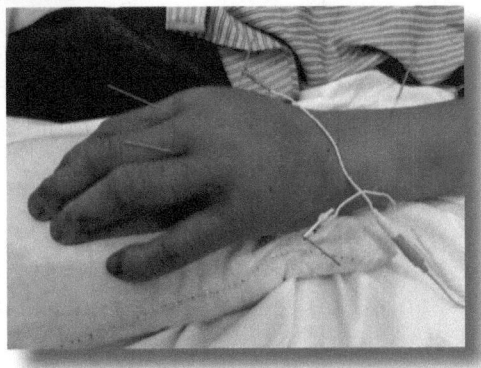

Emergency Acupuncture Treatment for Penicillin Allergy

Background: Once, while travelling on a train from Chengdu to Kunming, Dr Diarra heard a broadcast requesting for medical help. When he arrived at the scene, Dr Diarra found a 24-year-old man suffering from severe penicillin allergies.

Diagnosis: The man was feverish and breathing rapidly and with difficulty. Skin allergies had broken

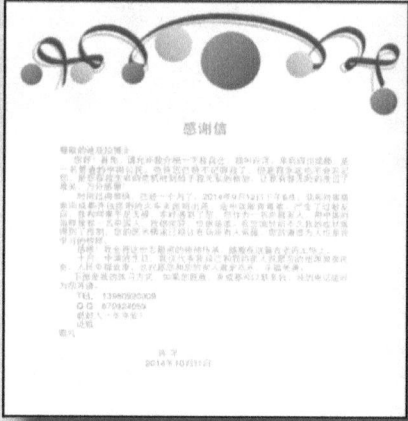

Figure 12: "Thank You" letter from patient

out on his feet, face and body. His facial complexion was also purplish red. There were a few biomedical doctors at the scene but they could do nothing. This was because biomedical treatment for penicillin allergies requires the use of corticosteroids. Unfortunately, the next stop was 3–4 hours away. At the rate that he was going, the man could possibly die within the next 1–2 hours.

Therapy: Dr Diarra needled the man's two *hegu* (合谷) and two *taichong* (太冲) acupuncture points. These four points are needled whenever the ailment encountered is unclear (*zabing*, 杂病). In addition, both his *quchi* (曲池) acu-points were also needled. This acupuncture technique is drawn from Through the Roof Needling Approach (*toutian liangzhenfa*, 透天凉针法).

Results: After 15 minutes, the patient's breathing and body temperature began to normalise. The rashes on his hands and face also started to subside, and his condition stabilised.

Acupuncture Treatment for Heat Stroke

Background: After a hot day at school, the author's son, Isaiah, came home feeling feverishly hot and drowsy. He also felt weak and could barely walk.

Diagnosis: The TCM physician diagnosed him as suffering from heatstroke.

Therapy: Isaiah's *baihui* (百会) and *fengchi* (风池) acupoints were needled. Bloodletting was also performed at the *shishuan* (十宣) acu-point of his index finger. Isaiah's headache and feverish symptoms subsided in 10–15 minutes and he regained his strength to walk.

Moxibustion

Moxibustion (*jiufa*, 灸法) is a form of thermotherapy that operates on the same logic as acupuncture, that is, to treat the exterior body as the means of affecting and healing the interior body. The substance that is commonly burnt is moxa or mugwort, because it is most easily ignited and produces heat gently.[56] Generally, moxibustion is administered either with a moxa-stick (Figure 13), a moxibustion box (Figure 14) or, sometimes, by burning moxa on top of a slice of ginger (*gejiangjiu*, 隔姜灸). Moxa therapy is helpful for treating common colds, arthritis, *qi* deficiency in organ systems (such as the heart, lungs, spleen, kidney and liver), hypertension, dampness, yang deficiency, giddiness, Cold disharmony, diarrhoea and other ailments.[57]

---

56   Xie, *Nomenclature*, 280.
57   刘红 (Liu Hong), 零基础学会艾灸 (*Learning Foundations of Moxibustion*) (江苏: 江苏凤凰科学技术出版社, 2015), 54–90.

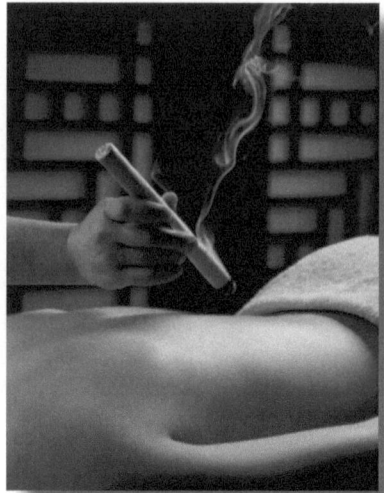

Figure 13: Moxibustion

Figure 14: Moxibustion Box

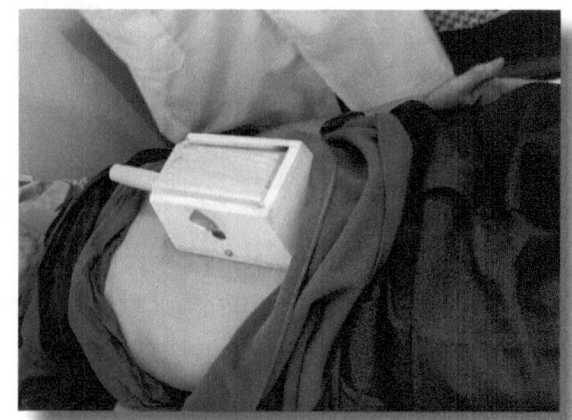

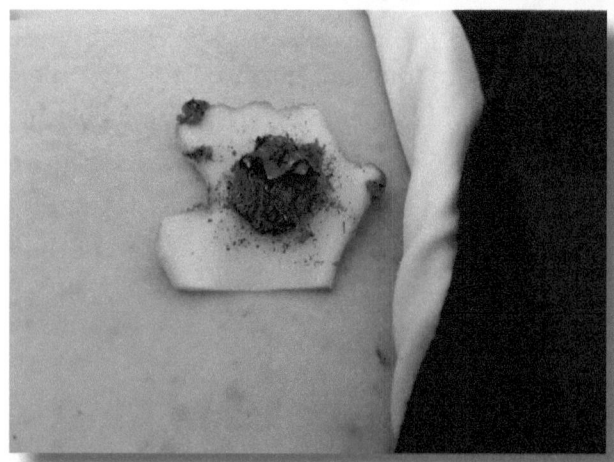

Figure 15: Burning Moxa on a Slice of Ginger

Moxibustion Treatment for Welder with *Yang Qi* Deficiency

Background: A 35-year-old male patient worked as a welder in a steel factory. Although this was a very hot work environment, he felt cold all the time and even had to wear a sweater while at work. When he returned home in the evenings, his wife had to prepare a very hot pail of water for his bath. When he consulted Dr Diarra, he complained of lower backaches (腰痛) and pre-ejaculation problems.

Diagnosis: The patient was suffering from kidney deficiency (*shenxu*, 肾虚) and *yang* deficiency (*yangxu*, 阳虚).

Therapy: Warm needling was administered to his *weizhong* (委中) and *sanyangjiao* (三阳交) acupuncture points. In addition, he also received ginger-base moxibustion (*gejiangjiu*, 隔姜灸), where a small pyramid of moxa is burnt on top of a slice of raw ginger placed at his *shenshu* (肾俞) and *mingmen* (命门).

Results: After the second day of treatment, he returned home for his bath. This time, he found the bath water too hot and scolded his wife for overheating the water. On consultation with Dr Diarra, they discovered that this was because his *yangqi* (阳气) had improved. After his seventh treatment, the patient recovered substantially and could go without his sweater at work.

Cupping (baguan, 拔罐)

In cupping therapy, cups made either of glass, plastic or bamboo are latched onto a specific area of skin (usually over an acupuncture point) by creating a vacuum in a cup. Generally, the vacuum is created by introducing a flame into the cup, followed by rapid withdrawal, or by suction. In a typical treatment, several vacuumed cups are positioned over one's back, legs and other parts of the body. In so doing, a Chinese physician is able to dispel dampness in the body, improve *qi* flow and even treat blood stasis.

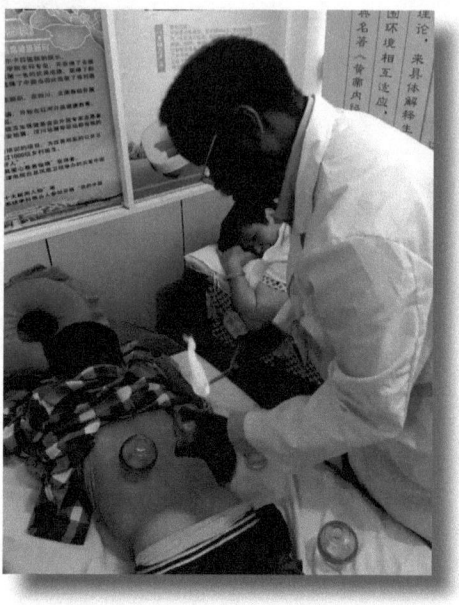

Cupping methods may differ—sometimes, a cup may be moved rapidly across one's back or face. Or it can be removed, vacuumed and repositioned rapidly. It is noteworthy that cupping is practised not only in Chinese medicine but is also in Greek, Islamic and European complementary medicine.

Chinese Therapeutic Massage (tuina, 推拿)

Like physiotherapy and chiropractic treatments, Chinese therapeutic massage, or *tuina* (推拿), is often used to treat musculoskeletal disorders (MSD) such as lower back pain, painful joints, sprains, cervical spondylosis (*jingzhuibing*, 颈椎病) and scoliosis (*jizucewan*, 脊柱侧弯). Where tuina differs from its Western counterparts is that it is also prescribed for giddiness, constipation, diarrhoea, chronic rhinitis (慢性鼻炎), myopia, fever, eczema and other forms of non-MSD ailments.[58] This is because many of these illnesses, as Chinese

---

58   刘明军 (Liu Mingjun), 推拿学 (*Chinese Massage Studies*) (北京: 人民卫生出版社, 2012), 159–249.

medical theory sees them, are due to a *qi* disharmony in the patient's organs and can be rectified, at least to some extent, by massaging the muscles and body.

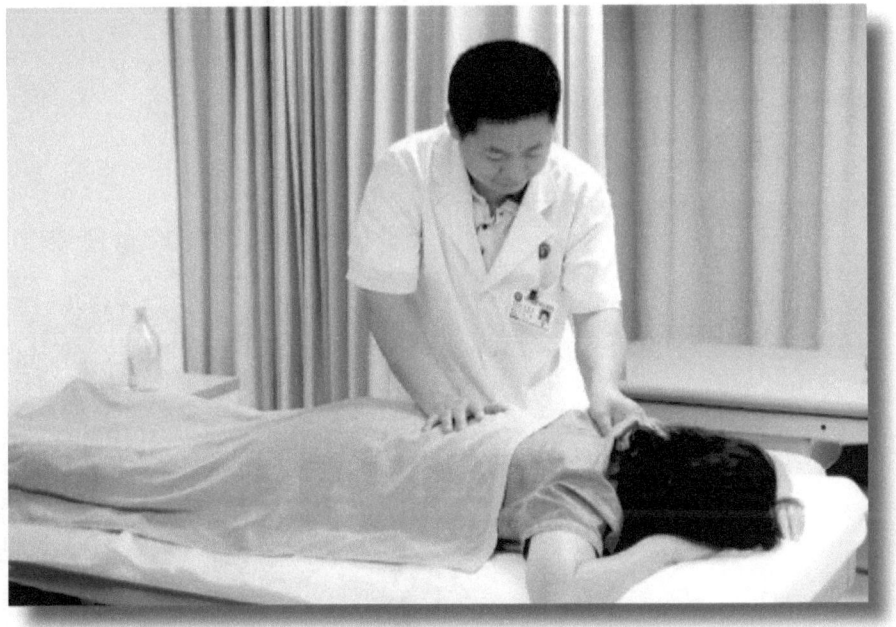

Figure 16: Chinese Therapeutic Massage

Other modern hybrid medical devices

In recent years, there has been much innovation in the TCM medical device industry. Several new devices have been introduced, often combining the therapeutic approaches of the traditional treatments mentioned above. The *Jingluo Jiudaoyi* (经络灸导仪), for example, mimics the moxibustion and acupuncture therapies by sending an electric current between two points of a body, usually on the spine. The *Fuyang Guan* (扶阳罐) likewise combines the therapeutic logic of tuina massage, cupping, moxibustion and acupuncture, with much success.

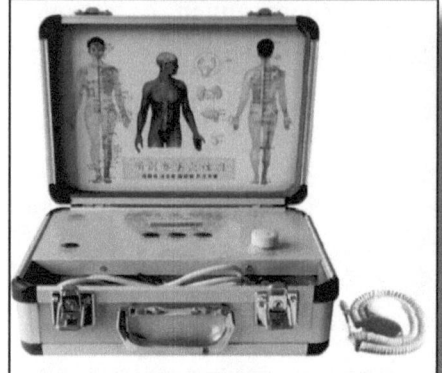

Figure 17: *Jingluo Jiudaoyi*

Figure 18: *Fuyang Guan* Treatment

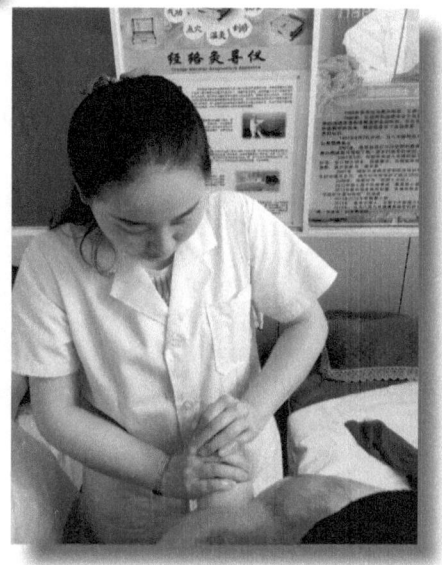

Chinese Healing Exercises

The earliest Chinese healing exercises were called *Daoyin* exercises (*daoyinshu*, 导引术), first practised by Han aristocrats as early as the second century BC.[59] Since then, these healing exercises have been developed in diverse ways and incorporated into different contexts, both religious and medical. The religious Daoists, for example, became avid proponents of these exercises, and incorporated them in their techniques for longevity.[60] The four eminent physicians

---

59   Tianjun Liu and Kevin W. Chen, *Chinese Medical Qigong* (London: Singing Dragon, 2010), 34.

60   Ibid., 46–47.

of the Jin-Yuan era likewise recognised the clinical value of these exercises and recommended them for a wide range of ailments. For example, Zhu Danxi, in his *Dan Xi's Experiential Therapy* (*danxixinfa*, 丹溪心法), teaches that "stagnation of *qi*, weakness, stiffness, cold, and heat can be treated with Dao Yin".[61] Besides religious and medical circles, *Daoyin* was also incorporated into martial arts by the Ming-Qing dynasties, thus giving rise to what is commonly known as internal

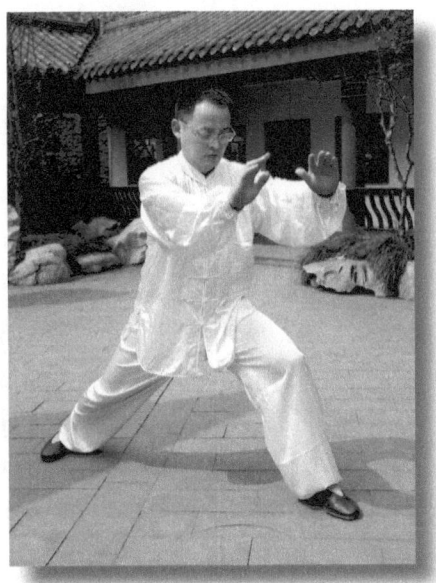

Figure 19: *Taiji* Boxing

martial arts (*neijiaquan*, 内家拳), such as Taiji Boxing (*taijiquan*, 太极拳), *Xingyi* Boxing (*xingyiquan*, 形意拳) and Bagua Palm (*baguazhang*, 八卦掌).

Over the last 50 years, *Daoyin* exercises have become known more popularly as Qigong Exercises (气功). Globally, they continue to be practised in diverse ways, as forms of medical therapy, non-religious "aerobic" exercises, in martial arts and also within religious contexts. With regards to Medical Qigong, it has proven successful in treating a wide range of ailments, such as pulmonary tuberculosis, coronary artery disease, chronic liver diseases, hypertension, peptic ulcers, myopia, tumours, depression and insomnia.[62] In most clinical encounters, however, it is still uncommon for Chinese physicians to prescribe Qigong exercises as part of their therapeutic strategies.[63] This being said, most Chinese physicians will regard regular Qigong

---

61   Ibid., 52.

62   Ibid., 367–509.

63   This is more common in TCM hospitals in China. As part of its development plan, a Chengdu TCM Hospital will build a park where Qigong exercises can be taught to its patients.

exercises as beneficial for one's health in general.

Having surveyed the history and medical benefits of Qigong, we turn to the actual practice itself. Qigong exercises may be categorised into active/moving forms (*donggong*, 动功) and still exercises (*jinggong*, 静功). The latter are generally meditative forms of exercise, while the former are essentially muscular stretching exercises aimed at conditioning one's muscles and meridians,

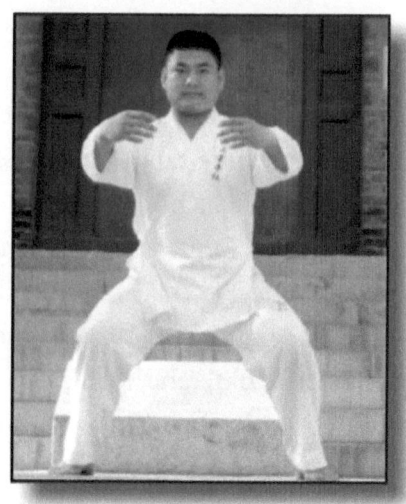

Figure 20: Stake Standing

making them supple. Where the active forms of Qigong differ from regular sports is their emphasis on coordinating one's movements and mental attention with one's breathing. The medical logic here is similar to that of *tuina*, namely, better muscular dexterity should improve the flow of blood and *qi* in the body and, therefore, the overall health of the practitioner's interior organs. Popular forms of such active exercises include the Eight Sectioned (or Eight Pieces of Brocade) Exercises (*baduanjin*, 八段锦), Six Words Formula (*liuzijue*, 六字诀), Muscle/ Tendon Changing Classic (*yijinjing*, 易筋经), Five Mimic-animal exercises (*wuqinxi*, 五禽戏) Stake Standing (*zhanzhuang*, 站桩) and even Taiji Boxing (*taijiquan*, 太极拳).[64]

---

64   For example, clinical trials for the *Baduanjin* Qigong exercise suggest that it can significantly improve sleep quality, premenstrual syndrome symptoms and knee osteoarthritis. Likewise, trials of *Taijiquan* found it to be helpful for improving aerobic endurance (and thus stroke recovery), and, quite possibly, alleviating oncological treatment symptoms. Mei Chuan Chen et al., "The Effect of a Simple Traditional Exercise Programme (*Baduanjin* Exercise) on Sleep Quality of Older Adults: A Randomized Controlled Trial", *International Journal of Nursing Studies* 49 (2012): 265–73; Huilin Zhang et al., "Baduanjin Exercise Improved Premenstrual Syndrome Symptoms in Macau Women", *Journal of Traditional Chinese Medicine* 34, no. 4 (2014): 460–64; Bing-chen An et al., "Effects of Baduanjin (八段锦) Exercise on Knee Osteoarthritis: A One-Year Study", *Chin J Integr Med.* 19, no. 2 (2013): 143–48; Ruth E. Taylor-Piliae et al., "Effect of Tai Chi on Physical Function, Fall Rates and Quality of Life Among Older

At this point, we should address a common concern of Christians. That is, whether Christians can practise Qigong, or would this practice expose Christians to the demonic realm? Generally speaking, most non-religious forms of active Qigong exercises, such as the Eight Sectioned Exercises and Taijiquan, are harmless and may be commended for their health benefits. Some Christians have even re-contextualised or, indeed, Christianised Qigong exercises into Praise Qigong Exercises (*zanmeicao*, 赞美操). For those interested in taking up active Qigong, we recommend that they do so under an experienced and reliable instructor who can guide and correct them over a prolonged period of time. It is best to avoid overseas instructors who offer short-term training but are not around to guide or correct the student. This is in order to avoid physical injuries due to improper training, such as injuries to the knees or spine.[65]

It should be noted that the silent or meditative forms of Medical Qigong exercises are usually more effective, but come with a higher degree of risk, both physical and spiritual. Physically speaking, when a practitioner experiences sudden shocks during his meditation (e.g., noises), he can easily injure himself. Consequently, an experienced instructor is necessary to guide his training. In other words, learning meditative Qigong without supervision is as dangerous as practicing demanding gymnastic exercises without supervision! Spiritually, higher levels of meditation have been recognised by all religious traditions, whether Christian, Buddhist or Daoist, as being able to sensitise the practitioner to the spiritual realm. The Christian Desert

Stroke Survivors", *Archives of Physical Medicine and Rehabilitation* 95 (2014): 816–24; Yingchun Zeng et al., "Health Benefits of Qigong or Tai Chi for Cancer Patients: A Systematic Review and Meta-Analyses", *Complementary Therapies in Medicine* 22 (2014):173—86.

65   With regards to still exercises, there have been rare cases where practitioners experience "Qigong deviation". This could range from minor symptoms such as headache, or shortness of breath to mental or emotional disorders. These deviations are due largely to improper practice, or training under inexperienced instructors. It is for this reason that one should carefully choose a reliable instructor. For treatment of deviation disorders, see Liu and Chen, *Chinese Medical Qigong*, 220–29.

Fathers of the fourth century, for example, were not unfamiliar with spiritual visions, whether divine or demonic. Much spiritual discernment is required, therefore, before one learns meditative Qigong. It is best to be learnt in a secular context, with an instructor trained in Medical Qigong and who does not emphasise the use of Qigong for gaining supernatural powers.[66] It is advised, however, that Christians avoid Qigong exercises that have incorporated Daoist or Buddhist teachings and rituals, since they may end up imbibing non-Christian ideas and rituals unknowingly.[67]

Qigong Practice and Longevity

Dr Deng Tietao (邓铁涛, 1916), TCM Emeritus Professor of Guangzhou TCM university (广州中医药大学), attributes his longevity to a regular practice of the Eight Brocade Exercises (*baduanjin*). He is 100 years old and esteemed nationwide as a National TCM Master Physician (*Guoyi Dashi*, 国医大师).

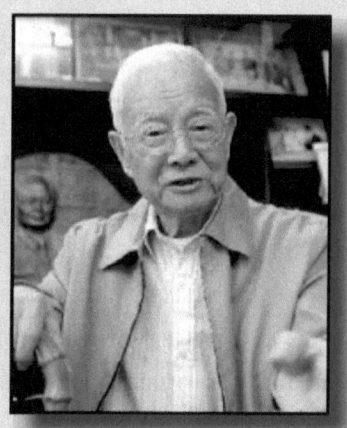

66   Medical Qigong classes are usually offered in TCM colleges in China. For the popularisation and eventual clampdown on Qigong practice (due to political reasons) in China, see David A. Palmer, *Qigong Fever: Body, Science, and Utopia in China* (New York: Columbia University Press, 2007).

67   For example, a TCM practitioner who provides bone setting, drug therapy, and acupuncture treatments, may also practice forms of religious healing. This could be summoning the aid of a deity to treat a particular ailment, or requiring a patient to drink a concoction of burnt talisman and water. In this case, even though the first three forms of treatment are secular or irreligious, one would be advised not to use this TCM physician, lest he received religious healing in the process. More will be said about discerning such treatments in Chapter 11.

Before we conclude, the following is another Emergency Treatment Case Study that Dr Diarra encountered while travelling on another train. This illustrates well how non-drug TCM therapy can help during occasions when drug therapies are not available.

TCM Emergency Treatment on a Train to Kunming

Background: Dr Diarra was on an overnight train from Liuzhou (柳州) to Kunming (昆明) when he heard a broadcast requesting medical help for three patients. When he arrived, he found himself in the company of five biomedical doctors and a nurse. There was a first-aid kit equipped with only a stethoscope, a thermometer and some cotton buds.

Diagnosis & Therapy 1: Patient A was a two-month-old baby girl. She had not been able to consume breast milk for the last five hours and was now seriously dehydrated, with signs of pneumonia, and a low body temperature of about 35°C. As the most serious case, she was treated first.

The nurse was instructed to moisturise a cotton bud with mineral water and drip the water into the baby's mouth. Meanwhile, Dr Diarra administered paediatric massage (小儿推拿) on her, by massaging both her palms and the lung meridian (肺经). This went on for 5 minutes each time, for 3–4 times in total. Forty minutes later, the baby began

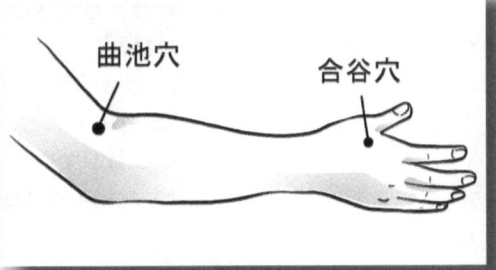

Figure 21: *Quchi* and *Hegu* Acu-points

to urinate, indicating that she was now hydrated, and her condition was stabilising. When the train reached Nanning (南宁), she was sent to the local hospital.

Diagnosis & Therapy 2: A 65-year-old woman (Patient B) had finished her hypertension medication while on holiday and was now on her way home. Unfortunately, her blood pressure had shot up to 185/115 mmHg (25/15 kPa). While treating A, Dr Diarra needled B's six acupuncture points: two at *hegu* (合谷), two at *taichong* (太冲), one each at *quchi* (曲池) and *taixi* (太溪). The needling technique he used is called "moving needle" (*xingzhen*, 行针), where the needle is rotated to stimulate the acu-points. After 30 minutes of treatment, the woman's blood pressure dropped to 150/95 mm Hg.

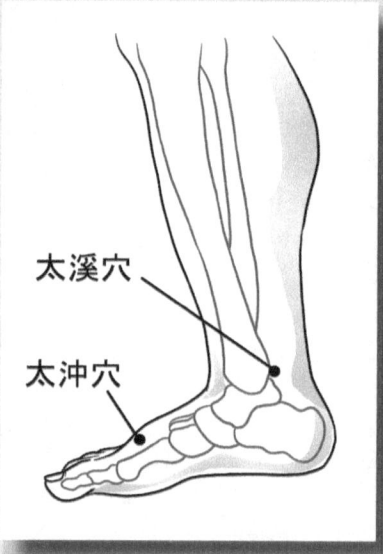

太溪穴

太冲穴

Figure 22: *Taixi* and *Taichong* Acu-points

Diagnosis & Therapy 3: A five-year-old boy was suffering from a 39°C fever and a bad sore throat. He was also crying and could not eat. To treat his fever, Dr Diarra administered bloodletting at the boy's *shaoshang* (少商) and *shangyang* (商阳) acu-points, located at the tip (near the nail) of his right-hand thumb and index finger. After an hour the boy recovered sufficiently and was able to eat his dinner.

Conclusion

Chinese medical theory is premised on the assumption that the body is constituted by a system of relationships between the different parts of the human body: the organs, blood, fluids, meridians, spirit and *qi*. Psychosomatic sicknesses occur whenever these relationships are not operating optimally, or as Chinese physicians would put it, there is a *qi* disharmony—an excess, a deficiency—or a *yinyang* imbalance in the body.

Over the last two millennia, Chinese medicine has developed two main approaches to medical diagnostics. The first is the method of Four Examinations, where a physician looks out for signs of disharmonies by observing the patient's face, skin and tongue; smelling her odours; enquiring about her medical history, dietary habits and lifestyle; and feeling her acupuncture points and meridian pulses. Second, the symptoms observed are then categorised according to the Eight Principal Patterns of interior versus exterior patterns, cold versus hot patterns, deficiency versus excess patterns, and *yin* versus *yang* patterns.

Having identified the primary patterns of disharmony, the physician has recourse to a wide range of therapies. Frequently, a drug formula would be prescribed, often supplemented by acupuncture, and other non-drug therapies such as moxibustion, cupping and Chinese massage. While medical Qigong is generally regarded as a legitimate form of therapy, it is often administered on its own, rarely in conjunction with the other forms of medical therapies.

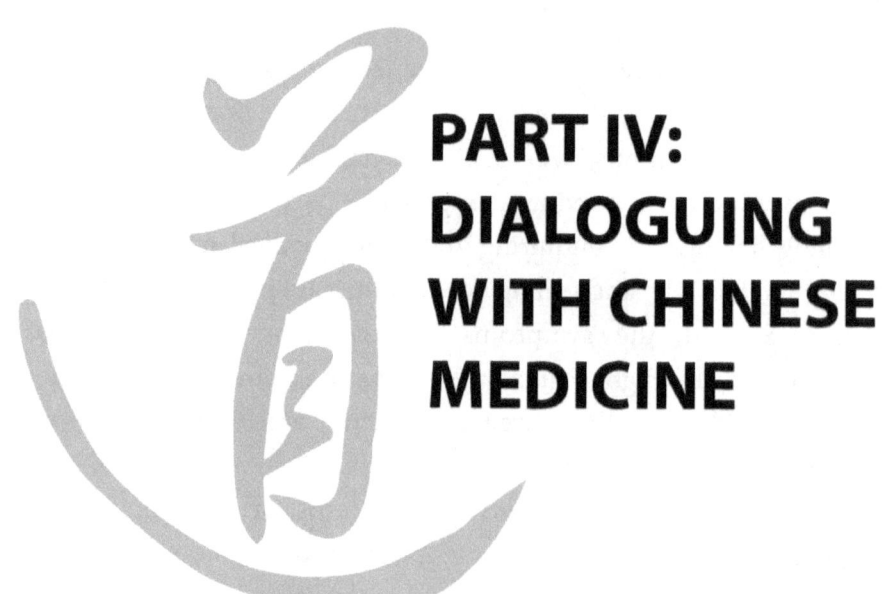

PART IV:
DIALOGUING
WITH CHINESE
MEDICINE

In the previous sections, we proposed a theological analytical framework for engaging Chinese medicine before examining the history of Western medicine, both Hippocratic and modern. The aim here is to discern the philosophical and epistemological assumptions we inherited from the West and to be more self-aware of how such biases operate in our evaluation of other indigenous cultures. Following which, we explored the history and philosophy of Chinese medicine, and how the metaphysical paradigms of both Chinese and Western influenced the way they conceptualised health, illness and therapy. Our study of Chinese medicine then concluded with a survey of Chinese medical theories and therapies, and how they are practiced presently. All these are to set the stage for Part 4, which is to engage in an in-depth dialogue with Chinese medicine. Chapter 10 will do so from the perspective of medical methodology, by considering the biomedical preference for clinical trials, and the extent to which this is useful for assessing the efficacy of TCM. Chapter 11 will bring Chinese medical philosophy and anthropology into dialogue with Christian theology. Our focus here is the degree to which the two traditions are compatible with one another, and how the questions posed by the former may enrich the broader Christian tradition.

10

BIOMEDICINE AND CHINESE MEDICINE IN DIALOGUE:

CONTEXT, ISSUES AND THE WAYS FORWARD

Thinking about Medical Efficacy

First, it was a sore throat. Then, it was sneezing, a stuffed nose and mild aches all over the body. "You must have caught a chill (*zhaoliang*, 着凉) last night," concluded David's grandfather. "No, grandfather," replied David, even as he tried to breathe through his congested nose. "Chills and cold temperatures don't give you colds. Rhinoviruses do!"[1]

What we have here is a classic clash of medical perspectives between Chinese and Western medicine.[2] In the previous chapters, we have seen how Western (both Greek and biomedical) and

---

1   As a website providing general information on common colds puts it, "there's no evidence that you get sick because you've been out in cold weather. And don't worry if you got overheated. It doesn't lead to a cold either". "Causes of Common Cold: Rhinovirus, Coronavirus, and More", accessed 7 July 2016, http://www.webmd.com/cold-and-flu/cold-guide/common_cold_causes.

2   Josephine Briggs, "The Art and Science of Traditional Medicine Part 1: TCM Today - A Case for Integration", *Science* 346, no. Suppl (2014): S7–9.

Chinese medicine evolved from fundamentally different epistemic paradigms. The former, being shaped by the Western interest in ontology, tends to conceptualise disease in ontological terms, that is, to enquire which natures or substances are the causes of a disease? Is it an imbalance in one's humours, a bug (whether it is a bacterium or a virus) or a flaw in one's genes or cells? The problem, so to speak, is to be found mostly in the "dot". Chinese culture, on the other hand, was never quite interested in ontological matters. Instead, its concern was always about how one entity is related to other entities in the cosmos, an idea well encapsulated in the theory of *yinyang*. The net result is that the cause of disease is always construed as a kind of physiological disequilibrium, whether this is due to an organ or *qi* deficiency, or environmental factors overwhelming one's body. The problem, in this case then, is to be found in the relationships between the dots.

The benefits of our current attempt at (medical) intercultural dialogue is clear. Besides reminding us that due respect to cultural peculiarities are essential for any effective cross-cultural communication, it should also assure Christians by now, I hope, that there are no religious (let alone, demonic) roots to secular Chinese medicine. All this is well and good. Nevertheless, what we have discussed so far does not quite answer some pertinent questions: Is Chinese medicine effective? Can it cure a patient? Should it be one of our viable medical options?

At first glance, these questions may not seem difficult to answer. For most people, their primary reference point would be their physicians, friends and relatives. If a physician recommends a particular therapy, or our friends and family undergo a specific medical treatment successfully, these therapies would be regarded as effective, whether they are biomedical or Chinese.[3] If we scrutinise things

---

3   Many may protest that they use biomedicine because it is scientifically proven. Practically speaking, only a handful of us will bother to research extensively about the clinical efficacy of a drug, a surgery procedure or a therapeutic option. Our primary reference point remains an authority, whether it is our physician, our friends or relatives.

further, the concept of medical efficacy is also not as straightforward as it appears. Let us return to our example of the common cold. When one suffers from a cold, one consults a General Practitioner (GP) who would diagnose the illness before prescribing a decongestant (antihistamine) for the blocked nose, cough suppressant (syrup) for the cough, and panadol or aspirin for the fever. These medications, however, are meant only to relieve the symptoms, not to kill the rhinovirus in his body. For the latter to happen, the patient must still wait for his body's immune system to do its work before he recovers entirely in a week or two. In other words, the medication is not curative but merely symptomatic relief. In this case, is the treatment effective then? Well, no, if we take efficacy as getting rid of the virus itself. On the other hand, most of us would regard the GP's treatment as effective since she not only diagnosed the ailment correctly, but also provided relief for his symptoms. In other words, when we talk about medical efficacy, we have in mind two things: a correct diagnosis of the illness, and either the cure of patient's illness, or the relief of his symptoms. For many who suffer from chronic diseases, such as arthritis or backaches, symptomatic relief is all that they can hope for, since a complete cure is not available.

For most biomedical physicians, therapeutic efficacy is even more narrowly defined: it must be established by empirical-statistical studies conducted through either observational studies or, more commonly, double-blind Randomised Controlled Trials (RCTs). Indeed, RCTs are generally regarded as the "gold standard" for measuring clinical efficacy of all forms of biomedical therapies. As we shall see, when Western medicine encounters its Chinese counterpart, the same rules of the game are expected of Chinese medicine. Consequently, our original question about TCM's efficacy can also be construed as: "To what extent is RCT a suitable measure of TCM's clinical efficacy?"

Answering this question will be the focus of this chapter. To begin, we shall survey the history of RCTs, before evaluating their assumptions, methodologies and limitations. As part of our survey, we shall also look at the development cycle of a biomedical drug. Thereafter, we shall consider how TCM theories and diagnostic approaches may be understood in relation to biomedicine, and how RCTs may be employed in TCM clinical trials profitably. Having done so, we shall examine the theoretical and practical characteristics unique to TCM, and the extent to which RCTs are suitable for assessing its therapeutic effectiveness.

Randomised Controlled Trials: A Short History

On 12 February 1941, a policeman by the name of Albert Alexander became the first patient to use penicillin. Four days after his treatment, he showed a marked improvement, with his temperature normalising, appetite improving and the abscesses on his face subsiding. Unfortunately for him, the supply of penicillin ran out the next day. It did not take long before his condition deteriorated once again, and the poor man succumbed to his illness a few weeks later.[4] Despite this setback, his physicians were convinced that penicillin was effective in treating bacterial infections. Over the next few months, they managed to persuade four pharmaceutical companies to mass produce the drug. So was born the first antibiotic, which would revolutionise medical therapy in the decades to come.

This penicillin experiment was quite typical of clinical trials in the early decades of the 20th century. Clinical procedures then were often no more than trial and error, while regulations were virtually non-existent. Parisian physicians, for example, were able to prescribe chlorpromazine to their schizophrenia patients just a few months after it was synthesised by the pharmaceutical company, Poulenc.[5] The same period, however, also saw a gradual improvement in clinical

---

4 James Le Fanu, *The Rise & Fall of Modern Medicine* (London: Abacus, 2014), 13–14.

5 Tests for drug toxicity and its pharmacology in the body, for example, were unheard of, ibid., 281.

trial procedures. In 1946, Sir Austin Bradford Hill was tasked to conduct the first RCT. Tuberculosis patients were assigned randomly to either a control or a test group, without the patients' knowledge (that is, a single-blind experiment). The first group received the standard treatment available, the antibiotic streptomycin, while the second received a combination of the same antibiotic with para-amino salicylic acid.[6] Within months of the trial, it was clear that the second treatment was far more effective.[7] Thus began the adoption of RCTs in clinical experiments. This comparison of a new treatment with another prevalent or mainstream therapy is now known as a *pragmatic trial*. Generally, its results help patients decide between different therapeutic alternatives, or aid policymakers in their "allocation of potentially limited resources for healthcare". That is, to decide whether to fund or insure a particular medical therapy.[8]

Over the next decade, RCTs gained popularity as the primary method for drug validation. In the 1950s, the procedure underwent yet another modification with the introduction of the double-blind technique. In a double-blind RCT, both the patients and the experimenters are kept in the dark as to who would be assigned the test drug and the placebo. The aim here is to prevent the researchers from influencing the patients unknowingly. The double-blind RCT method was first employed by Harry Gold and his colleagues when they evaluated the cardiac drug, khellin. In an earlier single-blind study, khellin was found to be dramatically better than the placebo pill. When Gold introduced the double-blind safeguards, the results

---

6   The randomisation is aimed at minimising selection bias. The error that a selection bias can introduce is well demonstrated in the 2016 Brexit referendum. A Singaporean parent asked his son (who was studying in London) whether the country will choose to remain in the European Union (EU). To which, the son replied that it was likely since all his friends voted to remain. The referendum result, however, was to leave the EU. As it turns out, a selection bias was operative here. This is because the son's friends were not only young adults (the majority of whom voted to remain), but were residents in London (the city most adamant against Brexit).

7   Le Fanu, *The Rise & Fall of Modern Medicine*, 41.

8   Volker Scheid and Hugh MacPherson, *Integrating East Asian Medicine into Contemporary Healthcare* (Edinburgh; New York: Churchill Livingstone Elsevier, 2012), 678.

proved otherwise. There was no significant difference between the test and control groups. Quite understandably, the double-blind technique quickly gained a reputation for being an effective means of eliminating placebo effects or bias in clinical trials.[9] This technique of comparing the tested drug with a placebo is known as an *explanatory trial*, and is used most often to

> enhance the internal validity [of the trial] by giving patients in the treatment group and patients in the placebo group an experience that is as closely identical as possible. This [also] makes it possible to identify more precisely which specific aspect of treatment (which is not delivered within the sham intervention) causes the effect.[10]

In 1962, news broke that thousands of babies in Europe and North America were born with malformed limbs. What they shared in common was that their mothers all used thalidomide to alleviate their morning sickness. Thalidomide was soon identified as the cause of the deformities and quickly banned.[11] After this tragedy, more stringent safety regulations were put in place and the double-blind RCTs became the "gold standard" not only to evaluate a drug's efficacy but also its potential toxicity and pharmacology in the body.

The mid-1980s saw the emergence of Evidence-based Medicine (EBM), which is "the process of systematically reviewing, appraising and using clinical research findings to aid the delivery of optimum clinical care to patients". Plainly speaking, EBM aids physicians in

---

9   More will be said later about the placebo effect. Ted J. Kaptchuk, "The Double-Blind, Randomized, Placebo-Controlled Trial: Gold Standard or Golden Calf?", *Journal of Clinical Epidemiology* 54 (2001): 541–49.

10   Scheid and MacPherson, *Integrating East Asian Medicine into Contemporary Healthcare*, 679–80.

11   "The Thalidomide Tragedy: Lessons for Drug Safety and Regulation | Helix Magazine", accessed 11 July 2016, https://helix.northwestern.edu/article/thalidomide-tragedy-lessons-drug-safety-and-regulation.

their decision making, so that they can "treat where there is evidence of benefit and not treat where there is evidence of no benefit". While personal experience, reasoning and clinical experience of fellow physicians are counted as valid evidence, EBM's bias is clearly for published evidence.[12] Among these, the most important remain the systematic reviews and meta-analyses of RCTs, which provide authoritative summaries of whether "the evidence for particular interventions is strong or not".[13] Given the rising healthcare costs in many developed countries, it is hardly surprising that EBM has become an important concern for both policymakers and insurance companies.[14]

Presently, the double-blind RCT is generally regarded as the "gold standard" for assessing the efficacy of a medical intervention. As Chinese medicine modernises and encounters biomedicine globally,

---

12   Jonathan Belsey, "What Is Evidence Based Medicine", *What Is Series*, 2009. 1–3.

13   As Sackett et al. put it, "because the randomised trial, and especially the systematic review of several randomised trials, is so much more likely to inform us and so much less likely to mislead us, it has become the "gold standard" for judging whether a treatment does more good than harm". Scheid and MacPherson, *Integrating East Asian Medicine into Contemporary Healthcare*, 668; D. L. Sackett and et al., "Evidence-Based Medicine: What It Is and What It Isn't", *British Medical Journal* 312 (1996): 71–72.

14   A good example is the National Institute for Health and Care Excellence's (NICE) decision not to continue funding the use of Kadcyla in the National Healthcare System (NHS). Kadcyla (*trastuzumab emtansine*) treats HER2-positive breast cancer and costs more than twice the amount of the mainstream therapy (*trastuzumab*) at £90,000 per patient. Understandably, this has caused a hug outcry among breast cancer patients and in the media, who argue that Kadcyla extends patient survival rates by a median of six months. What is often neglected in their criticisms, however, is that the mainstream therapies (usually *trastuzumab* and *lapatinib*) extend patient survival rates by a median of three months. In other words, Kadcyla only improves the survival rates by an additional three months. Yet, it would drastically increase the financial burden of the UK healthcare system. "Kadcyla Price Too High for Routine NHS Funding, Says NICE in Final Guidance | Press and Media | News | NICE", Press Release, accessed 19 August 2016,
https://www.nice.org.uk/news/press-and-media/kadcyla-price-too-high-for-routine-nhs-funding-says-nice-in-final-guidance.; Haroon Siddique, "NHS Cancer Patients Missing out on Innovative Drugs", *The Guardian*, 15 August 2016, sec. Society, https://www.theguardian.com/society/2016/aug/15/nhs-cancer-patients-innovative-drugs-breast-prostate-uk.; Ian E. Krop et al., "Trastuzumab Emtansine versus Treatment of Physician's Choice for Pretreated HER2-Positive Advanced Breast Cancer (TH3RESA): A Randomised, Open-Label, Phase 3 Trial", *The Lancet Oncology* 15, no. 7 (June 2014): 689–99, doi:10.1016/S1470-2045(14)70178-0.

RCTs are increasingly required of TCM as the means of validating its therapies. More shall be said about the use of RCTs in TCM research later. For now, we shall turn our attention to the developmental life cycle of a biomedical drug and how RCTs are employed in this context. This survey will be helpful in three ways. First of all, biomedical and TCM clinical trials share many common characteristics. To know one is to understand much also about the other. Secondly, the survey will also consider the limitations of RCTs in practice. This, hopefully, will nuance our common assumption that RCTs can be the unmitigated referee for therapeutic efficacy. Thirdly, the same knowledge will also provide us a context for discussing the extent to which RCTs are applicable to TCM research.

Developmental Life Cycle of Biomedical Drugs

The development of biomedical drugs usually begins with basic research. Through synthesising and screening thousands of drug molecules, a scientist identifies a molecule that can potentially target a specific physiological mechanism or process in the body. Thereafter, the potential drug candidate is put through several laboratory and animal tests to investigate its potency, toxicity and potential side effects.[15] If the drug proves viable, it is then subjected to clinical trials.

Typically, there are three phases to such trials. Phase 1 is usually conducted using "paid" healthy volunteers (maybe a dozen), either in the country where the drug will be marketed, or, increasingly, in Third World nations. In fact, whether it is Phase 1, 2 or 3, there is an increasing trend of pharmaceutical companies outsourcing these trials to clinical research organisations (CROs), such as Quintiles, Parexel and Covance, who often conduct the trials globally.[16] When a

---

15   Ben Goldacre, *Bad Pharma: How Drug Companies Mislead Doctors and Harm Patients* (Glasgow: Harper Collins, 2013), Kindle Location 1631.

16   This raises an ethical question. The Declaration of Helsinki, the medical code that frames most medical research, says that "research is justified if the population from whom participants are drawn would benefit from the results". This growing trend of conducting trials in third world

drug proves to have no significant side effects in Phase 1, it goes on to Phases 2 and 3 trials.[17] In Phase 2, the drug will be given to not more than a few hundred patients, while Phase 3 will administer the same to between 300 to 2,000 patients. Phase 3 is usually conducted using double-blind RCTs, either by comparing it with the best medication available for a particular disease, or more commonly, with a placebo. If a drug proves to be more effective than the placebo (even marginally by, say, 10%), and the clinical side effects seem tolerable, the results are likely to be published, typically in academic journals. Following this, the clinical findings would be submitted to the regulatory bodies for approval. It is to be noted that drug approvals are usually defined narrowly for use on a specific disease, say, to treat non-small-cell lung cancer. This does not mean that it is not effective against other forms of similar diseases. For this reason, it is not uncommon for physicians to administer the drug "off-label" to treat other similar diseases. So, in the case of our cancer example, a drug approved for lung cancer may also be tried out against other cancers such as liver or colorectal cancers.[18]

There are several qualifications to such drug approvals, however. First of all, approvals are based on drug efficacy and side effects that have been published. Truth be told, not all trials are published. Frequently, if a patient drops out of a trial (usually due to severe side effects), his results are excluded.[19] If some trials fail to demonstrate a

---

countries, which are unlikely to afford (or benefit from) the drug is thus problematic, unless the drug is made available to these countries eventually at sharp discounts. Ibid. Kindle Location 1656–88, 1732.

17   Only 20% of drugs will make it to the market eventually. Ibid., Kindle Location 1665.

18   Practically, it is financially exorbitant for a pharmaceutical company to test the efficacy of a drug on a whole host of diseases. For this reason, clinical trials are conducted on specific diseases, which become the basis for regulatory approval. This does not mean, of course, that the drug is not viable against other similar diseases. Ibid., Kindle Location 947.

19   Sometimes, the drop-out patient's data may be included as "Last Observation Carried Forward". This is controversial as last observations tend to be better than the original baseline and is likely to exaggerate the benefit of the drug. A more conservative way to include the drop-out patient's data is to use his "Baseline Observation Carried Forward", that is, his original symptoms instead. Ibid. Kindle Location 1118–24.

drug's efficacy, these results are sometimes not published, excluded or their primary outcomes switched with more positive secondary outcomes in the publications.[20] Quite often, approved drugs are experimented on "ideal patients". These are usually patients who suffer from fewer health complications and are, therefore, more likely to recover. This begs the question whether the approved drug will be equally effective when given to real-life patients, many of whom suffer from other medical problems, and are already on many other drugs that may interfere with the approved drug's efficacy.[21] There are yet other ways to window dress one's clinical results, such as shortening or lengthening the trials, bundling outcomes, comparing it with a useless treatment, or using too small a sample size.[22] Unfortunately, all these can do much to exaggerate the benefits of a drug, and can, therefore, mislead both physicians and patients.

Quite frequently, the "new" drugs that are launched are simply "me-too drugs", that is, similar versions of an already approved drug, which may or may not be as effective as the original product. This is because all the pharmaceutical company has to do is to prove that the new drug is more effective than a placebo—a rather low standard

---

20   Before a clinical trial begins, its primary outcomes (what the trial intends to measure) are defined in the research protocol. If a trial switches its primary outcome, it makes a mockery of the research protocols, which were designed to measure the original primary outcomes in the first place. A good illustration of this mischief is a 2009 study on the different clinical trials conducted on the applications of Gabapetin. Of these, half the trials were never published. This is always bad practice since most trials patients would have participated with the altruistic hope that their sacrifice would benefit the general public. An unpublished trial, unfortunately, is contrary to what is promised them and their expectations. Of the 12 trials that were published eventually, their research protocols specified a total of 21 primary outcomes. Unfortunately, only 11 of these were reported. Of the remaining primary outcomes, six did not appear at all while 4 were reported as if they were secondary outcomes. Ibid., Kindle Location 3015–28.

21   For example, a 2007 study "took 179 representative asthma patients from the general population, and looked at how many would have been eligible to participate in a group of asthma treatment trials. The answer was 6 per cent on average. ... Another study took six hundred patients being treated for depression in an outpatient clinic, and found that on average only a third of them would have been eligible to participate in thirty-nine recently published trials of treatments for depression". Ibid., Kindle Location 2413, 2673.

22   Ibid., Kindle Location 2716–3152.

to achieve actually.[23] Furthermore, drugs are often approved based on surrogate outcomes, such as a reduction in cholesterol levels, normalised blood pressures or improved blood tests, rather than real-life outcomes, e.g., heart attacks or death. Yet, the latter are the outcomes which both physicians and patients are more concerned about.[24] More importantly, some serious side effects are rare and may only occur, say, once in 1,000 cases. So, while these side effects may not occur during trials with the first 1,000 patients, they are likely to occur an average of 10 times once 10,000 patients have used it.[25]

RCT Methodological Assumptions and Limitations

Judging from the above, it should be clear that, while RCTs are commendable attempts at scientific-empirical studies of drug efficacy, their application remains vulnerable to a host of problems, ranging from design flaws, reporting issues to even unethical behaviour. Although these difficulties concern the use and practice of RCTs, there are yet a series of other limitations that impinge on the assumptions and methodology of RCTs. The issues we shall raise are particularly relevant for our purposes since they affect the extent to which RCTs are appropriate for validating TCM interventions. These limitations are as follows.

---

23   Comparisons with the most effective drug available (pragmatic trials) are less frequent. Such information, however, is more important for physicians and patients, since they will need it to decide whether to use the new or current drug. Ibid., Kindle Location 2031, 2717–39.

24   The most dramatic example of how surrogate outcomes can fail terribly is the Cardiac Arrhythmia Suppression Trial (CAST). Patients with abnormal heart rhythm are at higher risks of sudden death. Three anti-arrhythmic drugs were first tested whether they prevented these abnormal rhythms (surrogate outcome). They proved successful and were thus approved for use with heart patients. Later on, when a proper trial was conducted measuring real life outcomes, it had to be abandoned because it was discovered, to everyone's embarrassment, that the drugs increased the risk of death so much that the trial had to stop early. Unfortunately, more than 100,000 patients had fell victim to the drugs by then. Ibid., Kindle Location 2080–87.

25   Ibid., Kindle Location 2535.

RCTs generally test the efficacy of a single active ingredient or compound

As mentioned above, biomedical clinical research tends to look out for specific drugs against specific diseases (whether this is a cancer, virus or bacteria). The task of an RCT, therefore, is to assess the degree to which an identified drug module is effective against the targeted disease. To put it differently, RCTs are premised on a single-causality model. This requires it to assume all other factors in the experiment to be homogeneous and not impinge on the drug's efficacy. It is for this reason that patient profiles are narrowly defined (patients with complicated medical problems are usually excluded), drug dosages are pre-determined, while qualitative factors such as the patients' lifestyles, diets and so on are deemed the same. As we shall see, most of the latter factors are usually lumped together as a dummy variable known commonly as the placebo effect. More will be said later about the placebo phenomenon.

At this point, all we need to recognise is that RCTs are designed to assess single causalities. This then calls into question whether it can be satisfactorily applied in TCM drug trials. This is because, if a TCM trial is faithful to its theoretical assumptions, it would need to adjust the drug dosage or compounds according to the patient's body constitution and syndromes, and also account for the therapeutic benefits that non-drug therapies (such as massage, moxibustion or acupuncture) may have for a patient. In other words, a more complicated multi-causality model is actually required to properly assess TCM diagnoses and therapies.

Whether randomisation alone can eliminate all sources of bias

It is often assumed that the procedure of randomisation in RCTs guarantees "the test of significance ... against corruption by the causes of disturbance which have not been eliminated". To be sure, randomisation does reduce the problem of selection bias when it comes to allocating patients to the test and control groups. Having said this, to go further and claim that it eliminates all possible "causes of disturbances" is to be party to a quantification fallacy.[26] This is because there are "indefinitely many possible confounding factors".

> Even if there is only a small probability that an individual factor is unbalanced, given that there are indefinitely many possible confounding factors, then it would seem to follow that the probability that there is some factor on which the two groups are unbalanced ... might for all anyone knows be high.[27]

For example, the patients' lifestyles, diets, exercise regimens, and family support (which affects psychological well-being) can differ significantly. One cannot simply assume that the effects of these factors are homogeneous in both the test and control groups. Consequently, scientists should be circumspect about the value of randomisation. While it can safeguard an RCT against the experimenters' selection bias, it cannot ensure that the test and control groups would always be utterly similar and comparable.

Whether RCTs consistently give more conservative estimates of drug efficacy

It is often said that non-RCTs (such as observational studies)

---

26   A quantification fallacy is an error in logic where the quantifiers (either all, some or none) of the premises are in contradiction to the quantifier of the conclusion. For example, the advice, "experts agree that investors should buy stocks" is often interpreted as, "*all* experts agree (premise) that *all* investors should buy stock (conclusion)". This is a quantification fallacy, however, as quite a number of experts may not advise investors to do so. Consequently, it is more accurate to say, "*some* experts agree that *all* investors should buy stock". This nuance, however, would make the advice not all-encompassing and, thus, not helpful. The same may be said for randomisation. It is often assumed that "*all* randomisation eliminates *all* causes of disturbances" when, in all likelihood, "*all* randomisation eliminates some causes of disturbances (including selection bias)".

27   John Worrall, "What Evidence Is Evidence Based Medicine?", *Philosophy of Science* 69, no. 3 (2002): S316–30.

consistently provide higher estimates of drug efficacy, when compared to RCTs. Three recent systematic reviews, however, have made "a compelling case that poor methodology could either *overestimate or underestimate treatment effects*". When several randomised and non-randomised trials of the same medical intervention were compared, it was observed that some RCTs showed an increased efficacy, a few showed a decrease, while others showed no difference at all. It would appear then that "neither randomised nor non-randomised methodologies consistently [give] higher estimates of treatment effect, and that variations between random and non-random evidence may not be greater than those between different RCTs".[28]

Whether RCTs must necessarily provide more accurate clinical evidence

In the hierarchy of evidence, it is generally assumed that RCTs provide more accurate evidence than observational studies. Recent comparisons of observational studies with RCTs suggest otherwise, concluding that the outcomes of observational studies and RCTs can be "*remarkably similar*".[29] Rather than denying the value of RCTs, these studies suggest that it is possible to perform "accurate observational studies", and we need not necessarily privilege RCTs over well-controlled observational studies.[30] This conclusion is particularly relevant for TCM research, since TCM therapies tend to be more patient centred and lend themselves better to observational studies.

The presence of "masking bias" in RCTs

There may be an inherent "masking bias" within the RCT procedure itself. In 1990, the French conducted a clinical trial to study the

---

28   Kaptchuk, "Gold Standard or Golden Calf?", 542.

29   One was based on five meta-analyses of 99 reports and another on 19 treatment analyses (53 observational studies and 83 RCTs).

30   Kaptchuk, "Gold Standard or Golden Calf?", 543.

efficacy of naproxen, a pain-control and anti-inflammatory drug. Prior to the experiment, patients were randomly divided into two groups: those who were informed that they were participating in a trial, and those who were not. Both groups then underwent separate double-blind RCTs, where each test group received naproxen treatment, while the control groups received the placebo. The outcome of the experiment was surprising. For the patients who knew that they were participating in a trial, "both the naproxen and placebo were significantly more effective than in the unaware group".[31] Clearly then, the mere knowledge that one was undergoing a trial, at least in this case, yielded significantly improved results.[32]

The ambiguous conception of placebo effects

Before the advent of RCTs, placebos, such as bread pills and water, were deemed to have no therapeutic effects, and prescribed simply "to separate imaginary 'psychological' symptoms from real problems", or to comfort and reinforce the patient's faith in his recovery.[33] In 1955, the placebo effect was redefined by Henry Beecher (1904–1976). Placebos, he argued, can actually produce significant physical change in a patient, including "objective changes at the end organ which may exceed those attributable to potent pharmacological action". For this reason, if a clinical trial is to properly ascertain the active component of a drug, it must compare the drug with that of a placebo (or control group), so that the difference between the two can be determined.

This re-conception of the placebo effect is not without difficulty. This is because it assumes, in the first place, that "the placebo was a single and stable "power" that behaved in a consistent manner", whether in the active drug or in the sham therapy. In reality, this could hardly be possible, since the placebo practically assumes all

---

31   The trial was conducted before informed consent became mandatory practice.

32   Kaptchuk, "Gold Standard or Golden Calf?", 544.

33   Ted J. Kaptchuk, "Powerful Placebo: The Dark Side of the Randomised Controlled Trial", *Lancet*, 351 (1998): 1722–25.

sorts of "nonspecific effects" in the active arm of a clinical trial, or as Kaptchuk puts it, "a hodge-podge of non-linear, difficult to quantify, remnants collected under the rubric of the dummy control of an RCT". Realistically, such effects are unlikely to be the same in both the active and control arms of the trial. More importantly, these "non-specific" effects could well include many factors that contribute richly to the patient's health.[34] For example,

> nature taking its course; regression to the mean; routine medical and nursing care; regimens such as rest, diet, exercise, and relaxation; easing of anxiety by diagnosis and treatment; the patient-doctor relationship; classic conditioning and learnt behaviours; the expectation of relief and the imagination; and the will and belief of both patient and practitioner.[35]

In other words, the efficacy of a therapy may well be due to multiple causes, rather than the singular cause or active component regularly assumed in RCTs. Given the therapeutic benefits of these factors, surely there is a case for examining the placebo effects "in all its myriad facets", and their possible interactions with the active component of a drug, if any. Until this is achieved, "medicine", unfortunately, "will always have a limited perception of healing".[36]

In view of the above, it is clear that we should not regard the double-blind RCT as an unmitigated referee for validating all kinds of drugs and medical therapies. The RCT, as we have seen, is not without its imperfections, whether it is its inherent "masking bias" (the possibility that RCTs can either over- or underestimate the efficacy of a medical intervention), or its design flaws or poor implementation. Having said this, the blind RCT remains one of the most important

---

34   Ibid., 1723.
35   Ibid., 1724.
36   Ibid., 1725.

clinical methodologies that we have at hand. As a "standardised, explicit, replicable, and impersonal procedure that defines unambiguous and formal norms for medical researchers", concludes Kaptchuk, the blind RCT provides a "system of rules [that] minimises the need for personal trust and subjective judgment". Consequently, it is "the least subjective and most impersonal procedure ethically possible now" and may well be "the closest thing medicine has to a 'technology of trust'", where "'fairness' rather than 'truth'" is its central value.[37]

Chinese Medicine as Empirical Science

While the use of RCTs in TCM trials is a recent phenomenon, Chinese medical physicians have always been concerned with the empirical evidence for, and the efficacy of Chinese medical diagnosis and therapy.[38] Where they differ from the West is how these concerns are expressed. Medical treatises, such as the *Neijing Suwen, Nanjing* and *Shanghan Lun*, while steeped in the philosophies of *yinyang* and *qi*, were never mere works of philosophical speculation. Rather, they were clearly grounded in their authors' clinical experiences, and have stood the test of time. The *Shanghan Lun* is a good case in point. If it were not for its ability to alleviate the epidemics that broke out during the Song era, the treatise would never have been popularised by the Song authorities. As early as the Han dynasty, physicians were also known to have kept case records or histories (*yian*, 医案) of their patients and even publishing them occasionally. The Ming era, however, would see this interest developing significantly, with far more case histories published, based on either Ming or pre-Ming cases.[39]

In the last century, the modernisation of Chinese medicine,

---

37   Kaptchuk, "Gold Standard or Golden Calf?", 546–47.

38   Bridie Andrews, *The Making of Modern Chinese Medicine, 1850–1960* (Vancouver: UBC Press, 2014), 186.

39   李经纬 (Li Jingwei), 中医史 (*History of Chinese Medicine*) (Hainan: Hainan, 2007), 287–88.

along with the growing Western interest in alternative medicine and Chinese pharmacology, has seen more Chinese medical therapies subjected to the rigours of RCTs. Pragmatic trials, for example, have been conducted to assess the efficacy of acupuncture in treating back, neck and shoulder pains, as compared to mainstream therapies.[40]

In the area of pharmacology, the Chinese herb, *Mahuang* (麻黄, *Herba Ephedrae*), has been found to be a good source of ephedrine used in medications for colds and allergies, while another herb, *Huangqi* (黄芪, *Astragalus*), has been shown to be a good supplement for the body's telomerase, an enzyme necessary for promoting cell regeneration. While these discoveries are commendable, they "do little more than indicate that Chinese medicine is a useful source for Western drug discovery and new interventions".[41] To put it differently, these trials are still, in fact, biomedical trials, designed according to the assumptions and epistemic paradigm of modern medicine. What has yet to be demonstrated is whether

> TCM theory makes sense because it leads to systematic methods of diagnosis and therapeutic interventions that can alleviate and cure illnesses, as confirmed by clinical trials.[42]

Is this possible, given that Chinese medical physiology, theories and diagnostics are described largely in philosophical categories and metaphysical entities that are "mostly not measureable and even unobservable", let alone amenable to quantitative analysis? For the rest of this chapter, we shall explore this question from three angles.

Firstly, we shall consider how Chinese medical theories may be re-envisaged as heuristic models, "within which entities and con-

---

40   Ted J. Kaptchuk, "Acupuncture: Theory, Efficacy, and Practice", *Annals of Internal Medicine*, Complementary and Alternative Medicine Series, 136, no. 5 (2002): 374–83.
41   Hai Hong, *The Theory of Chinese Medicine: A Modern Explanation* (London: Imperial College, 2014), 2, 164.
42   Ibid.

cepts, and their mutual relationships, are presented in a manner that renders them applicable to the diagnosis and treatment of illnesses".[43] In doing so, we hope that those who are more familiar with biomedicine will have a better grasp of how TCM theories may relate to biomedical theories.

Secondly, we shall consider the major TCM diagnostic approaches and the extent to which they are amenable to empirical validation. Third, and finally, we shall examine how RCTs may be applied in assessing the efficacy of TCM therapies, before considering the limitations of RCTs in validating TCM theories and therapies in general.

Re-envisaging Chinese Medical Theories as Heuristic Models

Biomedical vs Chinese Medical Aetiologies

We begin with the different aetiological perspectives propounded by bio and Chinese medicine. For biomedical physicians, an aetiological cause must be "necessary and universal", in that "a cause must always have the same effect; the cause must also be necessary for its effect". To use tuberculosis (TB), or *feijieke* (肺结核), as an example, the presence of the *tubercle bacillus* bacteria in the bodies of TB patients would mean that the bacteria is "necessary and sufficient" for contracting TB. On the contrary, Hong Hai argues that the presence of the *tubercle bacillus* bacteria may be better understood as "the definition of the disease" rather than its cause. This is because the bacteria's presence

> says nothing about how the bacillus came to take hold in the patient's body, i.e., the factors that combine and are

---

43   Heuristic models are approaches of learning, discovery or problem solving by experimental or trial and error methods. While the results derived may not be perfect or optimal, they are usually sufficient for the immediate goals, such as diagnostics and therapy, in our case. Ibid., 19.

sufficient, along with exposure to the bacillus, to bring about the disease.[44]

Instead of this narrow view of causation, Hong proposes John L. Mackie's (1917–1981) INUS multi-causality model as a means of re-envisaging aetiology. Intrinsic to Mackie's model is the idea of the INUS condition, that is, "an insufficient, but non-redundant part of an unnecessary but sufficient condition (INUS)".[45] According to this model, the presence of the *tubercle bacillus* is but an INUS condition, which must operate in tandem with other "unnecessary but sufficient" factors, such as poor diet, stress or a weaker immune system, before the disease can take hold of a body.[46]

The INUS model, continues Hong, coheres very well with how Chinese medicine conceptualises aetiology. As Chinese physicians see it, diagnostic and therapeutic efficacy is the ability to identify and work with the factors that we can manage. By this scheme, the identification of the *rhinovirus* as the cause of the common cold (to use our introductory example) is of little value since this is a factor that we can hardly control. Bacteria and viruses are present everywhere and can never be eliminated entirely. A more fruitful therapeutic approach would be to focus on the factors that we can manipulate, instead. These factors are usually related to the patient's immediate environment or overall health, such as changing his diet, exercise regimen or the strengthening of his immune system.[47] Seen from this perspective then, the difference between bio- and Chinese

---

44   Ibid., 34.

45   Mackie gives the example of a fire that resulted from a short circuit in the house wiring. The short circuit alone would not have brought about the fire (that is, it is an *insufficient* condition). Neither was it *necessary* for starting a fire. Nonetheless, it was an essential (*non-redundant*) part of a set of conditions (such as presence of flammable materials, the absence of fire extinguishers and so on) that were sufficient to cause the fire. For a more detailed explanation of the INUS condition, see Lars-Göran Johansson, *Philosophy of Science for Scientists* (Cham: Springer, 2016), 125–29.

46   Hong, *Theory of Chinese Medicine*, 35–36.

47   Ibid., 41.

medical aetiologies comes down simply to differences in therapeutic focal points, with the former focused on eliminating what it sees as the pertinent INUS condition, while the other pays attention to other INUS conditions that it can control more readily.

TCM Organs and Meridians as Heuristic Models

As mentioned in the previous chapter, several entities in Chinese physiology do not have equivalence in modern physiology. These include the concepts of *qi*, phlegm and wind. Moreover, even when TCM organs are translated using biomedical terms, the functions attributed to the TCM organs often do not correspond to their biomedical counterparts. The Chinese spleen, for example, is seen as an important aspect of the digestive system, whereas the anatomical spleen is understood to be responsible for the body's immunity instead. The reason for this difference, as argued in the last chapter, is due to the fact that Chinese thought conceptualises physiology in functional or process terms, whereas Western medicine is more concerned with questions of ontology, and thus the physiological characteristics attributable to specific organs. Seen from this light, the vital organs in Chinese physiology should be understood heuristically, as denoting *clusters of functions* rather than anatomical attributes. Consequently, when a Chinese physician speaks of treating the spleen, what he means practically is the treatment of "a set of functions closely related to the biomedical concepts of digestion and absorption of food and water and the distribution of nutrients and liquids to the organs and tissues of the body". [48]

What about the meridians then? According to Chinese medicine, the meridians are a network of pathways that connects the *zang-fu* organs and transports the vital substances (*qi*, blood and *jingye*) throughout the body. When a physician needles a series of acupuncture points on specific meridians, he expects that what he administers to the body's exterior will have therapeutic effects on its interior

---

48   Ibid., 59–97.

zangfu organs. To date, both biomedical and TCM physicians have attempted to explain the healing effects of acupuncture according to their epistemic preferences. In biomedicine, acupuncture is most often applied to pain relief (acupuncture analgesia). Since pain is inextricably linked to the brain and nervous system, biomedical explanations for the efficacy of acupuncture have focused largely on how needling affects one's neurophysiological and neuropharmacological mechanisms, for example, how acupuncture triggers the production of endorphins and serotonin, both of which play important roles in pain relief.[49] On the other hand, engineering professor Wang Weigong postulates that acupuncture points actually resonate with different parts of the body and its organs. The healing effect of acupuncture, therefore, is to be found in how such resonance improves or restores the functional activity of the organs or one's body.[50]

In Hong Hai's opinion, the meridian system has no ontological reality and, thus, cannot be mapped out by electrochemical or other techniques.[51] As explained in Chapter 9, recent research employing CT Scans, MRI and other imaging technologies have proven otherwise, showing strong evidence for the existence of acupuncture points, and the *Du* meridian. Anecdotal clinical evidence also suggests that meridian lines, particularly the *Du* meridian, can sometimes be visible on a patient's body. Given these positive developments, it is likely that subsequent imaging technologies can shed more light on the existence of the other meridians in the near future.

Empirical Validation of TCM Diagnostic Approaches

Having reframed the major theories of Chinese medicine as heuristic

---

49   Endorphins help relieve pain and induce feelings of pleasure or euphoria while Serotonin is thought to be responsible for mood balance and a deficiency of which leads to depression. Ibid., 116.

50   王唯工 (Wang Weigong), 气的乐章 (*Qi as a Musical Movement*) (臺北市; 臺北縣三 重市: 大塊文化出版 大和书报总经销, 2002), 105–20.

51   Hong, *Theory of Chinese Medicine*, 118.

models and how they may relate to biomedicine, we shall now consider whether the TCM diagnostic methods are amenable to empirical validation. By this we mean "whether hypotheses regarding illnesses can be derived from these models and whether these are testable in principle, preferably also in practice".[52] To this end, we will consider three common methods of diagnostics: the *wuxing* or five phases model of physiological interaction, the climatic and emotional model for disease causation, and the use of Disharmony Patterns as a means of diagnosis and therapy.

Wuxing or Five Phases Diagnostic Model

The *wuxing* consists of five elements or phases—metal, wood, water, fire and earth. Since the Han dynasty, it has been commonly used as a paradigm for depicting either mutually generating (*xiangsheng*, 相生) or mutually conquering (*xiangke*, 相克) relationships. In the same period, this relational logic was transposed to secular medicine as a means of describing the mutually generating or conquering relationships between a body's *zangfu* organs. For example, the earth is identified with the spleen while the metal with the lung. Since the earth promotes or generates metal, it is assumed then that

> strengthening the spleen is one way of nourishing and tonifying the lung. A patient with weakness in his lung (functions) can be treated with a spleen tonic, which in turn strengthens the lung to overcome imbalances within that organ.[53]

In TCM clinical practice, this is, in fact, one of the most commonly used therapies for lung problems.

Having said this, Hong observed that "about half of the permutations of relationships among the organs implied by the five-

---

52   Ibid., 130.
53   Ibid., 131–32.

element theory are not used in clinical practice". As he saw it, the simple answer is that they have not been found to work.

> For example, a method of tonifying a weak spleen termed "strengthen fire to tonify the earth" (*yihuobutufa*, 益火补土法) would, by the five-element model, imply strengthening the mother heart organ [fire] to tonify the spleen [earth]. In practice, this is rarely done. Another source of "fire" is deemed to be the kidney which also has a warming function for the rest of the organs. In clinical practice, physicians strengthen kidney *yang*, rather than the heart, to tonify the spleen; this is not in accordance with the five-element model.[54]

Not all TCM physicians agree with Hong, however. As Diarra sees it, the *wuxing* model is complicated and not every TCM physician understands its wide range of applications well. This could be the reason why many of the *wuxing* permutations are not used in practice. Take, for example, a deficiency in the spleen (earth). To treat the ailment, it is quite common for a TCM physician to prescribe therapies that will strengthen the spleen. A more experienced doctor, however, would also recognise that a sick spleen can adversely affect the patient's liver (wood). Consequently, he would not only strengthen the patient's spleen, but also her liver (实肝), so as to prevent the organ from deteriorating. This precaution, in turn, will also have a secondary benefit on the patient's spleen.

Regardless of the positions taken for the *wuxing* model, the question remains as to how the model may be subjected to empirical validation? A good start, suggests Hong, would be to focus one's experiments on "those [*wuxing*] relationships among organs that are thought to be useful based on clinical experience".[55]

---

54   Ibid., 133.
55   Ibid., 134.

Climatic and Emotional Model of Aetiology

What about the climatic and emotional model (*liuying qiqing*, 六淫 七情) of disease causation? Underlying this aetiological model is the assumption that "protection against adverse climatic influences and moderation of one's emotions are the key principles for the cultivation of health". Or, to employ the INUS model discussed earlier, these aetiological theories provide guidelines for manipulating the INUS conditions that cause diseases, so that we can cultivate our health. This focus on disease prevention also means that the model is less useful for actual clinical diagnosis and provides few guidelines as to the therapy needed to treat a disease.[56] In practice, most TCM physicians would rely on the third and more prevalent mode of diagnosis—the differentiation of patterns or syndromes.

Disharmony Pattern Model for Diagnosis and Therapy

In a typical consultation, a Chinese physician would employ the Four Examinations (Observation, Smelling, Questioning and Touching/ Pulse Diagnosis) as the means for determining the different symptoms expressed by a patient. This complex of symptoms and signs are then interpreted according to the *Distinguishing of the Eight Principal Patterns* (thereafter, *Eight Principal Patterns*).[57] Based on this model, four pairs of disharmony patterns or syndromes (*zheng*, 证) may be discerned:

- Exterior versus Interior Patterns.
- Deficiency versus Excess Patterns.
- Cold versus Hot Patterns.
- *Yin* versus *Yang* Patterns.

It should be noted, however, that the Chinese medical syndrome is

---

56 Ibid., 137.

57 As mentioned in Chapter 9, this is but one of many TCM diagnostic paradigms. See the same chapter for more details on its diagnostic procedures.

fundamentally different from its biomedical counterpart. Whereas the latter sees "a combination of signs and/or symptoms that forms a distinct clinical picture indicative of a particular disorder", the TCM syndrome "may be associated with more than one disease, and a disease can exhibit different syndromes in the course of its progression (pathogenesis)". Thus, *qi* weakness is a common condition in coronary heart disease but may also be found in patients with stomach ulcers.[58] After the diagnosis is made and the patterns determined, a therapy is then prescribed to "treat a condition with opposing and balancing force", for example, "when there is heat, use cooling methods. When there is cold, use warming methods". In clinical practice, the therapies that can be employed include drug formulas, acupuncture, moxibustion, cupping, massage (*tuina*) or a combination of these methods.[59]

Among the models described above, Pattern Differentiation is most amenable to empirical testing. Specifically, it allows us to derive "hypotheses concerning appropriate therapies to be applied", which we can then test by the hypothetico-deductive method. As to how such a test might be conducted, Hong offers the following procedure.[60]

> Patients with a constellation of symptoms P are diagnosed with syndrome S and are treated by therapy method T which TCM prescribes based on the principle of syndrome [pattern] differentiation and corresponding treatment.

> Main Hypothesis: Syndrome S can be treated by use of therapy method T.

> Initial Condition: The patient exhibits the set of symptoms P.

---

58   Hong, *Theory of Chinese Medicine*, 137–38.
59   Ibid., 148.
60   Ibid., 163, 166–67.

Initial Condition: Syndrome S is identified ("differentiated") through TCM diagnosis of symptoms P.

Observational Prediction: Applying therapy T results in a reduction in the symptoms P in the patient.

In practice, how this works out may be as follows. Patients experiencing a constellation of symptoms, including "aching and weakness of the loins and knees, dizziness and tinnitus, night sweats, dry mouth and throat, afternoon flush in the cheeks, insomnia, thin rapid pulse, and a red tongue with little fur" (P) are identified. Based on these symptoms, the physician deduces that these patients suffer from a deficiency of kidney-*yin* (syndrome S). A drug cocktail, *Liuwei Dihuang Wan* (六味地黄丸), is then prescribed to treat this syndrome for a period of two weeks (T). The same group of patients are then randomised, divided into test and control groups, which are then prescribed with the test drug and a placebo respectively. If the improvement of symptoms in the test group proves to be significantly different from that of the control group, the main hypothesis can then be confirmed.

The Use of RCTs in Validating TCM Drug Formulas

What we have discussed thus far are hypothetical models for validating TCM diagnostic theories. The aim there is to establish that, at the very least, some of TCM diagnostic approaches can be empirically studied.[61] In this section, we turn to some of the research more commonly undertaken by TCM scientists. Currently, the types of TCM research conducted are quite varied, ranging from validating or systematising facial, tongue or pulse diagnoses, to RCTs on efficacy of therapies, such as acupuncture or drug formulas, on a

---

61   According to Hong Hai, however, most TCM clinical trial do not study these diagnostic approaches in the way described above. Ibid., 166.

variety of diseases.[62] For the purpose of illustration, we shall look at the application of RCTs on TCM therapies.

Typically, a TCM therapy, such as an acupuncture method or a drug formula, is passed down in the medical classics, such as the *Shanghan Lun*, or invented by an experienced TCM physician. A clinical trial occurs whenever a physician wants to examine an acupuncture method clinically, or a pharmaceutical company plans to mass produce a drug formula. In the case of a drug formula, where it differs from a biomedical drug is that the formula has already been prescribed to and well tested with patients for several years, with effective results and minimal side effects.[63] Consequently, there is a much higher chance that the drug will be effective on real trial patients even before the trials begin.

How then does a TCM drug trial proceed? As in the case of bio-medical trials, a TCM trial begins by specifying the research design protocols. Typically, these protocols define the disease to be treated (through a series of clinical symptoms), the ingredients to be used in the drug formula, how the concoction will be consumed, the demo-

---

62   See, for example, Yu-Feng Chung et al., "How to Standardize the Pulse-Taking Method of Traditional Chinese Medicine Pulse Diagnosis", *Computers in Biology and Medicine* 43, no. 4 (May 2013): 342–49.; Joyce K. Anastasi et al., "Tongue Inspection in TCM: Observations in a Study Sample of Patients Living with HIV", *Medical Acupuncture* 26, no. 1 (1 February 2014): 15–22; Chang Liu et al., "Computerized Color Analysis for Facial Diagnosis in Traditional Chinese Medicine" (IEEE, 2013), 613–14; Ted J. Kaptchuk, Keji Chen, and Jun Song, "Recent Clinical Trials of Acupuncture in the West: Responses from the Practitioners", *Chin J Integr Med* 2010 16, no. 3 (June 2010): 197–203.

63   In a normal TCM consultation, drug formulas will be prescribed to treat a patient's illness. These are usually based on or modified from classical formulas taught in the medical classics. Consequently, the formula would have been tested on hundreds of real-life patients before it undergoes clinical trials in anticipation of mass production. For example, Dr Diarra's teacher, TCM Master Physician, Sun Guangrong (孙光荣), has been prescribing a *Nine Taste Cooling and Qi Smoothening Drink* concoction (*jiuwei qingwen yiqiyin*, 九味清温益气饮) for more than two decades. The formula is effective for treating virus attacks, hand, foot and mouth disease, colds, and fevers with no specific causes (抗病毒、手足口病、感冒、无名发热). Should it be mass produced, it will have to undergo clinical trials to satisfy the approving authorities. The drug formula's success rate, however, would be much higher than that of a new biomedical drug, and its side-effects would be minimal.

graphic profile of the test patients, and the drugs or placebo that it will be compared with. In addition, the possible treatment outcomes will also be specified, that is, what constitutes complete recovery (治愈), improvement (好转) and no improvement (愈).[64] Apart from these requirements, a TCM trial protocol will further delineate the targeted disease by specifying the specific syndromes or patterns (证候分类) that the drug will treat. This criterion is unique to TCM trials since the possible patterns can only be derived from TCM pattern differentiation (辨证).

Take the common cold (感冒), for example. Both a biomedical and a TCM trial will identify its symptoms (诊断) as one or more of the several items in the following list:[65]

a. Running and congested nose, sneezing, cough, itchy throat.

b. Feeling cold and feverish, either without sweat or a little sweat, headache, body aches.

c. The symptoms could occur during any of the four seasons, but more commonly during spring or winter.

d. Normal or slightly lower white blood cell count, a decrease in neutrophils and an increase in lymphocytes.

a. 鼻塞流涕，喷嚏，咽痒或痛，咳嗽。

b. 恶寒发热，无汗或少汗，头痛，肢体酸楚。

64　TCM drug research protocols are specified in great detail in the *Criteria of Diagnosis and Therapeutic Effect of Diseases and Syndromes in Traditional Chinese Medicine* (中医病证诊断疗效标准). 国家中医药管理局， 中医病证诊断疗效标准 (*Criteria of Diagnosis and Therapeutic Effect of Diseases and Syndromes in Traditional Chinese Medicine*) (北京: 中国医药科技, 2012).

65　Ibid., 1.

c. 四时皆有，以冬春季节为多见。

d. 血白细胞总数正常或偏低，中性粒细胞减少，淋巴细胞相对增多。

The TCM trial protocol, however, will also include one of three pre-specified TCM syndromes or patterns from (a) to (c).[66]

a. Cold and Wind external pernicious influence: chills; fever; no sweat; headache and body aches; runny nose with clear nasal discharge; sneezing. Thin white fur on tongue; tight-floating or slow-floating pulse.

b. Hot and Wind external pernicious influence: fever; evil wind; migraine; blocked nose with yellow mucus; sore, reddish throat; cough. Sides and tip of the tongue are reddish; white or slight yellowish fur on tongue; floating and rapid pulse.

c. Heat and Dampness external pernicious influence: usually occurring during summer; migraine; blocked and runny nose; chills and fever; a body temperature that does not increase continually; little or no sweat; significant tightness of chest. Yellowish, greasy fur on tongue; moist and rapid pulse. A cold that arises from body deficiency, with dampness, stagnation and other symptoms.

a. 风寒束表：恶寒、发热、无汗、头痛身疼，鼻寒流清涕，喷嚏。舌苔薄白，脉浮紧或浮缓。

b. 风热犯表：发热、恶风、头胀痛，鼻塞流黄涕，咽痛咽红，咳嗽。舌边尖 红，苔白或微黄，脉浮数。

---

66   Ibid., 1 (Translation mine).

c. 暑湿袭表:见于夏季，头昏胀重，鼻塞流涕，恶寒发热，或热势不扬，无汗或少汗，胸闷泛恶。舌苔黄腻,脉濡数。临床尚有体虚感冒，以及挟湿、挟滞等兼证。

To illustrate how these protocols operate in practice, the following is a clinical trial conducted by Diarra to assess the efficacy of the Shuanghuang flower (双黄花) granule in preventing and treating acute respiratory tract infections (as compared to other mainstream therapies).[67]

Testing the efficacy of ShuangHuangHua drug formula for preventing and treating acute respiratory tract (ART) infections[68]

Trial Duration:
- March 2010 to Jul 2015

Patient profile:
- 3398 patients from Mali, Yunnan, Guangzhou, Kunming, Changsha and other cities. The Chinese patients were sub-divided according to their ethnic profiles (either Han or other minority tribes)
- Age group: 18-65 years old.
- 1903 (56%) female and 1495 (44%) male.
- All are volunteer patients.
- Patients with recognisable heart, kidney and liver medical problems, psychiatric problems, drug allergies, treated with other drugs, unable to adhere to the drug regime and other serious medical problems are excluded from the trial.

---

67   Diarra Boubacar, "Effect and Preventive Mechanism Study of ShuangHuangHua Granule on Acute Respiratory Tract Infections in Public Health Settings (超微双簧花颗粒防治人群呼吸道病毒感染的卫生学作用及相关机理的研究)" [Hunan TCM University (湖南中医药大学), 2015].

68   Ibid., 11–15.

Testing Procedure:

- SHH is administered in 10 g dosage (mixed with 100 ml water), 3 times a day, after food. Its efficacy is measured against 3 control groups:

  1. *Lianhua qingwen jiaonang* (莲花清瘟胶囊, thereafter LHQW), a TCM drug popularly used to treat ART.
  2. Moroxydine (ABOB), a biomedical drug commonly used to treat ART.
  3. A Placebo.

- The patients were divided into two groups and administered the above drugs using double blinded RCT. This is to test SHH's efficacy in preventing the onset of ART and its ability to treat patients infected with ART.

Highlights of clinical findings (based on 200 international/ Mali patients):

- For healthy volunteers, 92% of those who took SHH remained healthy, while LHQW, ABOB and the placebo protected 64%, 51% and 52% of its patients respectively. This implies that SHH is highly effective in preventing the onset of ART.
- For ART patients, SHH completely cured 85% of its patients, while LHQW, ABOB and the placebo cured 86%, 22.5% and 17% of their patients respectively. This implies that SHH and LHQW have comparable efficacies.

Overall findings (based on 200 international volunteers and patients):

- In terms of both prevention and treatment of ART, SHH was 90% effective, while LHQW, ABOB and the placebo were 71%, 42% and 30% effective respectively.

Methodological Issues in Validating Chinese Medicine

Now that we have a better sense of how double-blind RCTs may be applicable in TCM clinical trials, it is time to consider the methodological limitations of using RCTs in TCM research in general. For ease of illustration, we shall draw our insights primarily from the SHH clinical trial.

i) First of all, we should recognise that, no matter how fine-tuned the research protocols, the decision whether a patient's syndrome qualified for the SHH trial was largely dependent on the diagnostic skills of the TCM physician. For example, if the physician had misdiagnosed, and wrongly included a patient in the trial, the test drug would have been unlikely to cure the patient. What we would have ended up with is a false negative result.

ii) Secondly, in order for a patient to qualify for a TCM trial, she had to not only meet the specified symptoms, but also the pre-determined TCM syndromes or patterns. This second qualification clearly made it more difficult to find a sufficient number of patients who met both criteria. To complicate matters, it was also not uncommon for a patient to have more than one syndrome concurrently. Such a constraint only served to further restrict the number of patients who could qualify for a trial.[69]

iii) TCM syndromes often evolve or change quite quickly over the course of a patient's illnesses (as compared to biomedical pathogenesis). Consequently, the above trials had to assume or could only be "limited to those syndromes that are relatively stable and that do not change without intervention within the duration of the trial".[70]

---

69   Hong, *Theory of Chinese Medicine*, 168–71, 174–77.
70   Ibid., 169.

iv) The SHH trial presumed a fixed drug dosage administered against a specified target virus. Both conditions, quite clearly, conformed to the assumptions of biomedicine, rather than the patient-centric approach of TCM that is more commonly practised by physicians, where the drug formula's dosage and composition are adjusted according to the patient's body constitution, age, and "the severity of his symptoms and the appearance of other syndromes as his condition evolves". If one were to choose to be faithful to the therapeutic logic of TCM, it would mean prescribing customised drug formulas for each trial patient. This then raises the question of whether the individual trial results, even if they were successful, would be comparable and representative.

v) Finally, the placebo effects of some TCM therapies could well be higher than biomedicine and are still not properly understood. This was well illustrated in recent pragmatic and explanatory RCTs conducted to assess the efficacy of acupuncture for pain relief. While pragmatic trials suggested that acupuncture could be twice as effective as mainstream care, explanatory trials concluded, on the contrary, that "verum [traditional/genuine] and sham acupuncture had effects of identical magnitudes".[71] Scholars have differed on the reasons for this phenomenon. Some have questioned whether it was possible to administer sham acupuncture without the patient's knowledge, to begin with.[72] Kaptchuk, on the other hand, has highlighted evidence that demonstrates sham acupuncture to be superior to placebo pills in pain management. In addition, he draws attention to recent neurological studies that may well explain the verum and sham acupuncture dilemma. When acupuncture and sham acupuncture were administered to volunteers, the neuroanatomical correlates of

---

71   Kaptchuk, Chen, and Song, "Recent Clinical Trials of Acupuncture".
72   Vivienne Lo, "Introduction", in *Celestial Lancets: A History and Rationale of Acupuncture and Moxa*, by Gwei-Fjen Lu and Joseph Needham (London: Routledge, 2015), 141.

both the test and control groups were examined using functional magnetic resonance imaging (fMRI). As it turned out,

> needle stimulation inhibited incoming noxious stimuli with a peripheral-central *bottom up* somatosensory modulation, while sham acupuncture activated a *top-down* modulation of pain and worked through the brain's emotional circuitry.[73]

Likewise, a second study using positron emission tomography (PET) and a radioactive tracer in patients with fibromyalgia produced similar pain relief, but two very distinct brain mechanistic patterns. Specifically, verum acupuncture increased the availability of endogenous opioid receptors, while sham acupuncture produced decreased or no change in receptor availability while increasing the release of endorphins.

Notwithstanding the above difficulties, it remains necessary for Chinese medicine, I believe, to subject its diagnostic models and therapies to RCT validation, at least to some degree.[74] Without this, it would be difficult for Chinese medicine to deepen its engagement, dialogue and exchange of ideas with its Western counterpart. Finally, apart from RCTs, it is noteworthy that observational studies can also be a valuable source of clinical evidence for Chinese medical therapies. The potential for such studies is particularly promising in view of the large amounts of detailed and accurate patient records kept in the state-run TCM hospitals in China. Such data not only offers a substantial sample size for any clinical studies but can also lend itself to data-mining techniques and statistical analyses.[75]

---

73 Kaptchuk, Chen, and Song, "Recent Clinical Trials of Acupuncture", 200–1.

74 Hong, *Theory of Chinese Medicine*, 183.

75 Ibid., 183–84.

Chinese Medicine: A Viable Therapeutic Option?

We return now to our original question: whether Chinese medicine should be regarded as a viable medical option? The answer, as some readers may recognise by now, is not quite straightforward. If we base our decision mostly on the degree to which TCM therapies have been validated by biomedical clinical methods, the answer will be mixed. Some acupuncture therapies and drug formulas have been validated by RCTs, but most have yet to be. This does not mean that most TCM therapies are not based on empirical studies. On the contrary, they are. If they were not effective in healing thousands of Chinese over the last 2,000 years, they would not be recorded in the numerous medical classics, treatises and case histories to begin with. Furthermore, before one slights TCM therapies as less evidence-based (in biomedical terms) and, therefore, less reliable, let us remember that some of the common drugs that we use, because they have been well tested in real-life patients, have not been subjected to rigorous RCTs. Moreover, in some cases, some of these drugs have been found to be ineffective, as in the case of over-the-counter cough medication.[76] Then, there are the different clinical trial problems mentioned above that cast further doubts on the reliability of some biomedical trials. Seen from this perspective, is not the biomedical expectation that all TCM therapies be validated by RCTs overly stringent or, perhaps, even inequitable?

If we are to take the Chinese medical tradition seriously, and with respect, it should be clear that secular Chinese medicine has much to offer the world. Going by its therapeutic track record over the last 2,000 years, the anecdotal evidence that we gather from

---

76   RCTs of over-the-counter cough medications have concluded that "there is no good evidence for their effectiveness!" Knut Schroeder and Tom Fahey, "Systematic Review of Randomised Controlled Trials of over the Counter Cough Medicines for Acute Cough in Adults", *BMJ* (*Clinical Research Ed.*) 324, no. 7333 (9 February 2002): 329–31.; "Over-the-Counter (OTC) Medications for Acute Cough in Children and Adults in Community Settings | Cochrane", accessed 14 July 2016, http://www.cochrane.org/CD001831/ARI_over-the-counter-otc-medications-for-acute-cough-in-children-and-adults-in-community-settings.

Chinese medical writings, feedback from relatives and friends, and the growing body of RCT evidence, there is reasonable basis for one to use Chinese medicine. This openness to experimentation, or trying things out, has to be the case when we, with our finite knowledge, attempt to understand a discipline that is seemingly infinite in comparison. Interestingly, St Anselm's (1033–1109) dictum, "faith seeking understanding", is remarkably relevant here. For it is when we try out Chinese medicine "by faith", that we can "understand" whether it is truly effective. Indeed, of all people, Christians should be able to show the most empathy here. For we too recognise that it is only when we respond by faith to our limited knowledge of God, that we begin to encounter and understand the richness of His love, and the Christian tradition that we have received from our Christian forefathers.

Conclusion

The last century has seen the range of biomedical therapies grow by leaps and bounds. Alongside this development is a growing concern for establishing the necessary safeguards to assess and regulate this wide range of therapeutic options. It is within this context that the double-blind RCT came to be regarded as the "gold standard" and most important means of evaluating the diverse biomedical interventions. As Chinese medicine modernises, there are increasing expectations that it should likewise subject its theories and therapies to empirical validation, particularly using RCTs. To some extent, these requirements are already practised in TCM research. Notwithstanding this, we should recognise that RCTs are not without its own flaws. More importantly, the underlying premise of RCTs—that they were designed to assess the efficacy of standardised treatments for specific disease categories—does not auger well with several characteristics peculiar to Chinese medicine, such as the evolving nature of its disease syndromes, and its physicians' preference for prescribing individualised therapies specific to their patients' sicknesses. It is for this reason that large-scale observational studies should be concurrently employed as another means of TCM empirical studies.

Finally, as to the question whether one should use Chinese medicine as a viable therapeutic option, the decision, in the end, boils down to our grounds of authority. That is, whether we regard RCTs and biomedical methodologies as the sole arbiters and referees for clinical efficacy, or do we allow for the rich Chinese medical tradition to speak for itself.

11

CHRISTIAN PERSPECTIVES
ON CHINESE MEDICINE

Reviewing our Journey through East and West

In the course of this book, we surveyed 3,000 years of medical history and philosophy, both in the West and in China. We began with the classical Greek states, where we observed how Greek ontology played a formative role in the development of Hippocratic medicine. Due to the efforts of Galen, Hippocratic humoral medicine became dominant in the Roman Empire eventually, and was regarded as the *de facto* form of medicine, not only in the medieval West, but also in the Byzantine and medieval Islamic empires. During this period, the early Christians reflected extensively on the role and use of medicine among Christians. Generally speaking, they affirmed the value of Hippocratic medicine and adopted it readily for the Church's philanthropic causes. Indeed, Christians even played an important role in reintroducing Hippocratic medicine back to Western Europe, after the continent was plagued by centuries of wars and cultural decline.

The modern scientific revolution, however, cast so much doubt on Hippocratic teachings that, by the end of the 19th century, their influence was all but gone, having been supplanted by modern medical discoveries. Since then, the dual successes of the new aetiologies introduced by modern medicine, and its spectacular invention of a whole host of surgical and drug therapies have made biomedicine the new medical orthodoxy by which all other medical traditions would be judged.

Turning to the Chinese medical tradition, we saw that the Chinese too developed a secular form of medicine as early as during the Han dynasty (first century BC). Where they differed from the Greeks was their use of *yinyang* philosophy as the metaphysical paradigm for their medical discourse. This approach has held sway till this day, even with the recent incorporation of biomedical thinking into Chinese medicine. In our comparison of the Western and Chinese medical traditions, it is clear that the two diverge significantly in their understanding of human physiology, health, aetiology and medical therapy. This has been due largely to the different philosophical, epistemological and linguistic assumptions that they have brought to bear on these subjects. The Greeks and the West were preoccupied with the questions of ontology and epistemic certainty, while the Chinese by the network of relationships, or the *yin* and *yang*, that subsists in a human being and characterises his relationship with his environment.

Our journey thus far has spanned several disciplines and ventured into unfamiliar and often complex grounds, such as Chinese philosophy, cognitive linguistics and medical historiography. The reason, as we explained in Chapter 2, is simply this: this is an exercise in loving our neighbour (Mark 12:30–31); a careful attempt at understanding how the Chinese conceptualise medicine, and to represent them accurately. This, I believe, is the most important principle in any Christian cross-cultural engagement. Failure to do so not only creates unnecessary misunderstandings, but also renders such engagements futile exercises. Having said this, there is a second and equally important purpose for our investigation, namely, the findings we gather will also become the basis by which we reflect theologically about engaging and dialoguing with Chinese medicine.

This theological reflection will be the focus of our concluding chapter.

A Theological Framework for Evaluating Chinese Medicine

In Chapter 2, we asserted that all human knowledge is based on some form of empirical study, transcendental truths, or both. Where each of us differs is how we go about justifying the legitimacy of our empirical approaches or transcendental ideas. Being fashioned as images of God, we cannot help but desire that such knowledge be absolute. Being finite beings, however, our knowledge will always be limited and partial. This is also why, as a result of socio-political and environmental differences, the Western and Chinese medical traditions came to differ so drastically. Recognising this, however, tell us nothing about which aspects of a medical tradition are compatible with Christian belief. This is why a theological analytical framework is necessary.

Theologically speaking, human knowledge may be categorised in terms of the knowledge of God, and of the world. The knowledge of God can be sub-divided into three folds. The first is divine or religious knowledge that is contrary to Christian teachings—a result that is due, in no small measure, to humanity's estranged relationship with God, and our tendency to sin. The second is Special Revelation, or God's revelation of Himself through the history of Israel and Jesus Christ, and the Holy Scriptures. The third are features in our human knowledge of God that are compatible with Christian teaching. This is commonly known among theologians as General Revelation. Our evaluation of Chinese medicine can be construed, therefore, as a discernment of the degree to which Chinese medical philosophy and theory are compatible with General Revelation.

But how do we go about doing this? Two analytical models were introduced for this purpose. The first was the Wesleyan Quadrilateral which teaches that any theological reflection should be informed by (1) the teachings of the Bible; (2) the theological reflections and wisdom of our spiritual forefathers, or Christian tradition; (3) our reason (which involves a careful use of secular or non-Christian sources of knowledge); and (4) our spiritual experience. Among these, primacy must be accorded to the Scriptures.

The second model was Jackson Wu's model of contextualisation. According to Wu, religious knowledge may be envisaged as three overlapping spheres: biblical truth, theology and cultural context. Within these spheres, we have Areas C, D and F, which denote

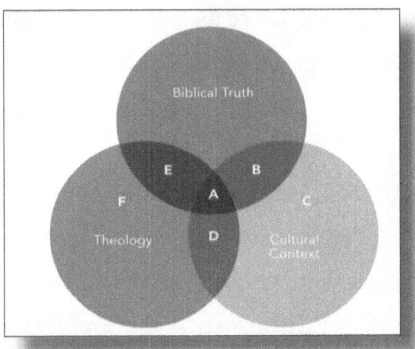

theological and/ or cultural ideas that are contrary to biblical teachings. Areas A and E, on the other hand, represent ideas that are compatible with Scriptures. When we examine Chinese medical teachings, we must discern which aspects of these teachings belong to the former category (and thus should be rejected), and which to the latter (and thus can be affirmed). What is unique and valuable about Wu's model, however, is his conception of Area B. Area B, as Wu explains, represents aspects of an indigenous culture that are compatible with "biblical categories and values", but not regarded as so by prevailing theologies.[1] What gives rise to Area B? How can an aspect of Chinese medical philosophy cohere with biblical teaching, but yet not Christian theology?

There are two reasons for this. The first is the fact that the structure and emphases of classical Christian doctrines were shaped mostly by

[1]   Jackson Wu, *Saving God's Face: A Chinese Contextualization of Salvation through Honor and Shame* (Pasadena, Calif.: William Carey International University Press, 2012), 51–53.

their historical contexts.[2] They were answers developed to address the pastoral or theological challenges that arose in the course of church history, using the biblical, theological and philosophical apparatus available to our spiritual forefathers. The Nicene Creed is a good example. To fend off Arian claims that Jesus Christ is but an exalted creature, the early Christians (known otherwise as the "Church Fathers") not only argued from Scriptures, but also employed the categories of Greek ontology. The net result was the Nicene Creed, where they declared Jesus Christ as not just the only begotten Son of God (to use the language of John 3:16), but also *homoousios* (of the same essence or nature) with the Father (using the categories of Greek ontology).

Chinese medical philosophy developed in a geo-political and social context that differed vastly from that of the West. The concerns that framed its questions about cosmology, anthropology and medical well-being were also quite different. It is hardly surprising then that the answers it came up with looked and felt very different from those formulated in classical theology. The second reason is related to the first. Namely, Chinese philosophical discourse is structured and guided by the ideas of *yinyang* rather than Greek ontology. The consequence of this is that metaphysically and linguistically speaking, its teachings would be quite dissimilar from classical theology, or, for that matter, Western philosophy in general. All this need not mean that such ideas must be incompatible with biblical teachings. Consequently, when we evaluate Chinese medicine, we must be attentive to aspects of Chinese medical philosophy that may cohere with biblical teachings, even if they sound foreign to our Western-trained ears initially.[3]

---

2   By "classical theology", I mean the orthodox Christian doctrine developed by the Church over the last 2,000 years in a predominantly Western context (whether, Roman, European, English or American).

3   James Houston adopts a similar approach in his exploration of how Japanese and Western Christians may mutually enrich one another. Cf. James Houston, *The Christian Life East and West: Toward the Mutual Enrichment of Japanese and Western Christianity* (Vancouver, B.C.:

Christian Perspectives on the Chinese Philosophy of *Yinyang*

Bearing in mind the above theological principles, how then do we evaluate Chinese medicine? A good place to start would be the metaphysical or philosophical paradigms assumed by the medical tradition: the theories of *yinyang, qi* and *wuxing*. We begin with the observation that Scriptures make no mention of these terms, and thus do not pronounce any explicit judgements on them.[4] Yet, might the Bible and our Christian tradition have something to say about these motifs? If we look deeper into what underlies these three philosophical ideas, it would be seen that they have a common concern for depicting cosmic and human reality as intrinsically relational and dynamic. That is, any impact or changes on an entity or node in the cosmos will have repercussions (positive or negative) on the other interlinking nodes.[5] More importantly, as the Chinese put it, the relationships between Heaven (*tian*, 天), which represents the divine, Earth (*di*, 地), which represents the land or the cosmos, and Humanity (*ren*, 人) must be coordinated and harmonised, in order that all may flourish. Seen from this light, it would seem that these philosophical motifs are analogous with or parallel Scriptural teachings on the relationship between God, Creation and humanity. The creation accounts of Genesis 1 and 2 clearly depict idyllic Creation as a state where humanity enjoyed a peaceful and fruitful coexistence with all other creatures and God—a *shalom*. The tragedy of Adam's Fall, unfortunately, fractured and soured all the relationships between God and man, human beings with one another, and our relationships with all other creatures. Turning to the New Testament, we find

---

Regent College Publishing, 2017).

4 The same may be said about the Greeks and Western preoccupation with ontology and mathematical epistemic certainty. The Bible says nothing about the veracity of describing the world in terms of circumscribed natures or essences.

5 In recent decades, non-Chinese secular sciences, most notably systems dynamics or Complexity theory, have also attested to the importance of conceptualising or modelling reality in terms of networks of relationships, rather than circumscribed or individualised natures.

that the healing of this three-fold relationship is an essential aspect of Christ's salvation. Christ died and rose again in order to heal the relationship between God and man. The proclamation of the Gospel, in turn, is intended to reunite humanity, and break down the "walls of hostility" between us (Eph. 2:14). Finally, the consummation of our salvation is regarded by Paul as a reconciliation of the world to God. It is for this reason that "creation waits with eager longing for the revealing of the sons of God", so that it will be "set free from its bondage to corruption and obtain the freedom of the glory of the children of God" (Rom. 8:19–21).

This is not to say that there are no problematic elements in the Chinese system, theologically speaking. A popular feature in *yinyang* theory is the assumption that the changing relationship between *yin* and *yang* is perpetual, and this is the way by which the cosmos re-generates itself eternally, without need of a Creator. This atheistic notion, nonetheless, is not intrinsic to the basic idea of *yinyang*. The latter does not fall apart or become invalid if the former is excluded. Certainly, *yinyang* perpetuity is not necessary for the theory and prac-tice of Chinese medicine. This being the case, *yinyang* theory can well be accepted as compatible with Christian revelation and teaching if these atheistic elements are excluded. Indeed, the Chinese often speak of a "Limitless" (*wuji*, 无极) generating or giving rise (*sheng*, 生) to the "Supreme Ultimate" (*taiji*, 太极), and the Supreme Ulti-mate giving birth to the "Two Poles" or *yinyang* (*liangyi*, 两仪), and these give rise ultimately to the eight trigrams (*bagua*, 八卦).[6] What this entails is a process where all things evolve and are created. Es-sentially, a conviction that "the one which is unknown or cannot be described" (*wuji*) is that which gives rise to all the varied, inter-relat-ed and complex entities of the world. If we postulate an ontological distinction between *wuji* and the rest of the processes, we can then

---

6   The earliest conception of this idea is found in the *Yijing*, or the Book of Changes, and *Yizhuan*, the earliest commentary on the *Yijing*. *Liangyi* is commonly regarded as a reference to *yinyang*.

regard *wuji* as God, who stands apart from all creation, acts to bring Creation into being, and continually sustains and transforms it. Making this suggestion is not a syncretistic compromise, or an attempt to "have our cake and eat it". Rather, such an attempt to reconceptualise or Christianise *yinyang* theory has many precedents in both Scripture and the history of Christian doctrine. The clearest example is, perhaps, the Apostle Paul's speech in Athens (Acts 17:23–28), where he not only employed the Athenian notion of "the unknown god", but went on to quote the philosophers, Epimenides of Crete and Aratus, favourably and as part of his Gospel proclamation at the Areopagus.[7]

> The God who made the world and everything in it … does not live in temples made by man … as though he needed anything, since he himself gives to all mankind life and breath and everything. And he made from one man every nation of mankind to live on all the face of the earth, having determined allotted periods and the boundaries of their dwelling place, that they should seek God, and perhaps feel their way toward him and find him. Yet he is actually not far from each one of us, for "in him we live and move and have our being"; as even some of your own poets have said, "For we are indeed his offspring."

Likewise, the word, *logos*, was commonly understood by the Greeks as a word, message or the principle of reason or creative order. It is for this reason that the Apostle John employed it to portray the Son as the *Logos* or Creator of the world. By doing this, however, John also redefined the word by investing it with new Christian meanings.

---

7   Paul's use of the two philosophers, of course, did not mean that he believes that all their teachings are similar to or compatible with Christian teachings. Rather, he employs what is compatible with Scriptural teachings in order that he may exemplify what he propounds in 1 Corinthians 9:22–23: "to the weak I became weak that I might win the weak. I have become all things to all people, that by all means I might save some".

Specifically, the *Logos* was reconceived as a personal being who put on flesh to dwell among humanity: Jesus Christ!

This Christian retrieval or reception of pagan philosophy was taken on board by the church fathers. A good example would be their use of Platonic philosophy. Although these early Christians rejected Plato's claim that matter is eternal and divine, they happily concurred with the philosopher that the cosmos was created and the goal of humanity was to become like god, or, in our case, Jesus Christ (Gen. 1:26, Col. 1:15).[8] As mentioned earlier, the Greek philosophers' preoccupation with ontology or nature was also brought to good use in the Trinitarian controversy, when the fathers affirmed Christ's full divinity using the *homoousios* formula.

In short, as Christians engage with indigenous cultures, like that of the Chinese, we need to intimate the approach of our spiritual forefathers. We need to be on the lookout for what coheres or does not cohere with biblical teachings (that is, Jackson Wu's Areas A and C). We also need to explore ways of redeeming, or indeed, transfiguring indigenous cultural ideas. For it is in this way then that an indigenous Christian learns how to affirm his cultural heritage, and to appropriate it to enrich the broader Christian tradition.

Conceptualising a Chinese Christian Anthropology

Practically speaking, how would such an endeavour look like? Are there aspects of Chinese medical philosophy that may come across as foreign to classical Christian theology, but actually offer theological insights congenial with biblical teachings? Besides the theory of *yinyang* discussed above, Chinese medical anthropology, I believe, is also a fertile ground for our reflections. Among the Chinese medical writings on this subject, the most representative summary is that presented in the opening chapter of the *Neijing Suwen*. When asked

---

8   *Timaeus* 28a.

why do the ancients managed to live beyond a hundred years, and did not weaken in their vitality, while the people of today waned and died even before the age of 50, Qibo replied that

> The people of high antiquity, those who knew the Way, they modelled [their behaviour] on yin and yang and they complied with the arts and the calculations. [Their] eating and drinking was moderate. [Their] rising and resting had regularity. They did not tax [themselves] with meaningless work. Hence, they were able to keep physical appearance and spirit together, and to exhaust the years [allotted by] heaven.

In contrast, the people of today are different because

> they take wine as an [ordinary] beverage, and they adopt absurd [behaviour] as regular [behaviour]. They are drunk when they enter the [women's] chambers. Through their lust they exhaust their essence, through their wastefulness they dissipate their true [qi]. They do not know how to maintain fullness and they engage their spirit when it is not the right time. They make every effort to please their hearts, [but] they oppose the [true] happiness of life. Rising and resting miss their terms. Hence, it is [only] one half of a hundred [years] and they weaken.[9]

This is a very rich passage, where several similarities with Christian teaching are observed. The first has already been discussed: that is, human beings should live in harmony with the cosmos. Or to express it in Christian terms, we should abide by the creative

---

9   Paul U. Unschuld and Hermann Tessenow, with Zheng Jinsheng, *Huang Di Nei Jing Su Wen: An Annotated Translation of Huang Di's Inner Classic — Basic Questions*, Vol. 1 (Berkeley: University of California Press, 2011), 30–33.

principles that God has planted in His Creation. The second is the *Neijing's* recognition that one's physical health and ethics are closely intertwined. Moral misbehaviour often leads to physical illnesses and premature death (John 5:14). The third is the text's implicit aspiration for immortal life, encapsulated in its esteem for the longevity of the "people of antiquity". To acknowledge these parallels, however, is not to say that there are no problematic elements here.

The most significant, I believe, is the absence of a biblical teaching of the Fall and sin in Chinese cosmology and anthropology. That is, a recognition of how sin has ruptured the harmonious relationships between humanity and Creation, and brought death, decay and destruction into every aspect of our lives. Not all is well in the world that we live in, and our human attempts to live in harmony with the *yinyang* will never quite resolve this problem. Although living according to the *yinyang* may prolong life or reduce the instances of sicknesses, it can neither eliminate sicknesses entirely, nor avoid the inevitability of death. Even TCM physicians acknowledge this readily! In a similar vein, while Chinese medical philosophy is on the right track in identifying longevity, or indeed, immortality, as a significant human desire, the solutions it provides will not get us there.

Related to this is the relationship that Chinese medicine posits between human morality and physical health. While it is true that Adam and his posterity would not have fallen ill had he remained faithful to God, this positive correlation between one's morality and physical health does not quite hold anymore. The picture that we get from Scriptures is far more complex. Job, for example, was plagued with boils not because of his sins, but his life had become the arena of a cosmic battle between good and evil (Job 2). The Apostle Paul likewise suffered from a "thorn in the flesh", not because he had sinned, but in order that he might learn how to accomplish all things by God's grace, and not his own strength (2 Cor. 12:9). In the case of the man born blind, he suffered this not because of his own sins or that of his parents, but in order that his healing might be an occasion to glorify God. The experiences of the church fathers, as mentioned in Chapter 3, attest similarly to the fact that those faithful to God still had to endure pain and suffering for all sorts of reasons. Consequently, if Chinese medical anthropology is to be accepted into the Christian fold, it must incorporate the complex dynamics introduced by Adam's Fall and sin. This is to recognise that while spiritual and moral progress often yield health benefits, there are also many exceptions to this principle. In truth, the relationship between physical and spiritual well-being is no longer a straightforward matter in our fallen world.

Having said all this, Chinese reflections on human flourishing do provide rich insights for how we can think about spiritual healing and Christian living. A good illustration of the former may be found in the way Chinese medicine conceptualises illnesses. According to Chinese medical theory, all kinds of illnesses, whether physical or emotional, are due to some form of disharmony or disequilibrium of yinyang (yinyang bupingheng, 阴阳不平衡) within one's body, or in the body's relationship with its environment. This aetiological metaphor, I think, can supplement our understanding of how sin is defined and operates in our lives.

Generally speaking, sin is understood as committing what is evil (whether in deed or thought), or omitting what is good. As the famous church father, Augustine of Hippo, puts it: sin is a privation, or absence of the good. That the early Christians would conceptualise sin as the corruption of "something" good, or the lack of goodness in "something" should not surprise us, given our appreciation of their ontological bias. While there is much to be commended about this approach to hamartiology (the doctrine of sin), I believe it can be enriched by incorporating the Chinese medical metaphor of yinyang disequilibrium.

Intrinsic to the idea of yinyang disequilibrium is the recognition that illnesses are not due entirely to individual causes, but a whole host of other factors, such as the environment we live in, the weather we come under, our level of stress at work, or even the health and well-being of our family members. Or, as Hong Hai put it, the state of our health is determined by multiple INUS conditions. This aetiological metaphor parallels very well with how sin actually takes hold of our lives. Adultery, for example, is unlikely to be caused just by the fleeting sight of a beautiful woman. On the contrary, it is more likely the result of multiple factors operating in tandem, such as loneliness, stress at work, poor relations with one's spouse, use of pornography and, perhaps, even parental alienation. Seen from this perspective, the "fleeting sight" is but the last factor that tips the balance for the man, causing a systemic breakdown in his self-control. The classical-ontological model of sin, unfortunately, does not lend itself well to representing this systemic dimension of our struggle with temptation and sin. The motif of *yinyang* disequilibrium, on the other hand, captures these dynamics very well, and, in so doing, provides fresh perspectives on how we can help others in their journey towards spiritual healing. That is, not just addressing the adultery itself, but to give attention to the other factors that may have contributed to the spiritual disharmony—as so many experienced counsellors know well!

Besides clarifying the systemic dimensions of sin, Chinese medical anthropology also offers much wisdom on how we can moderate our lives, so that we live in harmony with God's Creation. In the *Neijing*, the perfect or ideal human beings (*zhenren*, 真人) are described as "those who knew the Way", "modelled [their behaviour] on *yin* and *yang*", and led a moderate and regular lifestyle. Generally, this is understood as living according to the rhythms of creation, such as changes in seasons and the cycles of daily life. In practice, this involves a wide variety of disciplines and habits, such as resting and sleeping regularly at the appropriate hours (before midnight), coordinating our daily activities according to the seasons (more activity during the summer, less activity and more rest during winter) and eating fruits and grains according to what the seasons yield.[10]

10   With regards to the last example, TCM presumes that our bodies adapt best to the food

This is a sharp contrast, of course, with the experience of modern men and women (whether Christian or non-Christian).

Most of us live in technocratic societies where the rhythms of our lives are not only decoupled from the rhythms of Creation but dictated and driven by the demands of our technological systems and devices. Often, we push the limits of our bodies and deprive them of sleep by working long hours through the night; we work and exercise irrespective of changes in seasonal weather (for example, jogging during winter rather than resting and hibernating like all other creatures); and we import food from all over the world, with little regard to whether food grown from such lands are suitable for our bodies. By living so disharmoniously with God's Creation, we not only put undue stress on ourselves, but also generate an insatiable demand for the world's resources. The latter, of course, has given rise to the catastrophic levels of environmental destruction, and the severe challenges of climate change that we now face.

To be sure, the ascetic principles of TCM are not Gospel truth. Not all of them are true. Nevertheless, they are based on centuries of accumulated reflections on how human beings can flourish physically, emotionally and ethically. The early Christians, such as Basil of Caesarea, Augustine and John Chrysostom, did not reject Graeco-Roman ascetic practice entirely, but adapted it for Christian practice as and when they found it helpful. The same approach, I believe, is applicable to TCM ascetic principles. For example, Chinese medicine's exhortation that one should rest adequately according to the changing of the seasons, and its caution against excessive consumption and sexual practices can surely provide Christians with helpful handles for cultivating moderation in our lives. Another useful insight is the Chinese medical assumption that an intimate and bilateral relationship subsists between one's body and emotions. What happens to the body will affect the soul, and vice versa. This is a helpful reminder for many Christians who often neglect the one for the sake of another.

harvested at the prevailing season.

So, while they may participate actively in church ministries, they may also see no need to moderate their eating habits. The consequence of this is that their gluttony and resulting weight gain are likely to have a detrimental effect on their mental health and emotional states. Yet, if they were to take their cue from Chinese medical anthropology, they would realise, like the church fathers, that how and what we eat matters for our souls. When we moderate our stomachs, we reap much fruit for spiritual health.

Christian Perspectives on Chinese Medical Therapies

We turn finally to the therapies commonly employed in TCM practice. We begin with the observation that, ever since the rise of biomedicine, mainstream medicine has become entirely secularised. A biomedical physician prescribing some form of religious therapy is not only unheard of but legally proscribed. This is a sharp contrast to medical traditions in non-Western cultures, whether African, Indian or Egyptian. Here, secular and religious therapies often intermingled and were practised alongside one another since antiquity. The same can be said for classical Chinese medicine up until recently. For example, in his famous medical compendium, *Qian Jin Yi Fang* (千金翼方), the famous Tang physician, Sun Simiao, did not find it strange or incoherent to prescribe drugs against diseases supposedly caused by demonic spirits.[11] But things have changed radically since then. With the communist integration of Chinese and biomedicine in the mid-20th century, such religious aetiologies and healings have been all but abandoned. It would now be extremely difficult, if not impossible, to find such therapies offered in TCM hospitals and clinics, whether in China or overseas. This being said, there are rare occasions when TCM physicians, especially those among the Chinese diaspora, might offer both secular and religious therapies. For example, a TCM

---

11   Paul U. Unschuld, *Medicine in China: A History of Ideas* (Berkeley, CA; London: University of California Press, 1985), 35–46, 52–53.

sinseh might provide traditional bone setting treatments as well as religious healings that involve the summoning of a deity's aid, and the preparation of a concoction of water mixed with a burnt talisman.[12] Such syncretism, unfortunately, problematises Chinese medicine. For Christians who are unfamiliar with the medical tradition, apprehensive about the *yinyang* philosophy, and take for granted the authority of biomedicine, such rare cases alone would be sufficient to convince them to reject the use of Chinese medicine altogether.

Yet, given the distinctions we have made, it is possible to distinguish the different types of Chinese medical practice and therapies.

a. The first is the secular Chinese medicine offered by mainstream TCM hospitals and clinics. Here, the efficacy of their physicians' treatments is dependent entirely on their medical knowledge and skills, and not at all on some form of religious power.

b. The second type of TCM practice is the same as the first, except for the fact that the medical physician is known to be a non-Christian, whether Buddhist, Daoist or atheist. No matter the physician's religious affiliations, the efficacy of his treatments still does not depend on his faith, but only on his grasp of TCM knowledge and therapy.

c. The third category are those similar to the *sinseh* mentioned above, where secular and religious forms of healings are offered and often intermingle.

Which of these medical practices are acceptable for Christian usage then? The first should be perfectly legitimate, for the reasons laid out in the previous chapters. The same can be said for the second type

---

12   The term, *sinseh*, is often used in Singapore and Malaysia to refer to TCM physicians who learnt their practice through apprenticeship and received little formal training at TCM colleges.

of TCM physicians. Just as the faith of biomedical physicians do not improve or hamper their skills, likewise the faith of TCM physicians (or the lack of it). Rather, what counts here again is their mastery of their medical discipline. As for the third category, it is advisable for Christians to refrain from patronising such *sinsehs*. This is because the *sinseh* is unlikely to clearly distinguish the lines between secular and religious healings, the consequence of which is that one might subject oneself to the healing power of a foreign deity unknowingly.

What then is the theological rationale for the above distinctions, particularly for Categories 2 and 3? This would be made clear when we consider a claim that is popular within some Christian quarters: namely, that acupuncture therapy can expose Christians to demonic control. This is because they claim that demonic spirits can flow through the acupuncture needles into a Christian's body. To address this question, some deliberations on the Christian understanding of human nature, or Christian anthropology, are called for. Earlier, we established that a great part of what it means to be human must be understood through our nature as images of God (Genesis 1:26). The coming of Christ, however, introduced a new dimension to this doctrine. Through the Incarnation, the Son of God put on flesh (*sarx*), or human nature, in order to become our Mediator with God (1 Tim. 2:5), our Representative (Matt. 4:1–11) and our Exemplar (1 Cor. 11:1).[13] Indeed, Christ is fully human, but He did not sin (Heb. 2:17, 4:15). Over the next few centuries, the church fathers reflected much and deeply about the mystery of the Incarnation. Among them was Gregory of Nazianzus (c. 329–390), one of the most important theologians of the early Church. In one of his reflections on the relationship between Christ's humanity and His salvafic work, he

---

13   By subjecting himself to 40 days of temptation, Christ reenacted the experience of the Israelites when they sojourned 40 years in the wilderness. Where He differed from them was that He was obedient to God entirely. In this way then, he proves to be the perfect Israel and, thus, a worthy Representative of humanity.

declared that "the unassumed is unhealed".[14] By this he meant that the Son of God must assume the whole of human nature in order to heal every single aspect of it. Or to put it negatively, if Christ were to take on a different human nature, he would not have been a proper Mediator, Representative or Exemplar on our behalf.[15] Half a century later, the church fathers elaborated on Gregory's insight by asserting in the Chalcedonian Creed (451) that Christ is not only fully human and fully divine, but that these two natures do not change or intermingle with one another.[16]

These teachings on Christ's two-fold natures are instructive. Most significantly, they highlight the fact that, even with the Fall of Adam, human nature *does not* change. This is because the natures which God creates can never be changed by creatures, including the Devil and his minions. Rather, the only thing that the Devil can do is to corrupt the goodness which God has bequeathed to us, to render it less than its original potential. Or to recapitulate Augustine's dictum: evil is the absence of goodness, or the diminution of its being. What does this mean for TCM? Basically this: a medical therapy, whether it is acupuncture, moxibustion, or antibiotics, can work only to the extent that it conforms with our created and unchangeable human nature, or the natural laws that God has invested in it. If a therapy contradicts this nature or its creative principles, it can only worsen a patient's sickness or, worse, kill him. If a medical therapy is shown to

---

14   Gregory of Nazinzus, *Epistle* 101.

15   That this is the case may be seen in the hypothetical example of Clark Kent (Superman), the Kryptonian. It would be plainly ridiculous to expect human beings to imitate him since he is ontologically different from us by being far more powerful (and bulletproof).

16   As the Chalcedonian Creed puts it, "the same Son, our Lord Jesus Christ, the same perfect in Godhead and also perfect in manhood; truly God and truly man, of a reasonable soul and body; consubstantial with us according to the manhood; in all things like unto us, without sin; begotten before all ages of the Father according to the Godhead, ... [He is], to be acknowledged in two natures, inconfusedly, unchangeably, indivisibly, inseparably; the distinction of natures being by no means taken away by the union, but rather the property of each nature being preserved, and concurring in one Person and one Subsistence". The Chalcedonian Creed is regarded as orthodoxy for Catholic, Eastern Orthodox and Protestant Christians.

be effective empirically, and this happens regardless of the practitioner or the patient's religious beliefs, there are strong grounds to regard the therapy as effective because it has conformed to or abided by our created human nature. Consequently, to ascribe a therapy to the work of the Devil, just because its diagnosis or therapy is framed in an unfamiliar religious or philosophical paradigm (like *yinyang*), betrays an inadequate understanding of Christian anthropology. More seriously, it gives too much credit to the Devil, and robs God of His rightful glory. This is because it is ultimately God whom we should thank for the effectiveness of a medical therapy.

A similar principle, I believe, was assumed in Paul's discussion of food offered to idols. Addressing the Corinthians' concern about eating food offered to idols, he begins with the premise that "an idol has no real existence", and "there is no God but one" (1 Cor. 8:4).[17] On this basis, he concludes that an idol has no bearing or effect on the food offered to it—"we are no worse off if we do not eat, and no better off if we do" (1 Cor. 8:8). In other words, regardless of the idolatrous practices or spiritual ideas associated with the food, they do not affect the food materially or ontologically. They still function according to their natures. If they are edible for humans, they remain edible even after they have been offered to idols, and do not affect the spiritual state of their consumer. In practice, many Christians already presume this in their daily lives, especially for those who live in multicultural societies, such as in Singapore or Malaysia. For example, for commercial reasons, most of the chicken sold in Singapore are *halal*.[18] That is, the chickens are slaughtered while they are still alive, and a Muslim prayer of dedication, called the *tasmiya* or *shahada*, is recited during the slaughtering process.[19] On a daily basis, Christians in such

---

17   In Greek, "no real existence" literally means "it is nothing in the world (*ouden ... en kosmō)".

18   *Halal* means permissible in Arabic.

19   "What Is Halal Meat?" *BBC News*, accessed 10 May 2017, http://www.bbc.com/news/uk-27324224.

societies consume lots of *halal* meat but are not affected by the prayers at all. In fact, they are unlikely to even give any thought to this.[20]

By extension of this Pauline food principle, and the Christological arguments above, it should be clear that a medical therapy, whether it is Western or Chinese medicine, should be regarded as theologically legitimate for Christian usage as long as it has been empirically verified, either by clinical trials or, in the case of Chinese medicine, historical practice.[21] Even when a non-Christian surgeon says a prayer to his gods before performing surgery, this should have no bearing on his surgical success. What matters are his surgical skills, which are part of the gifts and talents that God has endowed the physician. In a similar vein, one should not believe in a doctor simply because he is a Christian. His faith has no immediate bearing on his medical expertise and experience. This is why the TCM practice in Category 2 is acceptable for Christians.

An exception to the above Pauline principle, however, is 1 Corinthians 10:14–21. Here, the question at hand again is the consumption of food offered to idols. In this case, Paul advises Christians not to participate in pagan rituals and feasts, and partake of the food served there. The reason is not because the food itself has become harmful to a Christian, or the idol has real existence. Rather, the problem lies in the Christian's willing and intentional participation at the "table of the demons", since this puts him in communion with the demons.

> Therefore, my beloved, flee from idolatry. ... for yourselves what I say. The cup of blessing that we bless, is it not a participation in the blood of Christ? The bread that we break, is it not a participation in the body of Christ? ... Consider

---

20   Unfortunately, many Christians actually refrain from consuming food offered to idols. This is not because of their concern for stumbling a fellow Christian, but their fear of the idolatrous practices associated with the food. Besides the practical incoherence of their behaviour, they are actually contravening Paul's teachings in 1 Corinthians 8.

21   The theologically legitimacy of a therapy, however, says nothing about its therapeutic efficacy. The latter must still be ascertained through empirical study or practice.

the people of Israel: are not those who eat the sacrifices participants in the altar? What do I imply then? That food offered to idols is anything, or that an idol is anything? No, I imply that what pagans sacrifice they offer to demons and not to God. I do not want you to be participants with demons. You cannot drink the cup of the Lord and the cup of demons. You cannot partake of the table of the Lord and the table of demons. (1 Cor. 10:14–21)

In other words, context and intention matters even when we are engaged in an ordinary activity, such as eating or receiving medical therapy. If we engage in such activities as part of our intentional participation in a pagan ritual, we would be found to be in fellowship with other religious deities and subjecting ourselves to their influence.

When we transpose this principle to Chinese medicine, the reason for our advice against Category 3 TCM physicians becomes clear. Christians should avoid Chinese medical, or for that matter, any form of therapy, if its efficacy is dependent on the healing powers of a foreign deity. In practice, such religious therapies are easily identifiable as they usually involve some form of religious ritual, such as the summoning of a deity to write a protective talisman on a patient's back. In all cases, their efficacy has no empirical basis beyond their religious context—they only work when specific spiritual powers are summoned. Although such *sinsehs* may still regard these as Chinese medical therapies, they would not be recognised as such by mainstream TCM physicians. It is for this reason that Christians can be well assured they will not receive such treatments if they seek medical help at the secular TCM hospitals and clinics.

Conclusion

In the opening chapter, we highlighted three concerns or objectives for our book. The first is apologetic, where we seek to ascertain the theological legitimacy of Chinese medicine. In the light of our investigations and analyses, we hope that our readers are now convinced that TCM philosophy and theory are either neutral ideas that have no bearing on the Christian faith, or, at times, are even compatible with Christian teachings. Consequently, there is no good reason to reject the medical tradition, or worse, demonise it. Indeed, to do so is to set up an unnecessary stumbling block before Chinese non-Christians, and to become a hindrance to the proclamation of the Gospel. Secondly, our study has also shown that, over the last 2,000 years, Chinese medicine has come up with different approaches to healthcare, diagnosis and therapy. Some have proven to be equally effective as, if not more so than, those of their biomedical counterpart.

In view of how we have addressed the theological concerns, we hope that Chinese medicine can now become an additional avenue of medical care for Christians, and, in so doing, widen the range of therapeutic options available to them. Our final concern is that of contextual theology. Namely, how might Chinese medical philosophy, to the extent that it abides by General Revelation, enrich the Christian tradition? In the course of this chapter, we explored how the theory of *yinyang*, the Chinese conceptions of health and disease, and ascetic practice, can contribute to our theological reflections and spiritual formation. These proposals are, by no means, exhaustive. In all likelihood, Chinese medical philosophy can shed further light on the philosophical and existential questions of the Chinese. In so doing, it provides fresh impetus and opportunities for us to contextualise biblical teachings that can better answer the questions and concerns of the Chinese.

Apart from the above, I hope that our study has been helpful in deepening our self-knowledge, drawing attention, in particular, to the intellectual biases we often bring to inter-cultural dialogues. More importantly, I pray that this exercise has also provided Christians with a theological framework and guidelines that can be of use in engaging indigenous cultures, in order that Christians may function more effectively as ambassadors and mediators between Christianity and other cultures; in order that misunderstandings between the two can be reduced; and that more may be drawn to the love and salvation of our Lord Jesus Christ, our ultimate Healer!

BIBLIOGRAPHY

A Decade in Medicine. Nature Reviews. London: Macmillan, 2015.

"A Long Way from Everything: The Search for a Grand Unified Theory". Accessed 7 November 2017. https://newatlas.com/einstein-quantum-field-theory-relativity-gravity/42389/.

"A Pill for Every Ill?—BBC News". Accessed 1 March 2016. http://www.bbc.com/news/health-30418580.

"A Pill for Every Ill: Two Million Brits Have Become Addicted to Prescription Drugs | Features | Lifestyle | *The Independent*". Accessed 26 February 2016. http://www.independent.co.uk/life-style/health-and-families/features/a-pill-for-every-ill-two-million-brits-have-become-addicted-to-prescription-drugs-1764497.html.

"About Cognitive Linguistics - Cognitive Linguistics". Accessed 4 January 2018. http://www.cognitivelinguistics.org/en/about-cognitive-linguistics.

Alexander, Denis. *Rebuilding the Matrix: Science and Faith in the 21st Century*. Grand Rapids, MI: Zondervan, 2003.

Algra, Keimpe. *The Cambridge History of Hellenistic Philosophy*. Cambridge: Cambridge University Press, 1999.

Amundsen, Darrel W. *Medicine, Society, and Faith in the Ancient and Medieval Worlds*. Baltimore; London: Johns Hopkins University Press, 1996.

An, Bing-chen, Ying Wang, Xin Jiang, Hai-Sheng Lu, Zhong-Yi Fang, You Wang, and Ke-Rong Dai. "Effects of Baduanjin (八段锦) Exercise on Knee Osteoarthritis: A One-Year Study". *Chin J Integr Med* 19, no. 2 (2013): 143–48.

Anastasi, Joyce K., Michelle Chang, Jessica Quinn, and Bernadette Capili. "Tongue Inspection in TCM: Observations in a Study Sample of Patients Living with HIV". *Medical Acupuncture* 26, no. 1 (2014): 15–22. https://doi.org/10.1089/acu.2013.1011.

Anderson, Neil T., and Michael Jacobson. *The Biblical Guide to Alternative Medicine*. Ventura, CA: Regal, 2003.

Andrews, Bridie. *The Making of Modern Chinese Medicine, 1850-1960*. Vancouver, BC: UBC Press, 2014.

Angell, Marcia. *The Truth about the Drug Companies: How They Deceive Us and What to Do about It*. New York: Random House, 2004.

"Antibiotics. Side Effects & Types of Antibiotics". Patient. Accessed 3 March 2016. http://patient.info/health/antibiotics-leaflet.

Awad, Mark M., and Alice T. Shaw. "ALK Inhibitors in Non–Small Cell Lung Cancer: Crizotinib and Beyond". *Clinical Advances in Hematology & Oncology: H&O* 12, no. 7 (July 2014): 429–39.

"Bacteria That Can Lead to Cancer | American Cancer Society". Accessed 13 January 2018. https://www.cancer.org/cancer/cancer-causes/infectious-agents/infections-that-can-lead-to-cancer/bacteria.html.

Borrell-Carrió, Francesc, Anthony L. Suchman, and Ronald M. Epstein. "The Biopsychosocial Model 25 Years Later: Principles, Practice, and Scientific Inquiry". *Annals of Family Medicine* 2, no. 6 (2004): 576–82. https://doi.org/10.1370/afm.245.

Brashier, K. E. *Ancestral Memory in Early China*. Cambridge, MA: Harvard University Press, 2011.

Brooke, John Hedley. *Science and Religion: Some Historical Perspectives*. Cambridge; New York: Cambridge University Press, 1991.

Bruun, Ole, and Stephan Feuchtwang. *Fengshui in China: Geomantic Divination between State Orthodoxy and Popular Religion*. Copenhagen, Denmark: NIAS Press, 2011.

Bynum, W. F. *History of Medicine: A Very Short Introduction*. Oxford; New York: Oxford University Press, 2008.

———. *Science and the Practice of Medicine in the Nineteenth Century*. Cambridge: Cambridge University Press, 1994.

Chang, Rhonda. "Making Theoretical Principles for New Chinese Medicine". *Australian and New Zealand Society of the History of Medicine*, Health and History, 16, no. 1 (2014): 66–86.

Chen, Mei Chuan, Hseuh Erh Liu, Hsiao Yun Huang, and Ai Fu Chiou. "The Effect of a Simple Traditional Exercise Programme (Baduanjin Exercise) on Sleep Quality of Older Adults: A Randomized Controlled Trial". *International Journal of Nursing Studies* 49 (2012): 265–73.

Chia, Roland. "Vestiges of the Divine". *Ethos Institute for Public Christianity*, November 2016. http://ethosinstitute.sg/vestigesofthedivine/.

Chung, Yu-Feng, Chung-Shing Hu, Cheng-Chang Yeh, and Ching-Hsing Luo. "How to Standardize the Pulse-Taking Method of Traditional Chinese Medicine Pulse Diagnosis". *Computers in Biology and Medicine* 43, no. 4 (May 2013): 342–49. https://doi.org/10.1016/j.compbiomed.2012.12.010.

Consortium, International Human Genome Sequencing. "Finishing the Euchromatic Sequence of the Human Genome". *Nature* 431, no. 7011 (2004): 931–45. https://doi.org/10.1038/nature03001.

Crislip, Andrew. *Thorns in the Flesh: Illness and Sanctity in Late Ancient Christianity*. Pennsylvania: University of Pennsylvania Press, 2013.

Csikszentmihalyi, Mark. *Readings in Han Chinese Thought*. Indianapolis, IN: Hackett Pub. Co., 2006.

"CT Scans Capture Acupuncture Point Discovery". Accessed 11 August 2016. http://www.healthcmi.com/Acupuncture-Continuing-Education-News/1418-ct-scan-acupuncture-point-discovery.

Dawkins, Richard. *The Selfish Gene*. Oxford; New York: Oxford University Press, 1989.

De Bary, William Theodore, Irene Bloom, and Wing-tsit Chan. *Sources of Chinese Tradition*. Vol. 2. New York: Columbia University Press, 1999.

Diamond, Jared. *Guns, Germs, and Steel: The Fates of Human Societies*. New York: W.W. Norton & Co., 1997.

"DNA Scientists Write "Book of Life"". *Mail Online*. Accessed 9 June 2016. http://www.dailymail.co.uk/news/article-176587/DNA-scientists-write-book-life.html.

Drake, Stillman. *Galileo: A Very Short Introduction*. Oxford; NY: Oxford University Press, 2001.

"DrugBank: Statistics". Accessed 1 March 2016. http://www.drugbank.ca/stats.

"Ebm.Pdf". Accessed 3 March 2016. http://www.medicine.ox.ac.uk/bandolier/painres/download/whatis/ebm.pdf.

Enders, Giulia. *Gut: The Inside Story of Our Body's Most Under-Rated Organ*. Vancouver, BC: Greystone, 2015.

Engelhardt, Ute. "Longevity Techniques and Chinese Medicine". In *Daoism Handbook*, edited by Livia Kohn, 74–103. Leiden: Brill, 2000.

Epstein, Robert. "Your Brain Does Not Process Information and It Is Not a Computer – Robert Epstein | Aeon Essays". *Aeon*. Accessed 21 March 2017. https://aeon.co/essays/your-brain-does-not-process-information-and-it-is-not-a-computer.

Ferngren, Gary B. *Medicine & Health Care in Early Christianity*. Baltimore, MD: Johns Hopkins University Press, 2009.

———. *Science and Religion: A Historical Introduction*. Baltimore, MD.: Johns Hopkins University Press, 2002.

Forum on Microbial Threats. *Ending the War Metaphor: The Changing Agenda for Unravelling the Host-Microbe Relationship—Workshop Summary*. Washington, D.C.: National Academies, 2006.

Fu, Louis. "The Protestant Medical Missions to China: The Introduction of Western Medicine with Vaccination", *Journal of Medical Biography*, 21 (2013): 112–17.

Galen, and Mark Grant. *Galen: On Food and Diet*. London: Routledge, 2000.

Gallagher, James. "Moments of Joy "Can Damage Heart"". *BBC News*, 3 March 2016, sec. Health. http://www.bbc.com/news/health-35710232.

Gawande, Atul. "The Problem of Extreme Complexity", in *The Checklist Manifesto: How to Get Things Right* (London: Profile Books, 2009).

Goldacre, Ben. *Bad Pharma: How Drug Companies Mislead Doctors and Harm Patients*. Kindle. Glasgow: Harper Collins, 2013.

Goldschmidt, Asaf Moshe. *The Evolution of Chinese Medicine: Song Dynasty, 960-1200*. London; New York: Routledge, 2009.

Grant, Hardy. "Geometry and Medicine: Mathematics in the Thought of Galen of Pergamum 4", *Philosophia Mathematica*, s2-4, no. 1 (1989): 29–34.

Gunter, W. *Wesley and the Quadrilateral: Renewing the Conversation*. Nashville, TN: Abingdon Press, 1997.

Halwani, T, and M Takrouri. "Medical Laws and Ethics of Babylon as Read in Hammurabi"s Code", *The Internet Journal of Law, Healthcare and Ethics*, 4, no. 2 (2006).

Hankinson, R. J. *The Cambridge Companion to Galen*. Cambridge; New York: Cambridge University Press, 2008.

Harper, Donald John. *Early Chinese Medical Literature: The Mawangdui Medical Manuscripts*. London: Kegan Paul International, 1998.

"Has the Era of Blockbuster Drugs Come to an End? | BioPharm International". Accessed 29 February 2016. http://www.biopharminternational.com/has-era-blockbuster-drugs-come-end.

Hildebrand, Stephen M. *The Trinitarian Theology of Basil of Caesarea: A Synthesis of Greek Thought and Biblical Truth*. Washington, DC: Catholic University of America Press, 2007.

Ho, Andy. "Pinning down Acupuncture: It's a Placebo." *The Straits Times*. 12 February 2011: 32.

Hong, Hai. T*he Theory of Chinese Medicine: A Modern Explanation*. London: Imperial College, 2014.

Houston, James. *The Christian Life East and West: Toward the Mutual Enrichment of Japanese and Western Christianity*. Vancouver, BC: Regent College Publishing, 2017.

Hussain, Amir. "Cordyceps 'likely led to post-op bleeding'". *The Straits Times*, 27 May 2016. http://www.straitstimes.com/singapore/courts-crime/cordyceps-likely-led-to-post-op-bleeding.

"Is the 2015 Nobel Prize a Turning Point for Traditional Chinese Medicine?" Accessed January 1, 2016. http://theconversation.com/is-the-2015-nobel-prize-a-turning-point-for-traditional-chinese-medicine-48643.

"JAMA Network | JAMA Oncology | Chemotherapy Use, Performance Status, and Quality of Life at the End of Life". Accessed 21 March 2016. http://oncology.jamanetwork.com/article.aspx?articleid=2398177.

Johansson, Lars-Göran. *Philosophy of Science for Scientists*. Cham: Springer, 2016.

Johnson, Mark. "Conceptual Metaphor and Embodied Structures of Meaning: A Reply to Kennedy and Vervaeke". *Philosophical Psychology* 6 (1993): 413–422.

———. *The Body in the Mind: The Bodily Basis of Meaning, Imagination, and Reason*. Chicago, IL: University of Chicago Press, 2013.

"Kadcyla Price Too High for Routine NHS Funding, Says NICE in Final Guidance | Press and Media | News | NICE". Press Release. Accessed 19 August 2016. https://www.nice.org.uk/news/press-and-media/kadcyla-price-too-high-for-routine-nhs-funding-says-nice-in-final-guidance.

Kaptchuk, Ted J. *Chinese Medicine: The Web That Has No Weaver*. Vol. Rev. and expanded. London: Rider, 2000.

———. "Acupuncture: Theory, Efficacy, and Practice". *Annals of Internal Medicine*, Complementary and Alternative Medicine Series, 136, no. 5 (2002): 374–83.

———. "Powerful Placebo: The Dark Side of the Randomised Controlled Trial", *Lancet*, 351 (1998): 1722–25.

———. "The Double-Blind, Randomized, Placebo-Controlled Trial: Gold Standard or Golden Calf?" *Journal of Clinical Epidemiology* 54 (2001): 541–49.

Kaptchuk, Ted J., Keji Chen, and Jun Song. "Recent Clinical Trials of Acupuncture in the West: Responses from the Practitioners". *Chin J Integr Med* 2010 16, no. 3 (June 2010): 197–203.

Kohn, Livia. *Chinese Healing Exercises: The Tradition of Daoyin.* Honolulu, HI: University of Hawai'i Press, 2008.

———. *Introducing Daoism.* London; New York: Routledge, 2009.

Kövecses, Zoltán. *Metaphor: A Practical Introduction.* 2nd ed. New York: Oxford University Press, 2010.

Krop, Ian E., Sung-Bae Kim, Antonio González-Martín, Patricia M LoRusso, Jean-Marc Ferrero, Melanie Smitt, Ron Yu, Abraham C F Leung, and Hans Wildiers. "Trastuzumab Emtansine versus Treatment of Physician"s Choice for Pretreated HER2-Positive Advanced Breast Cancer (TH3RESA): A Randomised, Open-Label, Phase 3 Trial". *The Lancet Oncology* 15, no. 7 (June 2014): 689–99. https://doi.org/10.1016/S1470-2045(14)70178-0.

Kuriyama, Shigehisa. *The Expressiveness of the Body and the Divergence of Greek and Chinese Medicine.* New York: Zone Books, 1999.

"Lab Mice Can"t Help Us in the Fight against Cancer | Comment | Voices | The Independent". Accessed 4 March 2016. http://www.independent.co.uk/voices/comment/lab-mice-cant-help-us-in-the-fight-against-cancer-8316756.html.

Larchet, Jean-Claude. *The Theology of Illness.* Crestwood, NY: St. Vladimir's Seminary Press, 2002.

Lakoff, George, and Mark Johnson. *Metaphors We Live By.* Chicago, IL: University of Chicago Press, 1980.

Le Fanu, James. *The Rise & Fall of Modern Medicine.* London: Abacus, 2014.

Liang, Qichao. "The Origin of Yinyang and Wuxing". In *The Debate on Ancient History (*古史辯*)*, edited by Jiegang Gu, Vol. 5. Shanghai: Shanghai Guji Press, 1982.

Link, Perry. *An Anatomy of Chinese: Rhythm, Metaphor, Politics.* Cambridge, MA: Harvard University Press, 2013.

Liu, Chang, Changbo Zhao, Guozheng Li, Fufeng Li, and Zhi Wang. "Computerized Color Analysis for Facial Diagnosis in Traditional Chinese Medicine", 613–14. IEEE, 2013. https://doi.org/10.1109/BIBM.2013.6732569.

Liu, Tianjun, and Kevin W Chen. *Chinese Medical Qigong.* London: Singing Dragon, 2010.

Lo, Vivienne. "The Influence of Nurturing Life Culture on the Development of Western Han Acumoxa Therapy". In *Innovation in Chinese medicine*, edited by Elizabeth Hsu. Cambridge; New York: Cambridge University Press, 2001.

Lo, Vivienne. "Introduction". In *Celestial Lancets: A History and Rationale of Acupuncture and Moxa*, by Gwei-Fjen Lu and Joseph Needham. London: Routledge, 2015.

Lo, Vivienne, and Michael Stanley-Baker. "Chinese Medicine". In *The Oxford Handbook of the History of Medicine*, edited by Mark Jackson. Oxford: Oxford University Press, 2013.

Lloyd, G. E. R. *Adversaries and Authorities: Investigations into Ancient Greek and Chinese Science.* Cambridge: Cambridge University Press, 1996.

————. *Disciplines in the Making: Cross-Cultural Perspectives on Elites, Learning, and Innovation*. Oxford: Oxford University Press, 2009.

————. *Being, Humanity, and Understanding: Studies in Ancient and Modern Societies*. Oxford: Oxford University Press, 2012.

Lloyd, G. E. R., and Nathan Sivin. *The Way and the Word: Science and Medicine in Early China and Greece*. New Haven, CN; London: Yale University Press, 2002.

Logan, F. Donald. *A History of the Church in the Middle Ages*. London; NY: Routledge, 2002.

Luther, Martin. *The Epistles of St. Peter and St. Jude: Preached and Explained*. New York: Anson D. F. Randolph, 1859.

Lyons, Kate. "Interest in Cupping Therapy Spikes after Michael Phelps Gold Win." *The Guardian*, August 8, 2016, sec. Sport. http://www.theguardian.com/ sport/2016/aug/08/cupping-therapy-interest-spikes-michael-phelps-rio-olympics.

Lynch, Joseph H. *The Medieval Church: A Brief History*. London; New York: Longman, 1992.

Maciocia, Giovanni. *The Foundations of Chinese Medicine: A Comprehensive Text for Acupuncturists and Herbalists*. Edinburgh: Elsevier Churchill Livingstone, 2005.

————. *The Psyche in Chinese Medicine: Treatment of Emotional and Mental Disharmonies with Acupuncture and Chinese Herbs*. Edinburgh: Churchill Livingstone, 2009.

Magazine, Elle Metz BBC News. "Why Singapore Banned Chewing Gum". *BBC News*. Accessed 21 March 2016. http://www.bbc.com/news/magazine-32090420.

"Malian Doctor All for TCM Healing—Global Times." Accessed January 4, 2016. http://www.globaltimes.cn/content/828560.shtml.

Martzloff, Jean-Claude. *A History of Chinese Mathematics*. New York: Springer, 2006.

Mayer, Wendy. "Shaping the Sick Soul: Reshaping the Identity of John Chrysostom". In *Christians Shaping Identity from the Roman Empire to Byzantium: Studies Inspired by Pauline Allen*, edited by Geoffrey D Dunn. Leiden: Brill, 2015.

McDermott, Gerald. *A Trinitarian Theology of Religions: An Evangelical Proposal*. Oxford: Oxford University Press, 2014.

McGuckin, John Anthony. *Westminster Handbook to Patristic Theology*. Louisville, KY: Westminster John Knox Press, 2005.

McKie, Robin. "Stunning Gene Therapy Breakthrough Driven by Great Dedication and Graft | Robin McKie". *The Observer*, 17 December 2017, sec. Science. http://www.theguardian.com/science/2017/dec/17/stunning-gene-therapy-breakthrough-riposte-to-truth-tarnished-times.

Merrill, Eugene H. *Deuteronomy*. Nashville, TN: Broadman & Holman, 1994.

Mettinger, Arthur. "Contrast and Schemas: Anonymous Adjectives". In *Issues in Cognitive Linguistics: 1993 Proceedings of the International Cognitive Linguistics Conference*, edited by Christoph Eyrich and Leon de Stadler. Berlin: De Gruyter Mouton, 2011.

Morgan, Graeme, Robyn Wardy, and Michael Barton. "The Contribution of Cytotoxic Chemotherapy to 5-Year Survival in Adult Malignancies", *Clinical Oncology*,

16 (2004): 549–60.

Nauert, Charles G. *Humanism and the Culture of Renaissance Europe*. Cambridge; NY: Cambridge University Press, 1995.

Nisbett, Richard E. *The Geography of Thought: How Asians and Westerners Think Differently... and Why*. New York: Free Press, 2003.

Noble, Denis. *The Music of Life: Biology beyond Genes*. Oxford; New York: Oxford University Press, 2008.

Nutton, Vivian. *Ancient Medicine*. London: Routledge, 2005.

O'Mathuna, Donal and Walt Larimore. *Alternative Medicine: The Christian Handbook*. Grand Rapids, MI: Zondervan, 2001.

"Over-the-Counter (OTC) Medications for Acute Cough in Children and Adults in Community Settings | Cochrane". Accessed 14 July 2016. http://www. cochrane.org/CD001831/ARI_over-the-counter-otc-medications-for-acute-cough-in-children-and-adults-in-community-settings.

Palmer, David A. *Qigong Fever: Body, Science, and Utopia in China*. New York: Columbia University Press, 2007.

Paton, William. "The Evolution of Therapeutics: Osler's Therapeutic Nihilism and the Changing Pharmacopoeia". *Journal of the Royal College of Physicians* 13 (1979): 74.

Porter, Roy. *Medicine: A History of Healing*. London: Michael O'Mara, 1997.

———. *The Greatest Benefit to Mankind: A Medical History of Humanity from Antiquity to the Present*. London: Fontana, 1999.

Pritzker, Sonya. "The Role of Metaphor in Culture, Consciousness, and Medicine: A Preliminary Inquiry into the Metaphors of Depression in Chinese and Western Medical and Common Languages". *Clinical Acupuncture and Oriental Medicine* 4 (2003): 11–28.

"Reading the Book of Life". *BBC*, 30 May 2000, sec. Human genome. http://news.bbc. co.uk/2/hi/in_depth/sci_tech/2000/human_genome/760893.stm.

Rechavi, Oded, Gregory Minevich, and Oliver Hobert. "Transgenerational Inheritance of an Acquired Small RNA-Based Antiviral Response in *C. elegans*". *Cell* 147, no. 6 (9 December 2011): 1248–56. https://doi.org/10.1016/j. cell.2011.10.042.

Reisser, Paul C, Dale Mabe, and Robert Velarde. *Examining Alternative Medicine: An Inside Look at the Benefits & Risks*. Downers Grove, IL: InterVarsity Press, 2001.

Rhee, Helen. *Loving the Poor, Saving the Rich: Wealth, Poverty, and Early Christian Formation*. Grand Rapids, MI: Baker Academic, 2012.

Rosenberg, Alex. *Philosophy of Science: A Contemporary Introduction*. London: Routledge, 2003.

Sackett, D. L. et al. "Evidence-Based Medicine: What It Is and What It Isn't". *British Medical Journal* 312 (1996): 71–72.

Sample, Ian. "Motherly Love May Alter Genes for the Better". *The Guardian*, 14 February 2007. http://www.theguardian.com/science/2007/feb/14/ medicalresearch.genetics.

Sanders, Sean, ed. "The Art and Science of Traditional Medicine Part 1: TCM Today - A Case for Integration". *Science* 346, no. Suppl (2014): S4–25.

"Sars in Singapore: Timeline, Singapore News & Top Stories — *The Straits Times*". Accessed 21 March 2016. http://www.straitstimes.com/singapore/sars-in-singapore-timeline.

Sauer, Uwe, Matthias Heinemann, and Nicola Zamboni. "Getting Closer to the Whole Picture". *Science* 316, no. 5824 (2007): 550–51.

Scanlon, Valerie C, and Tina Sanders. *Essentials of Anatomy and Physiology*. Philadelphia, PA: F.A. Davis, 2015.

Scheid, Volker. *Chinese Medicine in Contemporary China: Plurality and Synthesis*. Durham, NC; Oxford: Duke University Press, 2002.

———. *Currents of Tradition in Chinese Medicine, 1626-2006*. Seattle: Eastland Press, 2007.

Scheid, Volker, and Hugh MacPherson. *Integrating East Asian Medicine into Contemporary Healthcare*. Edinburgh; New York: Churchill Livingstone Elsevier, 2012.

Shahar, Meir. *The Shaolin Monastery: History, Religion and the Chinese Martial Arts*. Honolulu, HI: University of Hawaii Press, 2008.

Shapiro, James Alan. *Evolution: A View from the 21st Century*. Upper Saddle River, NJ: FT Press Science, 2011.

Schroeder, Knut, and Tom Fahey. "Systematic Review of Randomised Controlled Trials of over the Counter Cough Medicines for Acute Cough in Adults". *BMJ (Clinical Research Ed.)* 324, no. 7333 (2002): 329–31.

Siddique, Haroon. "NHS Cancer Patients Missing out on Innovative Drugs". *The Guardian*, 15 August 2016, sec. Society. https://www.theguardian.com/society/2016/aug/15/nhs-cancer-patients-innovative-drugs-breast-prostate-uk.

Smith, Gregory A. "How Thin Is a Demon?"", *Journal of Early Christian Studies*, 16, no. 4 (2008): 479–512.

Stackhouse, John. *Making the Best of It: Following Christ in the Real World*. Oxford; New York: Oxford University Press, 2011.

Studtmann, Paul. "Aristotle"s Categories". In *The Stanford Encyclopedia of Philosophy*, edited by Edward N. Zalta, Summer 2014., 2014. http://plato.stanford.edu/archives/sum2014/entries/aristotle-categories/.

Tanner, Harold Miles. *China: A History Volume 2*. Indianapolis, IN: Hackett, 2010.

Taylor, Geraldine. *Pastor Hsi (of North China); One of China's Christians*. London: Morgan & Scott, 1904.

Taylor-Piliae, Ruth E., Tiffany M. Hoke, Joseph T. Hepworth, L. Daniel Latt, Bijan Najafi, and Bruce M. Coull. "Effect of Tai Chi on Physical Function, Fall Rates and Quality of Life Among Older Stroke Survivors". *Archives of Physical Medicine and Rehabilitation* 95 (2014): 816–24.

"TCM Service | Bethel Community Services." Accessed January 4, 2016. http://www.bethelcs.org.sg/services/tcm-service/.

Temkin, Owsei. *Hippocrates in a World of Pagans and Christians*. Baltimore; London:

Johns Hopkins University Press, 1991.

"Tennis Wiz Novak Djokovic Uses Holistic Chinese Medicine to 'Serve to Win' | Examiner.com." Accessed January 1, 2016. http://www.examiner.com/article/tennis-wiz-novak-djokovic-uses-holistic-chinese-medicine-to-serve-to-win.

"The McKeown Thesis — *The Lancet*". Accessed 11 February 2016. http://www.thelancet.com/journals/lancet/article/PIIS0140-6736(08)60292-5/fulltext.

"The Spleen (Human Anatomy): Picture, Location, Function, and Related Conditions". Accessed 14 June 2016. http://www.webmd.com/digestive-disorders/picture-of-the-spleen.

"The Thalidomide Tragedy: Lessons for Drug Safety and Regulation | *Helix Magazine*". Accessed 11 July 2016. https://helix.northwestern.edu/article/thalidomide-tragedy-lessons-drug-safety-and-regulation.

Tong, Daniel. *A Biblical Approach to Chinese Traditions and Beliefs*. Singapore: Genesis, 2003.

"Traditional Chinese Medicine to Play Important Role as Singapore Population Ages: PM Lee." *Channel NewsAsia*. Accessed October 30, 2017. http://www.channelnewsasia.com/news/singapore/traditional-chinese-medicine-to-play-important-role-as-singapore-9244600.

Udias, Augustin. *Jesuit Contribution to Science*. Switzerland: Springer, 2015.

Unschuld, Paul U. *Huang Di Nei Jing Su Wen: Nature, Knowledge, Imagery in an Ancient Chinese Medical Text*. Berkeley, CA; London: University of California Press, 2003.

———. *Medicine in China: A History of Ideas*. Berkeley, CA; London: University of California Press, 1985.

———. *What Is Medicine: Western and Eastern Approaches to Healing*. Berkeley, CA: University of California Press, 2009.

Unschuld, Paul U., Hermann Tessenow and Zheng Jinsheng. *Huang Di Nei Jing Su Wen: An Annotated Translation of Huang Di's Inner Classic - Basic Questions*. 2. Berkeley, CA: University of California Press, 2011.

Von Staden, Heinrich. "The Discovery of the Body: Human Dissection and Its Cultural Contexts in Ancient Greece", *Yale Journal of Biology and Medicine*, 65 (1992): 223–41.

Wang, Robin. *Yinyang: The Way of Heaven and Earth in Chinese Thought and Culture*. New York: Cambridge University Press, 2012.

Wang, Weigong (王唯工). *Qi as a Musical Movement* (气的乐章). 臺北市; 臺北縣三重市: 大塊文化出版 大和书报总经销, 2002.

Ward, Benedicta, and Anthony Bloom. *The Sayings of the Desert Fathers: The Alphabetical Collection*. Kalamazoo, MI: Cistercian Publications, 1984.

"What Are Meridians? Can We See Them?" Accessed 15 August 2016. http://www.acupuncturetoday.com/archives2004/mar/03lo.html.

"What Is Halal Meat? — *BBC News*". Accessed 10 May 2017. http://www.bbc.com/news/uk-27324224.

"What's Causing My Cold?" Accessed 7 July 2016. http://www.webmd.com/cold-and-flu/cold-guide/common_cold_causes.

Whitehead, Alfred North. *Science and the Modern World. Lowell Lectures, 1925.* New York: Macmillan, 1925.

Wild, S., G. Roglic, A. Green, R. Sicree, and H. King. "Global Prevalence of Diabetes: Estimates for the Year 2000 and Projections for 2030". *Diabetes Care* 27, no. 5 (2004): 1047–53.

World Health Organisation. "WHO Definition of Health". Accessed 31 August 2018. http://www.who.int/suggestions/faq/en/

Worrall, John. "What Evidence Is Evidence Based Medicine?" *Philosophy of Science* 69, no. 3 (2002): S316-30.

Wu, Hongzhou, ed. *Learning Chinese Medical Diagnosis in 100 Days* (一百天中医诊断). Shanghai: Shanghai Science and Technology Publishing, 2015.

Wu, Jackson. *Saving God's Face: A Chinese Contextualization of Salvation through Honour and Shame.* Pasadena, CA: William Carey International University Press, 2012.

Xie, Zhufan. *On the Standard Nomenclature of Traditional Chinese Medicine.* Beijing: Foreign Languages Press, 2003.

Yu, Ning. *The Contemporary Theory of Metaphor: A Perspective from Chinese.* Amsterdam/Philadelphia: John Benjamins, 1998.

———. "Metaphor, Body, and Culture: The Chinese Understanding of Gallbladder and Courage". *Metaphor and Symbol* 18, no. 1 (2003): 13–31.

———. *The Chinese Heart in a Cognitive Perspective: Culture, Body, and Language.* Berlin; New York: Mouton de Gruyter, 2009.

Zarkadakes, Giorgos. *In Our Own Image: Saviour or Destroyer?: The History and Future of Artificial Intelligence.* New York; London: Pegasus Books, 2016.

Zeng, Yingchun, Tai-Zhen Luo, Hua-An Xie, and Andy S. K. Cheng. "Health Benefits of Qigong or Tai Chi for Cancer Patients: A Systematic Review and Meta-Analyses". *Complementary Therapies in Medicine* 22 (2014): 173—86.

Zhang, Dainian, and Edmund Ryden. *Key Concepts in Chinese Philosophy.* Beijing: Foreign Languages Press, 2002.

Zhang, Huilin, Mingxia Zhu, Yang Song, and Meirong Kong. "Baduanjin Exercise Improved Premenstrual Syndrome Symptoms in Macau Women". *Journal of Traditional Chinese Medicine* 34, no. 4 (2014): 460–64.

Zhang, Yanhua. *Transforming Emotions with Chinese Medicine: An Ethnographic Account from Contemporary China.* Albany, NY: State University of New York Press, 2007.

Zhuangzi. *The Complete Works of Zhuangzi.* Translated by Burton Watson. New York: Columbia University Press, 2013.

陈仁寿　(Chen Renshou). 江苏中医：历史与流传派传承 (*Jiangsu Chinese Medicine*). Shanghai: Shanghai Science and Technology Publishing, 2014.

狄灵, 张晓乐, 杨成志, 李睿萍, 阮班云, 杨海侠, 孙万森, and 刘素蓉. "红外热像仪观测"督脉运行不畅"颈腰椎病红外热像随机平行对照研究". 实用中医内科杂志, no. 12 (2014): 1–3.

国家中医药管理局. 中医病证诊断疗效标准 (*Criteria of diagnosis and therapeutic effect of diseases and syndromes in traditional Chinese medicine*). 北京: 中国医药科技, 2012.

李彩风(Li Caifeng). 史上最简单, 白话中医入门 (*The Simplest Introduction to Chinese Medicine in History*). Xinbi: Popular Book, 2011.

李经纬 (Li Jingwei). 中医史 (*A History of Chinese Medicine*). Haikou: Hainan Chu Ban She, 2007.

李婷婷, 魏明, and 李洪娟."红外热像在中医学中的应用现状与展望", 北京中医药大学学报, 20, no. 4 (2013): 59–61.

刘红 (Liu Hong).零基础学会艾灸 (*Learning the Basics of Moxibustion*). 江苏: 江苏凤凰科学技术出版社, 2015.

刘明军(Liu Mingjun).推拿学 (*Chinese Massage Studies*). 北京: 人民卫生出版社, 2012.

王修齐 (Wang Xiuqi). "对医学的误解." 联合早报网, June 7, 2017. http://www.zaobao.com.sg/forum/views/opinion/story20170607-769141.

"习近平签署主席令, 《中医药法》正式颁布! （附全文）". Accessed 21 December 2017. http://mp.weixin.qq.com/s/9H1OrpFPs9tEmLPCJd5mlA.

"徐文兵-树立正确的人生观与价值观(上)_医道修行_新浪博客". Accessed 12 May 2016. http://blog.sina.com.cn/s/blog_62030a540101cfaz.html.

杨建宇. 明医薪传: 北京同仁堂中医大师孙光荣教授学术经验传承. 北京: 学苑出版社, 2010.

"與癌共存". *Apple Daily* 蘋果日報. Accessed 23 March 2017. http://hk.apple.nextmedia.com/news/art/20110821/15542977.

张仲景, 杨建宇, 吴厚新, and 李杨. 白云阁藏本伤寒杂病论. 河南: 中原农民出版社, 2013.

郑心锦 (Zheng Xinjin). "中医是哪门子科学？." 联合早报网, May 31, 2017. http://www.zaobao.com.sg/forum/views/opinion/story20170531-766526.

"中药疗效为何越来越低？真相往往很残忍！". Accessed 21 December 2017. http://mp.weixin.qq.com/s/8fFAKYsG3XVuKCCnpMUX9A.

"中医名家张锡纯的影响_生活养生网." Accessed 30 December 2015. http://www.shenghuoqq.com/zyys1/585.html.

"中医体质分类与判定自测表 - 中医药学百科". Accessed 15 January 2018. http://zhongyiyao.h.baike.com/article-1344880.html.

"河南举行仲景传人师承大典". Accessed 21 December 2017. https://kknews.cc/culture/jvx6b5l.html.

INDEX

GRACEW♥RKS

Graceworks is a publishing and training consultancy based in Singapore, dedicated to promoting spiritual friendship in church and society, and seeing lives transformed through books that present truth for life.

Our publications can be found on our online store, *www.graceworks.com.sg/store*. Paperbacks are also available on Book Depository and Amazon and eBooks on Kindle, iBooks, Google Play and Kobo.

You can contact us at *enquiries@graceworks.com.sg*, or follow us on Facebook (@GraceworksSG) and Instagram (graceworkssg).

www.ingramcontent.com/pod-product-compliance
Lightning Source LLC
Chambersburg PA
CBHW030358130626
46549CB00004B/1540